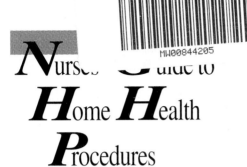

*N*urses' *G*uide to *H*ome *H*ealth *P*rocedures

*N*urses' *G*uide to *H*ome *H*ealth *P*rocedures

Joyce Young Johnson, PhD, RN, CCRN
Assistant Professor
Adult Health Nursing
College of Health Science
Georgia State University
Atlanta, Georgia

Jean Smith-Temple, MSN, RN
Clinical Assistant Professor of Nursing
Baccalaureate Nursing Program
Adult Health
The University of South Alabama
Mobile, Alabama

Patricia Carr, RN
Program Clinical Coordinator
Community AIDS Network
Sarasota, FL

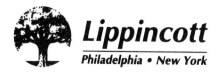

Lippincott
Philadelphia • New York

Acquisitions Editor: Susan M. Glover, RN, MSN
Editorial Assistant: Bridget Blatteau
Associate Managing Editor: Barbara Ryalls
Senior Production Manager: Helen Ewan

Production Coordinator: Patricia McCloskey
Design Coordinator: Kathy Kelley-Leudtke
Indexer: David Amundson

First Edition

9 8 7 6 5 4 3 2 1

Library of Congress Cataloging in Publications Data

Johnson, Joyce Young.
    Nurses' guide to home health procedures / Joyce Young Johnson, Jean Smith-Temple, Patricia Carr.
      p.   cm.
    Includes bibliographical references and index.
    ISBN 0-397-55468-0 (alk. paper)
    1. Home nursing—Handbooks, manuals, etc. I. Smith-Temple, Jean. II. Carr, Patricia A. III. Title.
    [DNLM: 1. Home Care Services—organization & administration—United States—handbooks. 2. Nursing Care—handbooks. WY 49 J68n 1997]
RT120.H65J64 1997
362.1'4—dc21
DNLM/DLC
for Library of Congress   97-19139
                                                                                CIP

Care has been taken to confirm the accuracy of the information presented and to describe generally accepted practices. However, the authors, editors, and publisher are not responsible for errors or omissions or for any consequences from application of the information in this book and make no warranty, express or implied, with respect to the contents of the publication.

The authors, editors and publisher have exerted every effort to ensure that drug selection and dosage set forth in this text are in accordance with current recommendations and practice at the time of publication. However, in view of ongoing research, changes in government regulations, and the constant flow of information relating to drug therapy and drug reactions, the reader is urged to check the package insert for each drug for any change in indications and dosage and for added warnings and precautions. This is particularly important when the recommended agent is a new or infrequently employed drug.

Some drugs and medical devices presented in this publication have Food and Drug Administration (FDA) clearance for limited use in restricted research settings. It is the responsibility of the health care provider to ascertain the FDA status of each drug or device planned for use in their clinical practice.

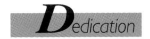

Dedication

To my husband, Larry, my daughter, Virginia, and my son, Larry Lee (L.J.), who help me make miracles with their encouragement, assistance, and love.

      Joyce (mommy)

To Richard for his love and support.
To Benjamin for sharing me during these special times.

      Jean

To my family and friends who are always with me.

To the nurses I've worked with and the patients we have learned from.

      Pat

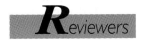

Reviewers

Lisa Burkhardt, MS, PT
Physical Therapist
Visiting Nurse Association of Fox Valley
Aurora, Illinois

Linda Larson, MS, RN
Case Manager, MCH
University of Maryland Medical System
Baltimore, Maryland

Sheila Ledermann, RN, CRNI
Home Infusion Coordinator
Visiting Nurse Association of Fox Valley
Aurora, Illinois

Sue Masoorli, RN
CEO/President
Perivascular Nurse Consultants, Inc.
Rockledge, Pennsylvania

Patricia L. Rafferty, RN, BSN
Director of Clinical Services
Mt. Washington Pediatric Home and Community Care, Inc.
Baltimore, Maryland

Elise Parsons-Johnson, RN, BSN, CETN
Enterostomal Therapy Nurse Coordinator
Visiting Nurse Association of Fox Valley
Aurora, Illinois

Joan Shaw, RN, BSN, CETN
Nurse Clinician
Visiting Nurse Association
Colchester, Vermont

Debra M. Walick, RN, BSN
Administrator
Advantage Home Health Care, Inc.
Channahon, Illinois

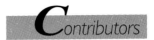
Contributors

Frankie R. Dunmore, RN, MSN
Assistant Professor
Alcorn State University School of Nursing
Natchez, Mississippi

Lorelei Papke, RN, MSN, CRNI
Manager, Clinical Nursing, IV Therapy Services
University of Michigan Medical Center
Ann Arbor, Michigan

Ola H. Fox, RN, C, MSN
Clinical Assistant Professor
University of South Alabama
Mobile, Alabama

Rosie Calvin, RN, DSN
Associate Professor
University of Mississippi
Medical Center
School of Nursing
Jackson, Mississippi

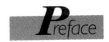

Preface

Nurses' Guide to Home Health Procedures is a quick-reference clinical support tool designed to serve practicing nurses in the home care setting as well as students in all types of educational programs. It explains the key steps necessary to perform nursing skills and provides cues to the critical thinking needed for client care.

This guide contains information about nearly 200 skills. A detailed table of contents and index are provided for easy reference to procedures. The procedures within the 12 chapters of *Nurses' Guide to Home Health Procedures* are organized in a modified nursing process format, with procedures listed at the beginning of each chapter for convenience. Chapter overviews review basic principles and concepts. Nursing procedures are organized as follows:

Equipment
Purpose(s) (includes examples of desired outcomes)
Assessment
Outcome Identification and Planning (includes client-centered goals and highlighted special considerations with general, geriatric, and transcultural aspects and hints about technique adaptations)
Implementation (actions with rationales)
Evaluation
Documentation (includes examples of charting)

Actions are presented concisely with clear illustrations to assist the user. Universal blood and body fluid precautions are considered whenever applicable. A pictogram next to the procedure title indicates that gloves should be worn. Icons mark transcultural considerations and special hints.

Nursing procedures have been organized to facilitate safe, expedient performance. *Nurses' Guide to Home*

Health Procedures should be used as a clinical reference; it is *not* intended for initial instruction of nursing procedures. The user should consult specific manufacturer's directions since equipment types change constantly. The equipment presented represent examples only.

The user should review principles in the chapter overview before proceeding to the nursing procedures. Procedures should be read in their entirety to ensure that all relevant health-care matters are considered during performance. Narrative documentation format will be used for charting examples, although many other forms of documentation may be used in the home health setting. Illustrations, tables, and appendices provide further support. Users should refer to these aids, as well as to related nursing procedures, as needed.

Joyce Young Johnson, RN, PhD, CCRN
Jean Smith-Temple, RN, MSN
Pat Carr, RN

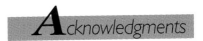
Acknowledgments

We would like to thank Susan Glover for her support and for helping us to get a fantastic start at making this project a success.

We would like to thank Barbara Ryalls and Bridget Blatteau for working so diligently and so closely with use to assure the quality of this book.

We would like to thank Dorothy Williams and Clyde Buchanan, Directors of Pharmacy at Crawford Long Hospital of Emory University, and Diane Williams at the Drug Information Center at the Medical College of Georgia Hospital and Clinics for providing essential information and assistance.

We would like to thank the nurses in Nutrition Support Services at Crawford Long Hospital of Emory University for providing invaluable assistance and expertise.

We would also like to thank the many other nurse colleagues and colleagues from other disciplines who provided us direction in the preparation of this guidebook.

*C*ontents

5 *Nutrition—Fluid and Nutrient Balance* **145**

Chapter 1

Basic Assessment and Planning

OVERVIEW

▶ Time spent in planning and organizing visits allows more concentration on care during visits and more efficient use of resources. When entering the home, have all needed supplies and documentation materials available and well organized.

▶ Detailed initial assessment of the client, the environment, and the support system contributes to an effective, individualized plan of care.

▶ The nurse is a guest in the client's home and must be aware of cultural patterns and family dynamics and make adjustments accordingly. The nurse should explain every action taken, and if uncertain of the client's or family's reaction, ask permission.

▶ Home health care is delivered on an intermittent or part time basis. It is essential to have support systems in place for each client so that care is consistent and adequate when home health personnel are not present.

▶ Continued evaluation of the client's progress toward independence in self care facilitates a successful client discharge from home care services and the re-establishment of functional personal life.

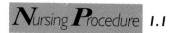

Preplanning and Organizing

☒ EQUIPMENT

- Client case record
- Area map
- Medical supplies
- Scheduling notebook

Purpose

Organizes, to the extent possible, a plan for caring for clients scheduled to be seen the next day.

Desired Outcomes (sample)

All scheduled clients will be seen and appropriate care given.

Assessment

Assessment should focus on the following:

Problems detected at prior visits
Special needs of the client

Outcome Identification and Planning

Key Goals and Sample Goal Criteria

The client will:

Be seen at an appropriate time and receive ordered care.

The nurse will:

See all clients scheduled.
Be prepared to complete all ordered procedures.

Special Considerations

 Transcultural

If the client's culture is unfamiliar, check within the Agency and
  community for people with specific knowledge of the culture,
  and obtain as much information as possible prior to making
  the visit.

HINTS

*Always carry a list of local physicians' phone numbers and
the name of a contact person in each office in case there are
questions about care.*
  *Know where the laboratories are in your area, what requisi-
tions and specimen containers are used by each lab, and how
quickly specimens need to get to the lab.*

IMPLEMENTATION

Organization and Scheduling

Action	Rationale
1. Review charts of clients to be seen the next day.	*Allows an opportunity to obtain missing or unclear information*
2. Determine special client needs, ie, timed specimens to be obtained, IV meds to be administered at a certain time.	
3. Use an area map to determine location of each client.	*Assists in reducing travel time between clients*
4. Determine approximate time frame for each visit, ie, 60–90 minutes for an initial visit, 30–60 minutes for a follow-up visit. If a specimen is to be obtained and taken to a lab, include the travel time to the lab in the total time for the visit.	*Allows for realistic scheduling of appointments, reduces chance of being late and keeping a client waiting*
5. Contact each client and set	*Increases nurse flexibility and*

Action	Rationale

an approximate time for each visit. Remind each client that the time is approximate and is affected by travel conditions, emergencies, etc.

eliminates the need to rush through one visit to get to another by allowing a "time window" for each visit

6. To the extent possible, take into account the client's preference for time of day, other appointments that the client may have, and the scheduling of other home care providers.

Increases client compliance by considering client's wishes, and helps avoid the scheduling of multiple providers on the same day, which could exhaust the client

7. List the day's scheduled visits, with client names and approximate times of visits in the scheduling notebook. Follow agency policy regarding advising the supervisor of the visit schedule.

Enables the supervisor to reach the nurse if new client information needs to be passed on

8. For each client to be seen, assemble the needed documentation, including admission documentation if needed, appropriate lab requisitions, visit notes, and client education materials. Complete the demographic portion of each form as completely as possible before the visit. (If using a computerized system, be sure that all pertinent information is downloaded into the laptop.)

Organizes the materials before the visit, which allows for efficient use of actual visit time, and better concentration on the client during the actual visit

9. Assemble any needed supplies and equipment for each client to be seen. Estimate and provide enough supplies for the client to use until the next scheduled visit. Do not overstock the home.

Ensures that proper supplies are available for each client. An adequate stock of supplies in the home reduces the need for extra visits to bring in supplies

10. If scheduling visits for a

Evens the nurse's caseload for

Action	Rationale
week or more for multiple clients, take note of the clients' physician appointments, and total number of visits scheduled for any one day of the week.	*the week, and allows the scheduling of clients in a certain area to be grouped on certain days to decrease travel time*

PERSONAL SAFETY

Action	Rationale
1. On area map, pinpoint location of each client to be seen.	*Determines if any client lives in an area previously considered unsafe. (Check with agency supervisor to determine which areas are considered unsafe.)*
2. Determine if any clients are to be seen at specific times.	*Allows the nurse to schedule visits during the day, as some areas may be unsafe at night.*
3. Be aware of agency policy concerning the use of escorts or law enforcement officers when making visits in unsafe areas.	*Permits time for advance notice and coordination if escorts are needed*
4. Be sure to let the client know when you plan to arrive.	*Allows the client to watch for the nurse's arrival and facilitates quick entry into the home*
5. At all times, if using a car, be sure it is in good working order. If using public transportation, have all schedules with you.	*Reduces the risk of being stranded in an unsafe area*
6. Always lock the car. Avoid leaving anything in the car in plain sight.	*Reduces the risk of theft*
7. Be observant. Survey the area when approaching the client's home. Drive at a normal rate of speed, and if illegal or dangerous activity appears to be occurring, keep driving to a safe area and notify the agency and client.	*Avoids driving through unfamiliar neighborhoods at a very slow rate of speed, which could indicate that the nurse does not belong in the area, and could attract unwanted attention*

Action	Rationale
8. When entering a home, observe for exits, weapons, dangerous situations.	*Allows the nurse to be aware of situations that may pose a threat to personal safety*
9. Before making any visits to clients in unsafe areas, be aware of agency policy and procedure. Be sure that the supervisor knows where you are going, and how long the visit is expected to take. Do not hesitate to terminate a visit if you feel that your personal safety is at risk.	*Promotes safety by providing agency back-up and support*

Evaluation

Were desired outcomes achieved?

DOCUMENTATION

According to agency policy and procedure.

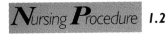

Nursing Procedure 1.2

Supplies and Equipment

EQUIPMENT

- Nursing bag
- Paper towels
- Handwashing soap
- Waterless handwashing solution
- Gloves—sterile and unsterile
- Sterile dressing supplies
- Venipuncture supplies
- Blood pressure cuff
- Stethoscope
- Alcohol wipes
- Antiseptic solutions
- Tape
- Syringes
- Supplies specific to area of practice

Purpose

Maintains an adequate stock of needed medical supplies.

Desired Outcomes (sample)

Needed supplies will be available in clean, usable condition.
Supplies will be restocked and rotated on a regular basis.
There will be minimal wastage of supplies due to soiling, loss of
package integrity, or deterioration.

Assessment

Assessment should focus on the following:

Types and amounts of items needed frequently, or unexpect-
edly.
Specific supplies needed for area of practice or current caseload.
Expiration dates, shelf life, and integrity of packaging of supply
materials.

Outcome Identification and Planning

Key Goals and Sample Criteria

The nurse will:

Have adequate supplies for each client.
Maintain supplies in good condition.

Special Considerations

HINTS

> *Supplies carried in the car are subject to extremes of tempera-*
> *ture that may cause deterioration. Examples are urinary*
> *catheters that become brittle, hydrocolloid dressings that dry*
> *out, and vacuum tubes for blood collection that lose vacuum*
> *at high temperatures. Supplies in the car are also subject to*
> *dust and water contamination. When stocking supplies, the*
> *nurse must consider exactly what supplies are needed and*
> *how the cleanliness and integrity of each item can best be*
> *maintained.*
> *Carry a supply of plastic bags that may be used for disposal*
> *of used supplies that are not considered biohazardous waste.*

IMPLEMENTATION

Nursing Bag Supplies

Action	Rationale
1. Keep paper towels, hand-washing soap, and water-less handwashing solution in the outside pocket of the nursing bag.	*Adheres to the principle that the outside of the bag is considered contaminated*
2. Carry items in the nursing bag that may be needed unexpectedly, or are used frequently for a number of clients. These may include sterile gauze pads, veni-puncture supplies, tape, syringes, blood pressure cuff, stethoscope, gloves,	*Allows for frequently needed supplies to be accessible and easily located. Reduces the weight of the nursing bag*

Action	Rationale
alcohol wipes, and anti-septic solutions.	
3. Any item that is removed from the inside of the nursing bag must be cleaned before it is returned to the bag.	*Adheres to the principle that the inside of the nursing bag is considered "clean"*
4. The bag should be checked and restocked at intervals. The specific items carried will depend on the nurse's area of practice and typical client caseload.	*Allows the nurse to have needed supplies available and in good condition. Allows for checking of expiration dates, soiling, or damage*
5. For all supplies, a written note should be made when the last item is used, and the item should be restocked as soon as possible.	*Eliminates extra trips to the agency office for needed supplies by giving a nurse a written reminder*
6. The stock supplies in the nursing bag should not be used to meet a specific client's ongoing supply needs. Supplies for any particular client should be separate from the nurse's stock.	*Eliminates forgetting to charge supplies used to a specific client, and reduces the risk of running out of supplies*
7. When in a home, place the nursing bag on a clean, dry surface. If necessary, place a paper towel under the bag. If there is no suitable area in the home to place the bag, take into the home only those items needed for the visit.	*Helps to avoid contamination of clean supplies*

Car Supplies

Action	Rationale
1. For supplies carried in the car, assign specific areas for clean, sterile, and con-taminated items.	*Maintains cleanliness and avoids contamination*

Action	Rationale

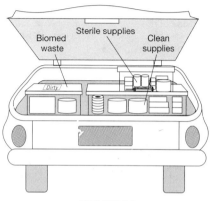

FIGURE 1.2

2. Place supplies in washable plastic containers, such as file bins, with lids. Do not place supplies directly onto the trunk carpet. Label bins with type of supplies in each.

   Maintains cleanliness, allows for easy removal of supplies. Covered bins prevent water and dust contamination

3. Depending on the nurse's area of practice, supplies kept in the car may include Foley catheters, extra dressing supplies, extra syringes, drainage bags, paper towels, antiseptic solutions, etc. The nurse should carry the smallest amount possible of each item (Fig. 1.2).

   Ensures that supplies carried in the car will be used quickly
   Reduces the risk of deterioration of supplies due to extremes of temperature and water and dust contamination

4. All supplies maintained in the car should be checked on a regular schedule. Soiled or outdated supplies should be discarded, and all dated supplies should be rotated.

   Maintains sterility, cleanliness, material integrity, and proper condition of supplies

Evaluation

Were desired outcomes achieved?

DOCUMENTATION

Agency policies vary as to how the use of supplies is to be documented. Check the agency policy and procedure.

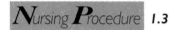 **1.3**

Environmental Assessment and Management

☒ EQUIPMENT

- Pen
- Comprehensive assessment form (agency specific)
- Client history
- Completed physical assessment
- Client problem list or care plan
- Physician's orders for care

Purpose

Determines strengths and weaknesses of client environment in relation to physical condition and care required.

Desired Outcomes (sample)

The client will receive care in a safe and supportive physical environment.

The client will actively participate in the adaptation of the environment to current needs.

Assessment

Assessment should focus on the following:

Safety of the client in the current environment

Status and adaptability of the environment to accommodate client functional limitations

Adequacy of environment for delivery of care ordered

Outcome Identification and Planning

Key Goals and Sample Goal Criteria

The client will:

Be safe and adequately cared for in the home environment

Adapt the environment to improve safety

Special Considerations

All nurses working in the home should be knowledgeable in
the procedures and resources available to immediately remove a client from an unsafe environment before performing
the environmental assessment.

Once the need for adaptation of the environment is determined,
it may be necessary to enlist the help of the social worker,
community resources, volunteer groups, client family and
friends to implement adaptations.

  Transcultural

The culture and belief system of the client is reflected in the
home environment. Assess the environment in the context of
the client's culture, not the nurse's. If unfamiliar with possible
cultural implications, check within the agency for a resource
person, or consult a text on cultural differences.

HINTS

> *Economic: Adaptations of the home environment may require
> structural changes or additions. The nurse must be aware of
> community resources, volunteer groups, and other sources for
> help that are available without cost or on a minimal cost
> basis.*
>
> *Economic: Certain items needed for care, such as oxygen
> concentrators that operate on electricity, may increase the
> client's monthly electric bill. Consider these factors when
> assessing the suitability of the environment for care. Use
> social services, community resources if necessary.*

IMPLEMENTATION

Action	Rationale
1. Review the client physical assessment, the care ordered, client history, and community assessment (Display 1.3).	*Provides a basis for determining if the environment can support the needs of the client*
2. Explain that a "walk through" of the home is necessary to ensure that client needs may be met. Ask permission to look around the home.	*Increases client cooperation and enhances client control*

DISPLAY 1.3   **Sample Assessment Form**

NAME _____   DATE _____

ENVIRONMENTAL ASSESSMENT

NEIGHBORHOOD

Appears safe _____   Avoid after dark _____   Escort needed _____

Comments _____

PHYSICAL SETTING

Adequate space _____   Barriers to entry _____

Stairs inside home _____   Narrow doorways or halls _____

Inadequate floor, roof, or windows _____   Pets _____

Possible substance abuse by client/family _____

Comments _____ _____

SAFETY

Inadequate lighting _____   Unsafe gas/electrical appliance _____

Inadequate heating _____   Inadequate cooling _____

Lack of fire safety devices _____   Unsafe floor covering _____

Inadequate stair railing _____   Lead based paint _____

Unsafe wiring _____

Comments _____

SANITATION

No running water _____   No toileting facilities _____

Inadequate sewage disposal __   Inadequate food storage __

No cooking facilities _____   No refrigeration _____

Cluttered/soiled living area _____   No trash pickup _____

Insect infestation _____   Rodents present _____

Comments _____

SIGNATURE _____

Action	Rationale
3. Assess barriers to entrance and exit from the home, such as steps or stairs that must be climbed to get in or out of the home. If needed, suggest ramps or alternative exits.	*Promotes client safety; alerts client that current physical limitations may hinder his or her ability to get in and out of the home*
4. Assess internal barriers to client mobility, such as stairs that must be climbed, narrow hallways, uneven floors. If needed, work with client to find paths through the home that avoid or overcome these barriers, ie, set up temporary bedroom downstairs, obtain narrow walker or wheelchair if needed.	*Enhances client safety and mobility. Promotes client participation in making needed changes*
5. Assess electrical safety— how electricity is supplied (power company, generator, no electricity in the home). Assess electrical cords and outlets for fire hazards, and cords on floor presenting hazards to ambulation. Assess adequacy of electrical system to support equipment needed for care, such as infusion or feeding pumps.	*Allows for adaptation of environment to promote safety. Allows nurse and client to consider alterations to care delivery if needed (eg, if electricity unreliable, consider manually controlled infusion without pump)*
6. Assess adequacy of heating and cooling systems in the home. If needed, advise on safe heating units, fans. Assist client in using community resources to obtain needed equipment.	*Evaluates possible adverse affect of excessive heat or cold on client's physical condition and medical progress*
7. Assess adequacy of plumbing system and availability of running water.	*Identifies obstacles to good hygiene, infection control*
8. Assess fire safety, presence	*Promotes safety*

Action	Rationale
of smoke detectors, and client plan for exit in case of a fire.	
9. Assess general cleanliness and adequacy of lighting for provision of care. Assess capability for refrigeration.	*Optimizes setting for provision of care*
10. Assess kitchen environment for safety, cleanliness, possible safety hazards, adequacy of food storage and preparation areas. Assess client ability to function in kitchen setting. Consider providing home health aide to assist with kitchen upkeep and food preparation. If client has new physical limitation, consider occupational therapy referral to instruct in skills for independent and safe use of kitchen.	*Promotes infection control, good nutrition*
11. Considering client current functional limitation, assess bathroom for safety and accessibility of tub, shower, toilet. Obtain order for adaptive equipment, and consider physical therapy for client instruction in safe techniques.	*Promotes client safety*
12. Assess for presence of insect infestation, presence of rodents. Assist in arranging for treatment of environment, if needed.	*Impacts on client hygiene, ability of nurse and client to perform clean or sterile procedures*
13. Assess communication devices, telephone, intercom system, presence of	*Determines client ability to contact help in an emergency*

Action	Rationale
emergency call system.	
14. Assess presence, habits, care of pets in the home.	*Alerts home care providers to presence of pets. Evaluates possible impact of pets on client health*
15. With client assistance, assess ability to move through the home, get in and out of chairs, get in and out of bed, etc. Suggest use of blocks to elevate furniture, suitable chairs, etc. Consider if physical therapy referral for transfer training is appropriate. If it is, obtain order.	*Determines client ability to safely perform activities of daily living in current home situation*
16. Ask client if he or she feels comfortable and secure in the home at this time.	*Determines client comfort level, desire to stay in the home setting*
17. Review suggested alterations to the home setting, and set a timetable for completion.	*Assists client in setting goals, enhances client independence*

Evaluation

Were desired outcomes achieved?

DOCUMENTATION

The following should be noted on the client assessment:

- Safety hazards noted and actions taken to resolve
- Adaptations needed to ensure safe and adequate care
- Client ability to assist with environmental assessment
- Client response to assessment, feelings about remaining in the home, response to suggestions for adaptations
- Contact with other disciplines, resources regarding adaptations

Sample Documentation

DATE	TIME	
5/21/98	1136	Environmental assessment completed with client cooperation. See assessment form. Suggestions to client re: need for smoke alarms, removal of scatter rugs in hallway, need for shower grab bars, and elevated toilet seat. Client agreeable to adaptations, has concerns about financial factors. Client will contact family in regard to assistance with finances, wishes to stay in the home. Nurse to assess progress in making adaptations next visit and contact social worker if additional community resources needed.

☒ *Nursing Procedure* **1.4**

Support System Assessment

☒ EQUIPMENT

- Pen
- Comprehensive assessment form
- Client history
- Completed physical assessment
- Client problem list or care plan
- Physician's orders for care

Purpose

Determines extent of emotional support, physical assistance, and assistance with care that can be provided to the client by others.

Desired Outcomes (sample)

The client will be emotionally and physically supported.
The client will have sufficient support to meet care needs when home health personnel are not present.

Assessment

Assessment should focus on the following:

Client relationship with family, friends, others in community
Client wishes regarding information given to others
Availability, willingness, and ability of others to assist with client care

Outcome Identification and Planning

Key Goals and Sample Goal Criteria

The client will:

Be comfortably supported and assisted with care
Be in control of information disseminated to others

Special Considerations

 Transcultural

Cultures vary widely in response to illness and to support of a person who is ill. In some cultures, offering assistance is considered insulting. In other cultures, everyone involved with the client is expected to know all details of care and the disease process. In still other cultures, certain disease processes are considered "shameful" and the client may be reluctant to risk any possibility of disclosure to another person. It is the responsibility of the nurse to be aware of cultural factors that influence the client, assess the support system in a nonjudgmental manner, and make every effort to provide resources that may support the client both emotionally and physically.

HINT

When assessing the client support system, provide the client with privacy to enable him or her to answer questions honestly. In some instances, the nurse will be unable to accurately assess the support system until the client has developed trust in the particular nurse.

Indications of abuse or neglect may be noted during an assessment of the support system. All nurses working in home health should take classes in recognizing signs of abuse, and be knowledgeable in actions to take.

IMPLEMENTATION

Action	Rationale
1. During any visit, observe the interaction between the client and others in the home.	*Provides insight into client relationships with others*
2. Initially, and on an ongoing basis, ask the client who is to be notified in an emergency, and with whom information concerning the client's condition may be discussed.	*Preserves the client's right to confidentiality*
3. Explain to the client that it is necessary to know who is available to assist with care, run errands, etc.	*Enhances client cooperation*

Action	Rationale
4. If the client lives with others, inquire as to who can help with care, be responsible for decisions, provide emotional support, etc. Questioning must be done in a nonjudgmental manner, and questions about personal relationships, family matters, etc., must be avoided unless there will be an impact on care.	*Elicits information without violating the client's right to privacy*
5. Assess for indications of abuse—client appears fearful, appears to be restricted to one room in home, has bruising or injuries that cannot be explained; family members will not allow client to be alone with nurse, or appear very hostile to nurse's presence. Suspicions of abuse must be reported to the appropriate agency. Check agency policy and procedure.	*Identifies problem that will impact client safety; allows for interventions necessary to protect client*
6. If client lives alone, inquire about available friends, neighbors, family members who could provide assistance—note on assessment form.	*Determines the existence of extended support*
7. Once support individuals have been identified, ask client what information may be shared with them.	*Protects client confidentiality*
8. Ask support individuals what help they can provide. Ask about help with care, errands, transportation, meals, emotional support. Approach support individuals in a nonjudgmental manner to elicit honest responses.	*Determines if support individuals are able, willing, and available*

Action	Rationale
9. If no support system is identified, refer to social worker for assistance with use of community resources. Provide client with information on transportation services, grocery delivery, housekeeping services, etc. Assist client in use of services. Advise client of local groups that may provide help. Consider using home health aides to assist with care, if appropriate.	*Provides a basis of support if no specific individuals can be identified*
10. Review the results of the support system assessment with other agency personnel involved in the care of the client.	*Prevents breach of client confidentiality, and provides consistency of care*

Evaluation

Were desired outcomes achieved?

DOCUMENTATION

The following should be noted on the client assessment:

• Whom to notify in an emergency
• Who has access to client information
• The availability, willingness, and ability of support persons
• The name, address, phone number, and relationship to the client of each support person

Sample Documentation

DATE	TIME	
10/01/98	0330	Support system assessment completed. Client lives alone, has several friends and neighbors willing to help with care. Has daughter out of state who is to be kept informed of care and condition. See assessment form for specific information.

*N*ursing *P*rocedure *1.5*

🖐 *Client Assessment*

❎ EQUIPMENT

- Pen
- Appropriate assessment form
- Gown or loose clothing
- Drape or sheet
- Blood pressure cuff
- Stethoscope
- Penlight
- Sphygmomanometer
- Thermometer
- Scales
- Watch with second hand
- Measurement tape
- Cotton balls
- Nonsterile gloves

Purpose

Determines strengths and weaknesses of physical and mental health status

Desired Outcomes (sample)

Signs and symptoms of underlying mental or physical alterations do not go undetected and undocumented.

Assessment

Assessment should focus on the following:

Medical diagnosis
Source of information
Information obtained on health history
Need for partial versus in-depth assessment

Outcome Identification and Planning

Key Goals and Sample Goal Criterion

The client will:

Have no undetected signs and symptoms of altered physiologic or mental status

Special Considerations

Acutely ill clients may require a more in-depth assessment of certain systems.

Assessment in acute situations should be prioritized to address life-threatening areas immediately, with assessment of other areas undertaken as soon as possible thereafter.

After initial detailed assessment is obtained for baseline data, an abbreviated assessment of problem areas noted from initial assessment may be performed as needed. A detailed assessment may need to be performed periodically, depending on agency policy and client state of health.

Geriatric

Normal developmental stage and physiologic changes must be taken into consideration when assessing the client.

Although most of the information in the history may be obtained from the client, the caregiver's or significant other's perspective regarding illness and care will be valuable throughout treatment plan.

A complete assessment must be completed on the client initially with abbreviated updates on each visit.

Transcultural

- When interviewing clients for whom English is not their native language, secure an interpreter to reduce the potential for mistaken interpretations of client responses.
- Biocultural norms should be determined before judging whether findings are pathologic (ie, mongolian spots are a normal skin variation in children of African, Asian, or Latin cultural background, but may be pathologic in Caucasian children).
- Color changes in persons of color may be best observed in areas of minimal pigmentation—sclera, conjunctiva, nail beds, palms and soles, and the mucosal areas. Consider, however, that a bluish hue may be normal for persons of Mediterranean or African descent.

IMPLEMENTATION

Action	Rationale
1. Wash hands and organize equipment.	*Reduces microorganism transfer* *Promotes efficiency*
2. Explain procedure to client, emphasizing importance of accuracy of data.	*Decreases anxiety* *Increases compliance*
3. Provide for privacy.	*Decreases embarrassment*

Health History

Action	Rationale
4. Obtain health history by interviewing client using therapeutic communication techniques (see Procedure 2.5). Include the following areas:	*Provides baseline data for future reference when providing care*
- Biographical information (name, age, sex, race, marital status, informant)	*Identifies client*
- Chief complaint (as stated in client's own words)	*Explains why client sought health care and what problem means to client*
- History of present problem (date of onset, detailed description of problem: nature, location, severity, and duration as well as associating, contributing, and precipitating factors)	*Defines details of manifestations of problems* *Helps define diagnosis*
- Past medical and surgical history (date and description of problems, previous hospitalizations, doctor's name, allergies as well as current medications and time of last dose)	*Serves as baseline and guide for treatment decisions* *Identifies potential problems related to present complaints*
- Family history of mental and physical conditions	*Identifies hereditary factors that may affect health status*
- Psychosocial history (occupation; educational level; abuse of alcohol and other drug sub-	*Identifies psychosocial, spiritual, and educational factors that may contribute to state of health*

Action	Rationale

stances; tobacco use; religious preference; cultural practices)

- Nutritional information (diet, food likes and dislikes, special requirements, and compliance to diets, intake over past 24 to 72 hours, as indicated).

Identifies nutritional factors related to present state of health

- Review of body systems (client's self-report of conditions or problems)

Detects subjective cues that may further define problem

Physical Assessment

5. Assess general appearance.

Provides objective cues about overall health state

6. Obtain vital signs, height, and weight.

Provides objective data about health state

7. Assess the following in relation to neuromuscular status:

Detects cues to abnormalities of neurologic or muscular status

Level of Consciousness
- Awake, alert, drowsy, lethargic, stuporous, or comatose

Orientation
- Oriented to person, time, and place or disoriented

Sensory Function
- Able to distinguish various sensations on skin surface (ie, hot/cold, sharp/dull) and aware of when and where sensation occurred

Motor Function
- Muscle tone (as determined by strength of extremities against resistance), gait, coordination of hands and feet, and reflex responses

Range of Motion
- Structural abnormalities

Action	Rationale

such as burns, scarring, spinal curvatures, bone spurs, contractures

8. While proceeding from head to toe, inspect skin of head, neck, and extremities:

    - Note color, lesions, tears, abrasions, ulcerations, scars, degree of moistness, edema, vascularity

    - Measure size of all abnormal lesions and scars with tape measure

    - If pressure ulcer detected, see guidelines for staging pressure ulcers in Procedure 10.11.

9. Palpate skin, lymph nodes, pulses, capillary refill, and joints of head, neck, and extremities. Note temperature, turgor, raised skin lesions, or lumps:

    - Lymph node tenderness and enlargement (Fig. 1.5.1 identifies lymph node areas)

    - Pulse quality, rhythm, and strength (Fig. 1.5.2 identifies pulse sites)

    - Crepitus, nodules, and mobility

10. Complete assessment of head and neck including eye, ear, nose, mouth, and throat:

Eye

    - Pupillary status (size, shape, and response to light and accommodation)

    - Visual acuity

Rationale:

Detects skin abnormalities

Provides baseline data for comparison

Detects skin abnormalities and lymph enlargement

Determines quality and character of pulses

Detects cues to pathophysiologic abnormalities of eye, ear, nose, mouth, and throat

Action   Rationale

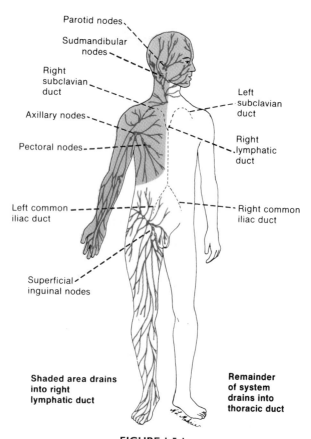

Parotid nodes

Sudmandibular nodes

Right subclavian duct

Left subclavian duct

Axillary nodes

Right lymphatic duct

Pectoral nodes

Left common iliac duct

Right common iliac duct

Superficial inguinal nodes

Shaded area drains into right lymphatic duct

Remainder of system drains into thoracic duct

FIGURE 1.5.1

Action	Rationale

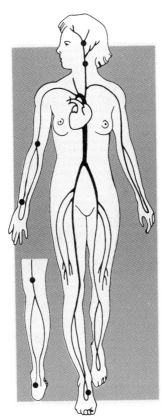

FIGURE 1.5.2

Action	Rationale

- Condition of cornea, conjunctival sac
- Abrasions, discharge, discoloration

Ear

- External ear structure (shape, presence of abnormalities on inspection and palpation)
- Hearing acuity (ability of client to respond to normal sounds)
- Presence of ear discharge and degree of wax buildup

Nose

- External and internal structure
- Presence of unusual or excessive discharge
- Ability to inhale and exhale through each nostril
- Ability to identify common odors correctly

Mouth

- Presence of lesions internally or externally
- Color of mucous membranes
- Abnormalities of teeth
- Unusual odor

Throat

- Presence of swelling, inflammation, or abnormal lesions
- Ability to swallow without difficulty

11. Inspect skin status of anterior and posterior trunk and extremities, including the feet.

   Detects skin abnormalities

12. Palpate chest, breasts, and back, noting:
   - Raised lesions on any

   Detects abnormal masses and lesions

Action	**Rationale**

area, tenderness on
   palpation
 - Symmetry of breasts
   and nipples; skin status;
   lymph nodes; presence
   of discharge, lumps, or
   nodules	

13. Assess cardiac status for the following:	*Detects cues related to patho- logic cardiac abnormalities*

- Unusual pulsations at
  precordium
- Character of first (S1)
  and second (S2) heart
  sounds
- Presence or absence of
  third (S3) or fourth (S4)
  heart sounds
- Presence of murmurs or
  rubs
- Auscultate heart sounds
  in the following areas
  (Fig. 1.5.3).

Aortic—at second or

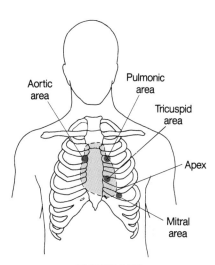

FIGURE 1.5.3

Action	Rationale

third intercostal space just to the right of sternum
Pulmonic—at second or third intercostal space just to the left of sternum
Tricuspid—at fourth intercostal space just to left of sternum
Mitral—in left midclavicular line at fifth intercostal space

14. Assess respiratory status: Note character of respirations and of anterior and posterior breath sounds in the following areas:
Bronchial—over trachea
Bronchovesicular—on each side of sternum between first and second intercostal space
Vesicular—peripheral areas of chest
Note: When auscultating breath sounds, use side-to-side sequence to compare breath sounds on each side (Fig. 1.5.4). Avoid auscultating over bone or breast tissue.

Determines if adventitious breath sounds (rales rhonchi, or wheezes) are present, indicating abnormal pathophysiologic alterations
Side-to-side comparison approach increases possibility of detecting abnormalities in a given client

15. Assess abdomen. PERFORM AUSCULTATION BEFORE PALPATION AND PERCUSSION OF ABDOMEN.
- Inspect size and contour.
- Auscultate for bowel sounds in all quadrants.
- Palpate tone of abdomen and check for underlying abnormalities (masses, pain, tenderness) and bladder distension.

Detects masses, abnormal fluid retention, or decrease or absence of peristalsis
Palpation and percussion set underlying structures in motion, possibly interfering with character of bowel sounds

Action	Rationale

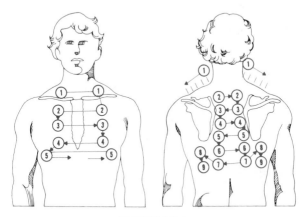

FIGURE 1.5.4

16. Assess genitalia and urethra.
    - Inspect for abnormalities in structure, discoloration, edema, abnormal discharge, or foul odor

    Detects abnormalities of genitalia and urethral opening

17. Restore or discard equipment properly.

    Removes microorganisms

18. Wash hands.

    Prevents spread of microorganisms

Evaluation

Were desired outcomes achieved?

DOCUMENTATION

The following should be noted on the visit note:

- Time of assessment
- Informant
- Chief complaint
- Information from client history
- Detailed description of assessment area related to chief complaint or need for visit
- Detailed description of abnormalities
- Reports of abnormal subjective data (pain, nausea, and so forth)
- Priority areas of assessment
- Assessment procedures deferred to a later time
- Ability of client to assist with assessment

Sample Documentation

DATE	TIME	
4/29/98	0830	Special visit for complaint of nagging chest pain in center of chest that started 24 hours ago. Denies nausea, headache, or radiation of pain to arms or back. No abnormal heart sounds detected. Vital signs: blood pressure, 130/90; pulse, 82; temperature, 98.8°F; respirations, 22. Noted irregular pulse. No jugular vein distention. Pulses in upper and lower extremities weak (1+). Skin slightly moist but warm. No lower extremity edema noted. Doctor notified regarding pain and irregular pulse.

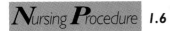

*N*ursing *P*rocedure 1.6

Blood Pressure by Palpation

☒ EQUIPMENT

- Blood pressure cuff
- Sphygmomanometer
- Sheet for recording
- Pen

Purpose

Obtains blood pressure measurement by palpation for pulse return (systolic pressure) when blood pressure cannot be obtained by auscultation

Desired Outcomes (sample)

Significant changes in blood pressure are detected at early stages.

Client shows signs of adequate tissue perfusion (brisk capillary refill; normal heart rate; warm, pink, and dry skin).

Assessment

Assessment should focus on the following:

Ordered frequency of readings, if any, or conditions that might indicate need for frequent readings (eg, cardiac failure, postoperative hemorrhage)

Extremity being used to obtain blood pressure (if arm cannot be used for brachial blood pressure, use leg for popliteal pressure)

Skin integrity of extremity being used

Initial and previous blood pressure recordings

Circulation in extremity in which readings are being obtained (skin color and temperature, color of mucous membranes, pulse volume, capillary refill)

Outcome Identification and Planning

Key Goals and Sample Goal Criteria

The client will:

Have no undetected significant changes in blood pressure
Show signs of adequate tissue perfusion (brisk capillary refill; heart rate normal; skin warm, pink, and dry)

Special Considerations

If blood pressure was audible previously and becomes palpable only, notify the physician and continue to monitor the client closely with blood pressure, pulse, and respirations every 5 to 10 minutes.

Readings reflecting a 20-mmHg change in blood pressure should be reported.

Systolic readings in popliteal area are usually 10 to 40 mmHg above brachial readings.

Although a diastolic pressure can be obtained by palpation, frequent errors occur in obtaining results.

If you are unable to palpate blood pressure, try using Doppler, if available.

If client has had a mastectomy or has a hemodialysis shunt or IV infusion, avoid taking blood pressure in the affected extremity.

Geriatric

Avoid leaving blood pressure cuff on elderly clients, because skin may be thin and fragile.

IMPLEMENTATION

Action	Rationale
1. Explain procedure to client and family.	*Decreases anxiety* *Promotes cooperation*
2. Wash hands and organize equipment.	*Reduces microorganism transfer* *Promotes efficiency*
3. Palpate for brachial or radial pulse.	*Finds pulse offering best palpable volume for procedure*
4. Place cuff on arm selected for blood pressure.	*Positions cuff for inflation*
5. Palpate again for pulse. Once pulse is obtained, continue to palpate.	*Relocates pulse for procedure*
6. Inflate cuff until unable to palpate pulse.	*Occludes arterial blood flow*

Action	Rationale
7. Inflate cuff until measurement gauge is 20 mmHg past the point at which pulse was lost on palpation.	*Clearly identifies point of pulse return*
8. Slowly deflate cuff at 2 to 3 mmHg per second.	*Prevents missing first palpable beat*
9. Note reading on measurement gauge when pulse returns.	*Identifies systolic blood pressure reading*
10. Repeat steps 5 through 9.	*Confirms readings*
11. Remove cuff (or leave on if readings are being obtained at frequent intervals).	*Promotes comfort*
12. Restore equipment.	*Prepares for next use*
13. Wash hands.	*Reduces microorganisms*

Evaluation

Were desired outcomes achieved?

DOCUMENTATION

The following should be noted on the visit note:

- Systolic blood pressure measurement upon palpation
- Extremity from which blood pressure was obtained
- Circulatory indicators (capillary refill, color of skin and mucous membranes, skin temperature, quality of pulses)
- Level of consciousness
- Follow-up reporting to physician

Sample Documentation

DATE	TIME	
3/4/98	0830	Blood pressure by palpation, 80 mmHg systolic from right arm. Client slightly lethargic at times. Skin cool to touch. Nailbeds and mucous membranes slightly blanched in color. Capillary refill, 5 seconds. Doctor notified. Ambulance phoned.

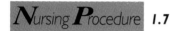 **1.7**

Apical–Radial Pulse Measurement

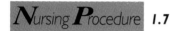 EQUIPMENT

- Pen
- Recording sheet
- Stethoscope
- Watch with second hand
- Second person (family/caregiver), if available

Purpose

Detects presence of pulse deficit that is related to poor ventricular contractions or dysrhythmias

Desired Outcomes (sample)

No undetected pulse irregularities or pulse deficit is experienced.

Assessment

Assessment should focus on the following:

Ordered frequency of readings with follow-up orders
History of dysrhythmias or cardiac conditions
Pulse characteristics
Previous pulse recordings
Medication regimen for cardiac drugs

Outcome Identification and Planning

Key Goals and Sample Goal Criterion
The client will:

Experience no undetected pulse irregularities or pulse deficit.

Special Considerations

Clients with ventricular (pump) pathologies, cardiac dysrhythmias, and chronic conditions such as diabetes and atherosclerosis, are particularly prone to pulse deficits, and should be checked every 24 hours for apical–radial pulse deficit.

Because procedure requires two persons, enlist and train a family member to assist. Teach family member(s) to perform the procedure between nurse visits.

IMPLEMENTATION

Action	Rationale
1. Explain procedure to client and family.	*Decreases anxiety*
2. Wash hands and organize equipment.	*Reduces contamination* *Promotes efficiency*
3. Have family, caregiver, or home health aide position themselves to take radial pulse (at radial artery).	
4. The nurse should place stethoscope on skin at apex (fifth intercostal space at midclavicular line) to obtain apical pulse. Maintain privacy.	*Locates apical pulse*
5. Place watch so that both people counting can see second hand.	*Facilitates accuracy in beginning and ending*
6. State "begin" when ready to start (nurse counting apical pulse will state when to begin and end counting).	*Prevents error in count, because nurse with stethoscope in ear cannot hear count call*
7. Both counters should count pulse for 1 full minute AT THE SAME TIME.	*Ensures accuracy of reading*
8. Call out "stop" when minute has passed. NOTE: If second counter not available, nurse should obtain radial pulse in a	*Ends 1-minute count*

Action	Rationale

one-minute period, followed immediately by the apical rate in the subsequent one-minute period.

9. Compare rates obtained. If a difference is noted between apical and radial rates, subtract the radial rate from the apical rate. — *Determines if pulse deficit exists. Pulse deficit will be the number obtained by deducting radial from apical*

10. Repeat steps 6 through 9. — *Verifies results*

11. Adjust clothing and adjust position for comfort. — *Restores privacy*

12. Wash hands. — *Reduces microorganisms*

13. Notify doctor if pulse deficit was noted. — *Initiates prompt medical intervention*

Evaluation

Were desired outcomes achieved?

DOCUMENTATION

The following should be noted on the visit note:

- Apical–radial pulse rate
- Quality of pulse
- Irregularities of pulse rhythm (if present)
- Calculated pulse deficit, if present
- Response to deficit
- Current cardiac drugs

Sample Documentation

DATE	TIME	
1/6/98	0830	Apical–radial pulse, 94 apical and 74 radial with pulse deficit of 20. Pulse irregular. Client states no dizziness, faintness, or chest discomfort. Doctor Britt notified.

Nursing Procedure *1.8*

Obtaining Weights at Home

☒ EQUIPMENT

- Portable floor scales
- Pen
- Graphic sheet or weight record

Purpose

Obtains body weight for periodic evaluation of nutritional or fluid status

Desired Outcomes (sample)

2 pounds per week weight loss indicated by daily scale readings.

1 kilogram weight loss noted by scale weight after 3 days of fluid restriction diet.

Assessment

Assessment should focus on the following:

Doctor's orders regarding frequency and specified time of weight
Medical diagnosis
Previous body weight
Rationale for home weight
Type and amount of clothing being worn (should be weighed in same type and amount of clothing)
Adequacy of scale function

Outcome Identification and Planning

Key Goals and Sample Goal Criteria

The client will:

Lose 2 pounds per week on a 1100-calorie diet
Lose 1 kilogram of weight during next 3 series of dialysis exchanges

Special Considerations

Always be sure to weigh client on the same floor surface in the same location to avoid changes caused by carpet, unlevel floor, etc.

If client is unable to stand independently or has drainage tubes which could become dislodged, secure adequate assistance with moving of client.

If client weight possibly exceeds weight capacity of scale, seek alternative means for weighing client.

IMPLEMENTATION

Action	Rationale
1. Explain procedure to client.	*Decreases anxiety*
2. Wash hands and gather equipment.	*Reduces microorganisms*
3. Place scales on flat, non-skid area on floor.	*Stabilizes equipment and prevents falls*
4. Calibrate (zero balance) scales according to manufacturer's directions.	*Controls accuracy of results*
5. Assist client into sitting, then standing position.	
6. Secure all tubes so that no pulling occurs during procedure. Have assistant hold tubes, if necessary.	*Prevents dislodgment and subsequent client injury*
7. Assist client onto scales, allowing client to stand until balance is achieved.	*Prevents falls*
8. Note weight on bathroom scale. For digital scale, press button on readout console to obtain weight in pounds or kilograms.	*Obtains weight*
9. Assist client back to bed or chair.	*Positions client*
10. Assist as needed to position of comfort.	*Facilitates comfort*
11. Restore or discard all equipment appropriately.	
12. Wash hands.	
13. Record weight immediately	*Avoids loss of data and re-weighing of client*

Evaluation

Were desired outcomes achieved?

DOCUMENTATION

The following should be noted on the visit chart:

- Weight obtained in pounds or kilograms
- Type (and number) of scale used for weight
- Tolerance of procedure

Sample Documentation

DATE	TIME	
3/9/98	0600	Weight after third day of fluid restrictions 82 kilograms. One kilogram weight loss noted since first day. Has voided 900 mL over last 24 hours. Will instruct on sodium restricted diet on next visit when family present.

Verbal Communication Skills

OVERVIEW

▶ Accurate, concise, and thorough verbal communication is a key skill in home care. The home care nurse acts as the eyes and ears of the physician, other care providers, payor sources, and the agency.

▶ The nurse must remember that most verbal communications with payor sources and other providers take place over the phone or over a fax machine. The person receiving the communication does not know the nurse, and must base judgments on the information given.

▶ Verbal communication involves a sender, a receiver, a message, and the environment in which the interaction takes place.

▶ Communication includes the attitude projected—gestures, voice tone, rhythm, volume, and pitch—in addition to words spoken.

▶ Effective communication is
  - *simple*—briefly and comprehensively relates data using commonly known and understood terms
  - *clear*—states exactly what is meant covering the who, what, when, where, why, and how of the matter

- *pertinent*—contains data that are important to the current situation and ties data to an apparent need to show significance
- *sensitive*—considers readiness of the receiver and adapts depth and breadth of data to meet receiver's needs
- *accurate*—includes factual information related with confidence and credibility

▶ Building effective communication skills requires a constant awareness of one's self as a sender and a receiver of messages.

▶ Communication approaches should be modified to meet the cultural needs of the client.

▶ Teaching is a part of all home health visits. Approaching each visit with a general plan that is also flexible to the client's perceived needs enhances learning and the nurse–client relationship.

▶ When caring for a client with multiple disciplines, eg, therapists, home health aides, etc., the nurse should be responsible for communicating with all individuals, to provide the client with a truly multidisciplinary plan of care.

Nursing **P**rocedure *2.1*

Verbal Communication in Home Care

▣ EQUIPMENT

- Pen
- Form to document verbal communication

Purpose

Provides for sharing of accurate information concerning client condition, plan of care, and changes needed in care among various care providers.

Desired Outcomes (sample)

All applicable care providers and payor sources will have accurate information concerning the client.

Changes in client condition will be effectively communicated.

Assessment

Assessment should focus on the following:

Identity and availability of care providers and payor sources involved in the client's care.

Information needed by various care providers, payor sources.

Desired method of communication, ie, phone or fax.

Outcome Identification and Planning

Key Goals and Sample Goal Criteria

The client's care will be:

Supported and enhanced by accurate and timely communication among care providers and payor sources

Special Considerations

Establish with the agency a method of routing information received from the physician's office. In some agencies, the field nurse is called directly by pager or by cellular phone, while in others, the supervisor is the go-between. All parties involved in the communication must have the same information.

When verbally communicating with any party, take a few minutes to review exactly what information is needed. A medical supply company about to make a delivery will need a correct address, while a payor source will need to know client condition, care being received, and expected duration of care. Being well prepared with accurate information indicates to the other party that you are acting with professionalism and competence.

HINT

> *It is rare that the home health nurse will speak directly with the physician during physician office hours. Establish a contact at the office who will reliably transfer information to the physician. Check with the office to determine the best time to leave non-emergent messages for the physician, and the best method. Some physicians prefer a call at certain times of the day, while others may prefer a faxed report.*

 Transcultural

When interacting with a client, the nurse must communicate in a way that is understood by the client. For those clients who speak another language, or who are hearing-impaired, family members may be used as interpreters. If an interpreter is not available, the nurse may use more visual tools, such as pictures and drawings, to enhance communication. Local community groups may be able to assist with materials in a specific language, or may, with the client's permission, be able to provide an interpreter.

IMPLEMENTATION

Action	Rationale
1. Before initiating a phone communication with any other party, determine what information is needed.	*Having needed information readily available increases the clarity and focus of the communication*

Action	Rationale
2. Have all related information with you at the time you make the call, and make the call in as quiet an environment as possible.	*Allows the nurse to answer questions, and to hear and understand the other party*
3. Clearly state who you are, the agency you represent, and what the call is about.	*Allows the party receiving the call to route you to the proper person*
4. Obtain the name of the person with whom you are speaking.	*Permits the nurse to follow-up with the same person if needed*
5. Give all information in a clear and concise manner. If giving a condition report, know current vital signs, symptoms, medications, etc.	*Reduces the need for additional calls by having all needed information*
6. If receiving a phone order from a physician, repeat it back to the physician for verification, and put it in writing immediately, to be sent out for physician signature.	*Reduces the chance of acting on a misunderstood order*
7. Document all verbal and phone communication concerning any client.	*Provides a clear picture in the client record and reduces the reliance on any individual's memory*

Evaluation

Were desired outcomes achieved?

DOCUMENTATION

Document all physician orders on the form specified by the agency.

Document all client communication on the form designated for that function by the agency. All documentation must be dated.

Sample Documentation

DATE	TIME	
5/07/98	0530	**Physician order** - "Continue current daily wound irrigation and wound care × 7 days." Phone order Dr. Jones/N. Smith R.N.
		Phone conference with insurance co. case manager - Spoke with Tom Bridges, case manager re: John James. Reported increased drainage from wound, need for continued skilled nursing visits daily × 1 week to observe healing, perform sterile irrigation, packing, and wound dressing as ordered by Dr. Jones. Approval received from Tom Bridges. N. Smith R.N.

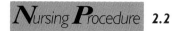

Nursing Procedure 2.2

Therapeutic Communication

☒ EQUIPMENT

- Calendars
- Clocks
- Picture or word boards
- Any items needed to add clarity to message

Purpose

Facilitates sense of well-being and control
Promotes beneficial nurse–client/family interaction

Desired Outcomes (sample)

Client evidences no sign of anxiety and communicates needs effectively.
Client complies with dietary, activity, or home care regimen.
Client discusses major stressors in current life.

Assessment

Assessment should focus on the following:

Client's age, developmental level, cultural or ethnic background, educational level
Physical and mental barriers to communication, such as poor sight or hearing, speech impediment, pain, and so forth
Client's use of nonverbal gesturing
Client's perceptions of people and situations
Sources of stress for client
Client's use of defense and coping mechanisms
Immediate environment (eg, noise, lighting, visitors)
Support systems (family, friends, community agencies)
(See Nursing Procedure 1.4 - Support System Assessment)

Outcome Identification and Planning

Key Goals and Sample Goal Criteria

The client will:

DISPLAY 2.2.1 **Considerations for Interactions With Special Clients/Families**

When interacting with an anxious client, recognize client's decreased ability to focus on and respond to multiple stimuli:
- maintain quiet, calm environment
- keep messages simple, concrete, and brief
- repeat messages often
- minimize need for extensive decision making
- monitor anxiety level, using verbal and nonverbal cues

When interacting with an angry client:
- use careful, unhurried, deliberate body movements
- provide an open, nonthreatening environment
- clear area of anger-provoking stimuli (persons, objects, etc.)
- maintain a nonthreatening demeanor, using open body language, soft voice tones, and so forth

When interacting with a depressed client:
- allow additional time for interactions
- emphasize use of physical attending
- avoid giving client time-limited tasks due to slowed reflexes
- monitor closely for cues of self-destructive tendencies
- keep messages simple, concrete, and brief
- minimize need for extensive decision making

When interacting with a client exhibiting denial:
- use direct questions to determine the situation triggering use of coping mechanism
- do not avoid the reality of the situation, but allow client to maintain denial defense; it often serves a protective function
- recognize that denial may be the first of a series of crisis phases, to be followed by phases of: increased tension, disorganization, attempts to reorganize, attempts to escape the problem, local reorganization, general reorganization, and possibly resolution
- be alert for cues that the phase is ending (ie, questions from client regarding the disturbing situation)

Communicate needs and their satisfactions effectively
Comply with dietary and activity regimen
Verbalize feelings about recent occurrences

Special Considerations

The nurse should anticipate questions and concerns when explaining factual information.

Encourage the client and family to prepare a list of questions or concerns during the time between visits.

Plan interaction times to ensure privacy and avoid interruptions.

When planning interactions consider the phase of the nurse–client relationship:

- *Orientation phase:* initial meeting of client and nurse; verbal contract is made
- *Working phase:* basic nurse–client trust established and relationship solidified through meeting of objectives
- *Termination phase:* preparation for discharge and ending of relationship

When interacting with clients consider their stage of coping or possible grief: denial, anger, bargaining, depression, and acceptance (see Display 2.2.1).

Avoid statements or behaviors that might result in barriers to communication (Display 2.2.2).

Geriatric

Elderly clients may have one or more communication barriers that may readily be removed once discovered; necessary dentures, hearing aids, and glasses should be acquired, if possible.

With increasing age, a client's speech and comprehension may be slowed, requiring more time for communication.

  Transcultural

- Use of an interpreter for clients whose native language is not English may reduce chances of miscommunication by client and nurse.

DISPLAY 2.2.2	**Blocks to Therapeutic Communication**

Giving advice
Using responses that imply approval or disapproval
Agreeing or disagreeing
Not listening attentively
Appearing distracted
Imposing judgment
Stereotyping
Providing false reassurance
Using clichés
Excessive probing
Questioning without basis
Responding defensively

- Clients of some cultures may view direct eye contact as offensive and intrusive. It is best to follow the cues of the client in developing a rapport.
- Sociocultural differences should be considered when interpreting a client's nonverbal behavior (ie, lack of eye contact may signify respect, not insecurity, and a shuffling gait may signify "cool" use of body language, not physical debilitation).

IMPLEMENTATION

Action	Rationale
1. Approach the client in a purposeful but unhurried manner.	*Facilitates controlled but nonthreatening interaction*
2. Identify self and relationship to client.	*Initiates orientation phase of nurse–client relationship*
3. Obtain family/client assistance and permission in arranging environment so that it is conducive to type of interaction needed.	*Eliminates environmental distractions*
4. Use physical attending skills throughout the interaction process:	*Exhibits nonverbal body language consistent with verbalizations*
- Face directly and lean toward client	*Conveys interest, attentiveness, sincerity, and nondefensiveness*
- Maintain eye contact and an open posture (do not cross legs or arms)	
5. Begin interaction using therapeutic techniques when eliciting or sharing information or responses:	*Facilitates purposeful and mutually beneficial interaction for nurse and client*
- Use open-ended statements and questions	*Allows ventilation of those feelings and concerns most important to client at the time*
- Restate or paraphrase client statements when indicated	*Confirms significance of client's comments*
- Clarify unclear comments	*Ensures intended message*
- Focus the statement when client tends to ramble or is vague	*Promotes concreteness of message*
- Explore further when additional information is needed	*Promotes more complete information gathering*

Action	Rationale
- Provide rationale why more information is needed, when appropriate	*Maintains professional integrity of interaction*
- Use touch and silence, when appropriate	*Conveys compassion and allows time for client composure*
6. Use active listening techniques:	
- Do not interrupt in the middle of comments	*Prevents distraction*
- Use verbal indicators of acceptance and understanding ("um-hmm," "yes")	*Expresses interest*
- Focus on verbal and nonverbal message	*Facilitates receipt of complete message*
7. When client communicates, note use of gestures as well as facial expression and elements of speech—tone, pitch, emphasis of words, etc.	*Facilitates receipt of complete message*
8. Note client's nonverbal gestures as you are speaking (facial grimacing, smiling, crossing arms or legs).	*Facilitates detection of cues indicating acceptance or non-acceptance of message*
9. Toward end of the interaction, summarize important aspects of the conversation.	*Avoids abrupt and incomplete closure*

Evaluation

Were desired outcomes achieved?

DOCUMENTATION

The following should be noted on the visit note:

- Date, time, and place of interaction
- Nature and significant highlights of the discussion
- Communication barriers (if any) and interventions used
- Significant nonverbal gestures

Sample Documentation

DATE	TIME	
7/04/98	0211	Client in bed and tearful; upset because husband has not been home in 3 days. States concern about husband's feelings regarding loss of her breast. Reach to Recovery support group discussed and contacted. Nurse will contact husband this P.M. Sister available to assist with dressing change at current time. Will request social services consult.

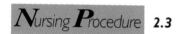

Client Education

⊠ EQUIPMENT

- Selected teaching tools (booklets, pamphlets, audiovisual materials, games, and so forth)

Purpose

Assists client in learning information necessary for participation in self-care
Reduces anxiety

Desired Outcomes (sample)

Client states purpose of procedure before beginning procedure.
Client demonstrates procedure correctly with 100% accuracy by discharge from home health services.
Client states solutions to potential complications of procedure by discharge from home health services.

Assessment

Assessment should focus on the following:

Client's or family's readiness to learn and ability to comprehend
Client's or family's age and educational level
Amount and accuracy of client's prior knowledge about content
Community resources for referral
Prior knowledge of significant others, if they are to be included
Presence of any communication barriers such as visual, hearing, or speech problems
Presence of any physical or emotional barriers (conditions or medications that alter mental state or cause pain or stress)
Environmental distractions (TV, noise, visitors not involved in client care)

Outcome Identification and Planning

Key Goals and Sample Goal Criteria

The client/learner will:

Demonstrate procedure using correct technique with 100% accuracy by discharge

State the purpose before beginning the procedure

State solutions to potential complications of the procedure by discharge from home health services

Special Considerations

Incorporate adaptations or modifications of procedures likely to occur in the home setting.

Individuals with similar problems are frequently helpful in facilitating client learning.

A list of support or referral groups may be available through home health agency and phone directory.

Geriatric

Because of delayed reaction times that occur with normal aging, elderly clients may require more response time during actual teaching and evaluation.

Consider response time when planning time frame.

 Transcultural

- Examples used for clarification or explanation of information may in some instances be understood more easily if they relate to some aspect of the client's culture. Pictures may be useful if a different language is spoken. Many facilities have access to interpreters of various languages if needed.
- It is important to find out how the client views health. Many clients of various cultures view illness as a curse or bad luck. This may affect the nurse's ability to engage the client successfully in active learning.

IMPLEMENTATION

Action	Rationale
1. Establish verbal contact with client or learner regarding teaching plans.	*Provides mutual goals for client and nurse*
2. Obtain client/family assistance to eliminate environmental distractions such as excess noise, poor lighting, uncomfortable room temperatures, cluttered rooms, excess visitor and staff traffic, and clini-	*Facilitates environment for communication and learning*

Action	Rationale
cal treatments and procedures.	
3. During assessment and along with client or learner, determine exactly what information is needed.	*Provides teaching focus* *Involves client* *Teaching is most effective when it occurs in response to specific needs expressed by the learner*
4. Determine nursing diagnoses based on assessment findings.	*Provides focus for goal-setting*
5. Set realistic, measurable goals with client and significant others.	*Allows client participation* *Provides focus for implementing teaching*
6. Develop teaching plan (Display 2.3) that specifically addresses: - Objectives to be met by the end of teaching session	*Facilitates optimal learning*

DISPLAY 2.3   **Preparation Guide for Development of a Teaching Plan**

Objectives to be met by end of session
Content
   What content will be taught to meet objectives?
   Will complex content need to be taught in divided stages?
Teaching methods
   What reading materials are needed?
   What audiovisual aids are needed?
   Will games or role-playing be used?
   Will support groups or group sessions be used?
   What equipment/supplies are needed?
   Will tours or visits to related agencies be helpful?
   How much time is needed to cover each section of
     material?
   Will practice time be needed?
   How much time is realistic for this client?
Evaluation methods
   How much time will be needed to evaluate learning?
   Will evaluation be:
     verbal?
     written?
     return demonstration?

Action	Rationale

- Content to be taught
- Methods of teaching
- Methods of evaluation
7. Obtain all necessary equipment.
8. Implement teaching plan.
9. Evaluate plan and implementation.

Provides questions to guide teaching plan preparation

Evaluation

Were desired outcomes achieved?

DOCUMENTATION

The following should be noted on the visit note:

- Extent to which each objective was met (fully, partially, not met)
- Nature of material taught
- Persons other than client included in session
- Client response to teaching
- Client concerns expressed during teaching
- Need for additional teaching or alternate method of teaching
- Need for revision of plans with client input

Sample Documentation

DATE	TIME	
6/11/98	0900	Client teaching done regarding importance of low-sodium diet in relation to managing hypertension. Client demonstrated selection of low-sodium foods with 80% accuracy from list. Participated actively in learning. Denies concerns in relation to topic at this time. Re-instruction session needed for family.

Chapter 3

Written Communication Skills

3.1 Plan of Care/Visit Plan
3.2 Progress Notes

OVERVIEW

▶ Written documentation in home care is a specialized skill, unlike nursing documentation in other health settings. The plan of care and visit plan for each client may be prepared by the nurse, and reviewed by the physician. Once signed by the physician, the plan of care becomes the client's physician orders, and any deviation from the plan of care must be documented in an additional physician order.

▶ Payor sources and regulatory agencies routinely use the documented plan of care, visit plan, and progress notes to determine compliance with various federal and state regulations, and to determine if payment is warranted.

▶ A plan of care and visit plan must clearly indicate what care is needed, what health care discipline is to provide that care, how long the care will be needed, and what limitations prevent the client from doing his or her own care, or going to another setting for the care. The plan of care, also called the plan of treatment, is the basic document of home health nursing. Mastering the skill of writing a clear, cohesive, complete, and accurate plan of care is essential to successful home health practice.

▶ Each progress note must indicate the extent of the client's functional limitations, what skilled care was provided, who provided the care, how the client responded to the care, the client's progress, the plan for further care, and progress toward discharge from services.

▶ Progress notes in a client record should reflect the client's progress toward the goals of care. In addition, each progress note must stand alone in indicating that the care performed was skilled care, requiring the services of a professional nurse.

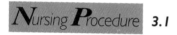 **3.1**

Plan of Care/Visit Plan

☒ EQUIPMENT

- Pen
- Client assessment
- Environmental assessment
- Support system assessment
- Specific physician orders

Purpose

Establishes a plan of care and schedule of visits for each individual client based on that client's physician orders, functional limitations, care needs, and general living situation.

Desired Outcomes (sample)

The plan of care will accurately reflect the client condition, need
for skilled care, specific physician orders, anticipated progress, criteria for discharge, supplies needed, visit schedule for
all disciplines, and environmental and support system factors.

Assessment

Assessment should focus on the following:

Client diagnosis
Client assessment information
Specific physician orders

Outcome Identification and Planning

Key Goals and Sample Goal Criteria

The plan of care/visit plan will accurately reflect the status and
needs of the client.
The plan of care/visit plan will include all necessary information to meet agency policy, regulatory requirements, and
payor source needs.

Special Considerations

If the client will need supplies such as dressing supplies, catheters, etc., be sure to note them on the plan of care. Many payor sources will only reimburse for supplies noted on the plan of care.

HINT

A plan of care, once signed by the physician, acts as physician orders for the client. The nurse must be able to complete the plan of care and turn it in to the agency for mailing to the physician in a timely manner.

 Transcultural

The culture of the client may impact on every aspect of his or her care. Take this into consideration when writing the plan of care and visit schedule.

IMPLEMENTATION

Action	Rationale
1. Use the agency-specific format for entering information for the plan of care. (Display 3.1)	*Complies with agency policy, regulatory and payor requirements*
2. Enter the client demographics correctly.	*Allows for accurate identification of the client*
3. Enter the name and number of a person to be called in an emergency	*Allows for rapid agency response in the event of a client emergency*
4. Enter the client diagnosis and procedure if applicable, being aware that all care provided must be related to the diagnosis and/or procedure.	*Relates the care needs to the diagnosis*
5. Note the client functional limitations that prevent the client from leaving home to obtain the needed care.	*Justifies the provision of home health services*
6. Note any safety modifications needed in the home environment.	*Indicates environmental assessment was done, and adaptations suggested*

Action   **Rationale**

Department of Health and Human Services Health Care Financing Administration	EFFECTIVE DATE:	A:_____	B:_____		Form Approved OMB No. 0938-0357
	**HOME HEALTH CERTIFICATION AND PLAN OF TREATMENT**				

1. Patient's HI Claim No.	2. SOC Date	3. Certification Period		4. Medical Record No.	5. Provider No.
		From: To:			

6. Patient's Name and Address (PRINT/Last Name First)

Phone:

7. Provider's Name and Address
NOTIFY IN EMERGENCY:
(Name:
(Relationship:
(Phone:

8. Date of Birth:	Ethnic:	9. Sex ___ M ___ F	10. Medications: Dose/Frequency/Route (N)ew (C)hanged

11.ICD-9-CM	Principal Diagnosis	Date	(Supv. Responsibility) PAYOR CODE: REFERRAL CODE:
12.ICD-9-CM	Surgical Procedure	Date	ECF:_____ DATES:_____ HOSP:_____ DATES:_____
13.ICD-9-CM	Other Pertinent Diagnosis	Date	

| 14. DME and Supplies | Medicare Covered? Yes_____ No_____ |
| | 15. Safety Measures: |

| 16. Nutritional Req. | 17. Allergies: |

18.A Functional Limitations

1	Amputation	5	Paralysis	9	Legally Blind
2	Bowel/Bladder	6	Endurance	A	Dyspnea with Minimal Exertion
3	Contracture	7	Ambulation	B	Other (Specify)
4	Hearing	8	Speech		

18.B Activities Permitted

1	Complete Bedrest	6	Partial Weight Bearing	A	Wheelchair
2	Bedrest BRP	7	Independent at Home	B	Walker
3	Up as Tolerated	8	Crutches	C	No Restrictions
4	Transfer Bed/Chair	9	Cane	D	Other (Specify)
5	Exercise Presc.				

19. Mental Status

| 1 | Oriented | 3 | Forgetful | 5 | Disoriented | 7 | Agitated |
| 2 | Comatose | 4 | Depressed | 6 | Lethargic | 8 | Other |

20. Prognosis

| 1 | Poor | 2 | Guarded | 3 | Fair | 4 | Good | 5 | Excellent |

21. Orders for Discipline and Treatments (Specify Amount/Frequency/Duration) RN Projections: RN Orders:	WRITE SIGNIFICANT CLINICAL FINDINGS ON REVERSE SIDE Injury Related to accident: Yes___ No___ Explain (where, how, date):_____ COMMENTS:
MSW Projections: MSW Orders:	
HHA Projections: HHA Orders:	Justification:

22. Goals/Rehabilitation Potential/Discharge Plans
GOALS:

REHAB POT.:

D/C PLAN:

23. Verbal Start of Care and Nurse's Signature and Date Where Applicable:	25. Date HHA Received Signed POT
24. Physician's Name (Last Name, First Name) CC: (Last Name, First Name)	26. I certify/recertify that this patient is confined to his/her home and needs intermittent skilled nursing care, physical therapy and/or speech therapy or continues to need occupational therapy. The patient is under my care, and I have authorized the services on this plan of care and will periodically review the plan.
27. Attending Physician's Signature and Date Signed	28. Anyone who misrepresents, falsifies, or conceals essential information required for payment of Federal funds may be subject to fine, imprisonment, or civil penalty under applicable Federal laws.

DISPLAY 3.1

7. Note client nutritional requirements.

Provides diet order, indicates possible need for diet instruction

8. Enter supplies needed.

Allows for planning of care and reimbursement from payor source

9. Detail specific visit plan for nursing skilled care to be provided. Include in-

Acts as a blueprint for care; once signed, becomes physician orders; allows the nurse to de-

Action	Rationale

struction to client as a skill, nursing assessment, specific nursing tasks. If home health aides are to be used, indicate specific tasks to be performed. Include in all visit plans the number of nurse and aide visits per week, and the number of weeks of care anticipated.

tail all nursing skills to be performed while the client is receiving home health services

10. Enter specific goals for the client that are measurable, and indicate when those goals are expected to be reached.

Specifies what the care to be provided is expected to achieve, and when

11. Enter specific discharge criteria for the client.

Indicates an end point for skilled care

12. Write a brief summary of the client condition. Include all factors that justify the care needed, and all factors that could interfere with the care process and the achievement of desired goals.

Provides a clear picture of the client's current condition and supports the need for care

Evaluation

Were desired outcomes achieved?

DOCUMENTATION

Documentation of the plan of care/visit plan varies according to agency. Some agencies use preprinted forms or checklists and some agencies use computer data entry. Regardless of the form, the documentation of the plan of care must follow certain principles. A completed plan of care should indicate the client demographics, functional limitations, and safety needs. There should be a clear relationship among the client diagnosis, the care disciplines required, and what those disciplines are to do. A specific plan for visit frequency and duration must be included. Specific, measurable goals for the client must be set, and a time frame for achievement of those goals established. Discharge plans must be noted, indicating when the client will be discharged, and any criteria for discharge must be specified. The narrative summary of the client condition must include all factors that impact on care, and must support all other information on the plan of care.

Sample Documentation
Documentation of the plan of care is agency specific.

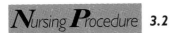 *3.2*

Progress Notes

☒ EQUIPMENT

- Pen
- Agency-specific progress note

Purpose

Documents each visit made by the nurse to the client.

Desired Outcomes (sample)

The progress note will accurately reflect the client's condition, the skilled care provided, the client's response, progress toward client discharge, and an ongoing plan for continued care.

The progress note will be completed in a timely manner.

Assessment

Assessment should focus on the following:

Relationship of progress note to plan of care

Outcome Identification and Planning

Key Goals and Sample Goal Criteria

The progress note will accurately reflect the client's functional limitations and physical condition, the care provided, the client's progress toward the goals stated on the plan of care, any discharge planning provided, and the nurse's plan for the next visit.

Special Considerations

Each progress note must indicate that the care performed requires the skills and judgment of a professional nurse. Care is not considered skilled simply because the client cannot do the care for him- or herself.

HINT

> *Always make it a goal to complete each progress note during or immediately after each visit. By doing this, you write the most accurate progress notes and avoid playing "catch up" with paperwork after your work day has ended.*

 Transcultural

While it is best to complete the note before leaving the client's home, in some cultures it is considered rude for the nurse to write and talk to the client at the same time. In these cases, complete the note after leaving the home, and before beginning the next visit.

IMPLEMENTATION

Action	Rationale
1. Note the client's functional limitations on each progress note.	*Supports the need for care in the home*
2. Record the physical assessment clearly, using approved abbreviations, measurements of wounds, and detailed description of abnormal findings.	*Provides a detailed picture of the client for other care providers reading the notes, and when placed on the client record with other notes, clearly indicates changes in client status*
3. Document the nursing assessment of the problem that is the focus of this visit.	*Allows the nurse to focus on the aspect of care that is the primary reason for this visit*
4. Document skilled care that is provided, including instruction. Skilled care provided must be that which is noted on the plan of care, or on additional orders obtained since the plan of care was written.	*Supports the need for the visit and ties the progress note to the plan of care*
5. Document the client response to the care or instruction provided.	*Indicates client participation in and understanding of care*
6. Document the plan for the next visit.	*Indicates ongoing planning or change in plan precipitated by*

Action	Rationale
	change in client condition or response to care
7. Document any discharge planning done.	*Indicates client progress toward self-care*

Evaluation

Were desired outcomes achieved?

DOCUMENTATION

Documentation on the progress note must include:

- Client functional limitations
- Client physical assessment
- Statement of problem that is the focus of the visit
- Skilled care provided
- Client response to care
- Planning for next visit
- Discharge planning

Sample Documentation

DATE	TIME	
12/23/98	1040	VS - T. 100°F, AP 100, RP 100, R24 BP - 102/64

Alert and oriented. Ambulates 6–8 feet with walker, non– weight-bearing R leg. Moderate pain with ambulation. Wound lateral right thigh 24 cm long, 9 cm wide, 4 cm deep, with 4-cm tunnel at upper wound margin. Odorless green-gray drainage, saturating two abdominal pads last 24 hours. Taking acetaminophen with codeine 1 tab q4 hours with good pain relief. Continued slow wound healing noted, needs skilled nursing care daily times 1–2 more weeks. With spouse observing, wound irrigated and dressed per plan of care. Client tolerates procedure well, expresses concern about continued temperature elevation. Spouse indicates readiness to participate in care. Will discharge care to spouse when wound status stabilizes.

Oxygenation

OVERVIEW

▶ One key to successful chest drainage and oxygen therapy is tube patency. Tubing must remain free of clots, kinks, or other obstructions to ensure proper equipment function.

▶ Agency policy and physician protocols vary regarding milking or stripping of chest tubes. Consult policy prior to intervening.

▶ Increasing restlessness or decreased level of consciousness are characteristic signs of hypoxia. Note associated signs or symptoms: elevated respiratory rate, tachycardia, or dysrhythmia.

▶ Improperly maintained artificial airway or tube cuff can cause trauma to mucous membranes, edema, and obstruction.

▶ High oxygen levels can be LETHAL to certain clients.

▶ **Remember "NO SMOKING" signs—OXYGEN IS HIGHLY COMBUSTIBLE.**

Transcultural

- The assessment of skin color is subjective and dependent on the sensitivity of the observer to color.
- For clients of African, Mediterranean, American Indian, Spanish, or Indian descent:
  - When caring for patients with highly pigmented skin, the nurse must first establish the baseline skin color.
  - Daylight is the best source for this assessment, but when not available, a lamp with at least a 60-watt bulb should be used.
  - Observation of skin surfaces with the least amount of pigmentation may be helpful. These include palms of hands, soles of feet, the abdomen and buttocks, and the volar (flexor surface) of the forearm.
  - The nurse should look for an underlying red tone, which is typical of all skin, regardless of how dark or light its pigment. An absence of this red tone may indicate pallor.
  - Nailbeds may be highly pigmented, thick, or lined and may contain melanin deposits. Nonetheless, for baseline assessment, it is important to evaluate how rapidly the color returns to the nailbed after pressure has been released from the nail.

Nursing **P**rocedures 4.1, 4.2

Chest Drainage System Preparation (4.1)

Chest Tube Maintenance (4.2)

EQUIPMENT

- Chest drainage system (bottles or disposable system)
- Suction source and set-up
- Nonsterile gloves
- Sterile irrigation saline or sterile water (500-mL bottle)
- Funnel
- 2-inch tape
- Sterile gauze sponges

Purpose

Removes fluid or air from chest cavity
Restores negative pressure facilitating lung re-expansion

Desired Outcomes (sample)

Respirations are nonlabored with breath sounds in all lobes.

Assessment

Assessment should focus on the following:

Doctor's orders for valve or type of drainage system (water-seal or suction) and amount of suction

Client's or caregiver's understanding of the purpose and location of chest tube(s) and maintenance procedures

Type of drainage systems available

Agency policy regarding use of saline or water in drainage system

Baseline data: breath sounds; respiratory rate, depth, and character; pulse rate and rhythm; temperature; blood gases; and chest drainage type and amount

Outcome Identification and Planning

Key Goals and Sample Goal Criteria

The client will:

Ventilate effectively, as evidenced by smooth, nonlabored respirations and a respiratory rate within client's normal limits

Show lung re-expansion by breath sounds audible in all lobes

Special Considerations

If the client has a small pneumothorax, a chest drain valve may be used instead of a drainage system. The valve might also be used with a glove or urine drainage bag or with a drainage system and suction. Maintenance of valve function and patency is essential.

Rules regarding clamping or not clamping chest tubes vary greatly among facilities and doctors. Investigate agency's policy BEFORE an emergency occurs.

Geriatric

Prolonged immobility can result in joint stiffening in geriatric clients and in increased frustration for hospitalized pediatric clients. Obtain rolling cart for drainage system and encourage ambulation as soon as it is allowed.

IMPLEMENTATION

Action	Rationale

Procedure 4.1 Chest Drainage System Preparation

Action	Rationale
1. Wash hands and organize equipment.	*Decreases microorganism transfer* *Promotes efficiency*
2. If chest drain valve (Heimlich valve) is present, verify that the valve is patent and flutters freely (Fig. 4.1.1). Valve will not flutter if: - the incorrect end of the valve is connected to the chest tube (see instructions embossed on the tube) - the valve is obstructed by exudate - the lung is fully expanded	

Action	Rationale

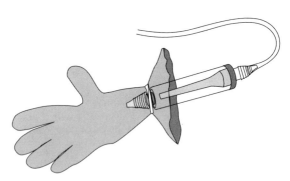

FIGURE 4.1.1

Connect chest drainage
system and suction or
drainage bag, as ordered,
to distal end of the valve.
3. Open saline or water container.
4. Unwrap drainage system
and stand it upright.
5. Fill bottle(s) or chambers   *Establishes proper amount of*
to appropriate level: *water-seal pressure*

One-bottle System
Place funnel in port or tubing leading to long rod
(straw) and fill bottle with
solution until end of rod is
2 cm below fluid level or
until marked fluid line is
reached (Fig. 4.1.2).

Two- or Three-bottle/chamber System
- Place funnel in tubing or
  port leading to suction-
  control chamber or bottle.
- Pour fluid into suction-   *Level of water controls amount*
  control port until des-   *of suction pressure*
  ignated amount is
  reached—per doctor's

Action	Rationale

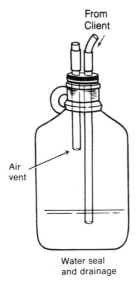

From
Client

Air
vent

Water seal
and drainage

FIGURE 4.1.2

orders, or to specific line
marked on bottle—usu-
ally indicating the 20-cm
water pressure level.
The suction-control bot-
tle in a two-bottle system
is the bottle with the long
rod (Fig. 4.1.3). The
closed-chamber drainage
system (Fig. 4.1.4) is more
commonly used than the
three-bottle system (Fig.
4.1.5). The bottles and
chambers of the systems
are similarly aligned. The
three-bottle systems have
a suction control bottle
with two short rods and

Action	Rationale

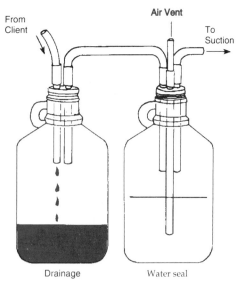

FIGURE 4.1.3

one long rod (see Figure 4.1.5).
Chamber systems have marked posts that correlate with the bottles of the three-bottle system (see Figure 4.1.3).
- Fill water-seal chamber or bottle of drainage system to the 2-cm level. (Tip of long rod should be 2 cm below fluid level. Rod may require adjustment in some two-bottle systems.)

6. Don gloves and connect drainage system to chest tube and suction source, if

Allows air to escape chest while preventing air reflux into chest
Stabilizes suction control altered by chest drainage

Action	Rationale

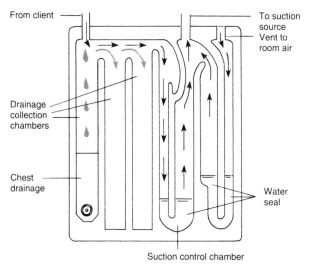

FIGURE 4.1.4

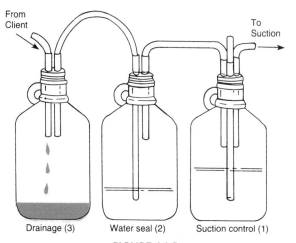

FIGURE 4.1.5

Action	Rationale

suction is indicated.
- Connect tubing from client to tubing entering drainage collection bottle or chamber. MAINTAIN STERILITY OF CONNECTOR ENDS.
- If changing drainage systems, ask client to take a deep breath, hold it, and bear down slightly while tubing is being changed quickly.   *Prevents air influx into chest while water seal is broken*
- If indicated, connect tubing from suction-control chamber to the suction source. (MOST ONE-BOTTLE SYSTEMS SHOULD NOT BE CONNECTED TO SUCTION.)   *Provides gravity drainage and water seal only*

7. Adjust suction-flow regulator until quiet bubbling is noted in suction control chamber.   *Regulates flow of suction, not pressure; vigorous flow is unnecessary unless large air leak is present*

8. Discard gloves and disposable materials.

9. Assist client to comfortable position.

Procedure 4.2 Chest Tube Maintenance

Chest Drain Valve Only

1. Monitor for patency.
2. Report absence of valve flutter to M.D. Assess breath sounds, chest excursion, and respiratory status.   *Absence of chest valve flutter could indicate obstruction of drainage and possible buildup of drainage in client's pleural cavity*

With Drainage System

1. Observe water-seal chamber for bubbling. Suspect air leak if bubbling is present and client has no known pneumothorax.   *Indicates air entering system (from client or air leak) Determines if air is entering system through loose tube connections*

Action	Rationale

Also suspect air leak if bubbling is noted and chest tube is clamped, or if bubbling is excessive. Check security of tube connections.

2. Instruct client or caregiver to monitor, 2–3 times per day depending on amount of drainage:
   - Note drainage in collection chamber/bottle.

     Detects hemorrhage or increased or decreased drainage
   - Monitor the drainage system for bubbling in suction-control chamber.

     Indicates suction is intact
   - Check for fluctuation in water-seal chamber with respirations.

     Indicates patent tubing (may not fluctuate if lung re-expanded)

3. If drainage slows or stops, consult agency policy and, if allowed, gently milk chest tube (or strip as last resort):

   Stripping tubes causes extreme pain and can cause hemorrhage

Milking
   - Grasp tube close to chest and squeeze tube between fingers and palm of hand (Fig. 4.2*A*).

     Pushes clotted blood toward drainage system
   - Move other hand to next lower portion of tube and squeeze.

     Exerts gentle increased suction to facilitate drainage
   - Release first hand and move to next portion of tube.
   - Continue toward drainage bottle.

Stripping
   - Place lubricant on fingers of one hand and pinch chest tube with fingers of other hand (Fig. 4.2*B*).

     Decreases pulling on tube while stripping
     Stabilizes tube to prevent dislodging
   - Squeeze tubing below pinched portion with lubricated fingers and slide

     Exerts increased suction to facilitate drainage (may disrupt tissue healing and cause

Action	Rationale

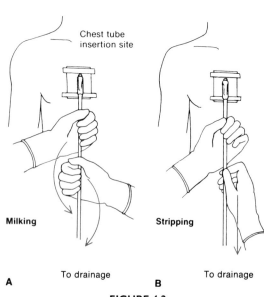

Chest tube
insertion site

Milking

Stripping

A   To drainage   **B**   To drainage

FIGURE 4.2

fingers down tube
toward drainage system.
- Slowly release pinch of
nonlubricated fingers,
then release lubricated
fingers.
- Repeat one to two times.
Notify doctor if unable to
clear clots from tubing.
Monitor for tension hemo/
pneumothorax.
4. Every visit (more fre-
quently if changes are
noted) monitor:
- chest tube dressing for
adequacy of tape seal
and amount and type of

*hemorrhage, so perform with
caution)*

*Facilitates prompt tube replace-
ment and avoids development
of hemothorax*

*Determines possible source of
air leak, hemorrhage, or tube
obstruction, and leakage at
tube insertion site*

Action	Rationale
soiling	
- breath sounds	*Indicates progress toward lung reinflation*
5. Instruct client or caregiver to monitor temperature two to three times a day. Use the following trouble-shooting tips in maintaining chest tube drainage.	*Facilitates detection of such complications as hemorrhage, tension pneumo/hemothorax and infection*

Troubleshooting Tips

If:

- *Drainage system is turned over and water seal is disrupted,* re-establish water seal and assess client.	*Prevents additional air reflux and determines presence of pneumothorax*
- *Drainage decreases suddenly,* assess for tube obstructions (ie, clots or kinks) and milk tubing.	*Determines if drainage has been blocked and re-establishes tube patency*
- Check that gravity drainage systems and suction systems are below level of client's chest.	*Ensures proper gravitational pull and negative water seal*
WATCH FOR TENSION HEMO/PNEUMO-THORAX.	*Indicates air or blood is entering chest cavity, increasing pressure on structures in chest cavity*
- Instruct client/family members to have emergency phone numbers posted prominently.	
- *Drainage increases suddenly or becomes bright red,* take vital signs, observe respiratory status, and notify doctor.	*Indicates possible hemorrhage*
- *Dressing becomes saturated,* reinforce with gauze, and tape securely. If permitted, remove soiled dressings without disturbing lubricating jelly gauze seal, and apply new gauze pads.	*Retains original seal around chest tube*
- *Drainage system is broken,*	*Prevents entrance of air into*

Action	Rationale
clamp tube with Kelly clamp or hemostat and replace system immediately, OR place end of tube in sterile saline bottle, place bottle below level of chest, and replace drainage system immediately.	*chest* *Establishes temporary water seal*
CLAMP CHEST TUBES FOR NO MORE THAN A FEW MINUTES (SUCH AS DURING SYSTEM CHANGE).	*Air can enter pleural cavity with inspiration and, if not able to escape, will cause tension hemo/pneumothorax*

Evaluation

Were desired outcomes achieved?

DOCUMENTATION

The following should be noted on the visit note:

- System function (type and amount of drainage)
- Time suction was initiated or system changed
- Client status (respiratory rate, breath sounds, pulse, blood pressure, skin color and temperature, mental status, and core body temperature)
- Chest dressing status and care done

Sample Documentation

DATE	TIME	
6/8/98	1100	Client alert and oriented; skin warm and dry. Chest tubes intact with dressing dry and intact. Disposable drainage system changed with no signs of air leak noted. Suction maintained at 20 cm. Drainage scant with 10 mL serous fluid this hour. Respirations, 12; nonlabored with breath sounds in all lobes. Pulse and blood pressure within client's normal range.

Nursing **P**rocedures **4.3, 4.4, 4.5**

🖑 *Postural Drainage (4.3)*

🖑 *Chest Percussion (4.4)*

🖑 *Chest Vibration (4.5)*

❌ EQUIPMENT

- Large towel (optional)
- Suctioning equipment
- Emesis basin or tissues and paper bag

Purpose

This three-part regimen, often referred to as *chest physiotherapy*, achieves the following:

Loosens secretions in airways
Uses gravity to drain and remove excessive secretions
Decreases accumulation of secretions in unconscious or weakened clients

Desired Outcomes (sample)

Respirations, 14 to 20, of normal depth, smooth, and symmetrical.
Breath sounds are clear in target areas; chest radiograph reveals clear lung fields.
Arterial blood gases are within normal limits for client.
Caregiver demonstrates accurate skill in and understanding of chest physiotherapy regimen.

Assessment

Assessment should focus on the following:

Bilateral breath sounds
Respiratory rate and character
Doctor's orders regarding activity/position restrictions
Tolerance of previous physiotherapy
Current chest radiographs

Outcome Identification and Planning

Key Goals and Sample Goal Criterion

The client will:

Ventilate with clear airways, evidenced by a respiratory rate within client's normal limits and clear breath sounds in all lobes

Special Considerations

Postural drainage should be omitted in clients with poor tolerance to lying flat (ie, clients with increased intracranial pressure or those with extreme respiratory distress)

Length of time of therapy or degree of head elevation should be altered for client tolerance.

Therapy should not be initiated until 2 or more hours after solid food intake (1 hour after liquid diet intake).

Performance of therapy prior to meals and at bedtime opens airways for easier breathing during meals and at night.

Do not percuss or vibrate over areas of skin irritation or breakdown, soft tissue, the spine, or wherever there is pain.

Always have suction equipment available in case of aspiration.

Geriatric

Pressure used in percussion or vibration must be modified to prevent fracture of the brittle bones of elderly clients.

HINT

Pillows and rolled linens may be used to achieve positions for clients without hospital or mechanical beds.

IMPLEMENTATION

Action	Rationale

Procedure 4.3 Postural Drainage

Action	Rationale
1. Explain and demonstrate procedure to client and family.	*Facilitates relaxation and cooperation*
2. Wash hands and organize equipment.	*Reduces microorganism transfer Promotes efficiency*
3. Administer bronchodilators, expectorants, or warm liquids, if ordered or desired.	*Loosens and liquifies secretions*

Action	Rationale
4. Encourage client to void.	*Prevents interruption of therapy*
5. Assist client into position to drain specific lung area (Fig. 4.3). To drain *upper lung segments/lobes*, position client:	
- Sitting upright in bed or chair; perform therapy to right and left chest (Fig. 4.3A)	*Drains anterior right and left apical segments*
- Leaning forward in sitting position; perform therapy to back (Fig. 4.3B)	*Drains posterior right and left apical segments*
- Lying flat on back, perform therapy to right and left chest (Fig. 4.3C)	*Drains anterior segments*
- Lying on abdomen, tilted to right or left side; perform therapy to right or left back (Fig. 4.3D)	*Drains posterior segments*
To drain *middle lobe,* position client:	
- Lying on back, tilted to left side in Trendelenburg's position; therapy to right chest (Fig. 4.3E)	*Drains middle anterior lobe*
- Lying on abdomen, tilted to left side, with hips elevated; therapy to right back (Fig. 4.3F)	*Drains middle posterior lobe*
To drain *basal/lower lobes,* position client:	
- Lying in Trendelenburg's position on back; perform therapy to right and left chest (Fig. 4.3G)	*Drains anterior basal lobes*
- Lying in Trendelenburg's position on abdomen; perform therapy to right and left back (Fig. 4.3H)	*Drains posterior basal lobes*
- On right or left side, in Trendelenburg's position; perform therapy to back (Fig. 4.3I)	*Drains lateral basal lobes*

Action	Rationale
- Lying on abdomen with therapy to right and left back (Fig. 4.3*J*)	*Drains superior basal lobes*
6. Maintain client in position until chest percussion and vibration are completed (approximately 5 minutes).	*Loosens secretions in target area*
7. Assist client into position for coughing, or position client for suctioning of trachea.	*Removes secretions from lungs accumulating in trachea*
8. Position client to drain next arget area and repeat percussion and vibration.	
9. Continue sequence until identified target areas have been drained.	*Completes drainage of congested lung fields*

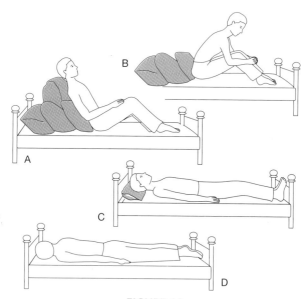

FIGURE 4.3

Action	Rationale

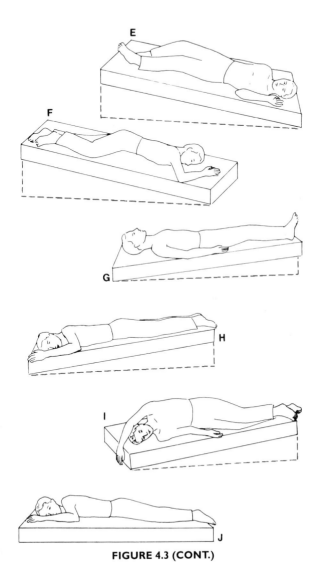

FIGURE 4.3 (CONT.)

Action	Rationale

Procedure 4.4 Chest Percussion

1. Assist client into position to drain target lung field and place towel over skin if desired (see Procedure 4.3).

   Decreases friction against skin

2. Close fingers and thumb together and flex them slightly, making shallow cups of your palms (Fig. 4.4).

   Allows palms to be used to trap air and cushion blows to chest

3. Strike target area using palm cups, holding wrists stiff, and alternating hands (a hollow sound should be produced).

   Delivers cushioned blows and prevents "slapping" of skin with flat palm or fingertips

4. Percuss entire target area using a systematic pattern and rhythmic hand alternation.

   Ensures loosening of secretions in entire target area

5. Continue percussion 1 to 2 minutes per target area, if tolerated.

   Facilitates maximum loosening of secretions from airway

6. Perform chest vibration to site (see Procedure 4.5), assist client to clear secretions, and position client for new target area (see Procedure 4.3).

7. Repeat percussion, vibration, and cough/suction sequence until identified lung fields have been drained.

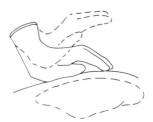

FIGURE 4.4

Action	Rationale

Procedure 4.5 Chest Vibration

1. Prepare and position client to drain target area.

2. Perform chest percussion to target area (Procedures 4.3 and 4.4).

   Facilitates the loosening of secretions

3. Instruct client to breathe in deeply and exhale slowly (may use pursed lip breathing).

   Uses air movement to push secretions from airways

4. With each respiration, perform vibration techniques as follows:
   - Place your hands on top of one another over target area (Fig. 4.5).
   - Instruct client to take deep breath.
   - As client exhales slowly, deliver a gentle tremor or shaking by tensing your arms and hands and making hands shake slightly.

     Provides gentle vibration to shake secretions loose

   - Continue tremor throughout exhalation phase.

     Moves secretions from lobes of lungs and bronchi into trachea

   - Relax arms and hands as client inhales.

5. Repeat vibration process for five to eight breaths, moving hands to different sections of target area.

   Facilitates loosening secretions over entire target area

6. Assist client in clearing secretions (through coughing or suction).

   Removes secretions drained into trachea and pharynx from lungs

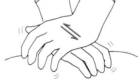

FIGURE 4.5

Action	Rationale
7. Position client for drainage of next target area.	
8. Repeat steps 2 to 7 until all targeted lung fields have been drained.	*Clears secretions from obstructed lung fields and prevents obstruction of airways*
9. Assess breath sounds in targeted lung fields.	*Evaluates effectiveness of therapy and need for additional treatment*
10. Assist client with mouth care.	*Removes residual secretions from oral cavity and freshens mouth*
11. Assist client to a position of comfort with chest elevated 45 degrees or more.	*Facilitates lung expansion and deep breathing*
12. Wash hands and chart procedure.	

Evaluation

Were desired outcomes achieved?

DOCUMENTATION

The following should be noted on the visit note:

- Breath sounds before and after procedure
- Character of respirations
- Significant changes in vital signs
- Color, amount, and consistency of secretions
- Tolerance to treatment (eg, state of incisions, drains)
- Replacement of oxygen source, if applicable

Sample Documentation

DATE	TIME	
1/12/98	1200	Postural drainage with chest percussion and vibration performed to right upper, middle, and lower lobes of lungs. Cough productive with thick, yellow sputum. Positioned in bed on left side with O_2 at 2 liters per cannula.

Nursing Procedure 4.6

🔖 *Nasal Cannula/Face Mask Application*

⊠ EQUIPMENT

- Oxygen humidifer (if ordered)
- Oxygen cylinder; concentrator
- Oxygen flow meter
- Nasal cannula or appropriate facemask
- Nonsterile gloves
- "NO SMOKING" signs
- Cotton balls
- Wash cloth
- Lubricating jelly

Purpose

Provides client with additional concentration of oxygen to facilitate adequate tissue oxygenation

Desired Outcomes (sample)

Respirations are 14 to 20, of normal depth, smooth, and symmetrical; lung fields are clear; no cyanosis.

Assessment

Assessment should focus on the following:

Doctor's order for oxygen concentration, method of delivery, and parameters for regulation (pulse oximetry)

Baseline data: level of consciousness, respiratory status (rate, depth, signs of distress), blood pressure, and pulse

Oxygen level in cylinder and presence of a full backup cylinder

Outcome Identification and Planning

Key Goals and Sample Goal Criterion

The client will:

Demonstrate adequate oxygenation as evidenced by alertness, full orientation, blood gases within acceptable level for client, and pink mucous membranes

Special Considerations

In most *acute* situations, placing client on oxygen is a nursing decision and does not require a doctor's order prior to initiation of therapy; check agency policy. Once oxygen is applied, notify doctor for future orders.

A face mask provides better control of inspired oxygen concentration than the nasal cannula.

The nasal cannula may be unsuitable for emergency oxygen delivery if high oxygen percentages are desired.

If client has history of chronic lung disease or extensive tobacco abuse, DO NOT PLACE ON MORE THAN 2 TO 3 LITERS OF NASAL OXYGEN (30% FACE MASK) WITHOUT A DOCTOR'S ORDER.

If problems are noted in oxygen equipment, contact medical equipment supplier for assistance.

"NO SMOKING" signs should be placed on door of client's home if oxygen is in use.

Clients may require extra-long tubing to permit movement from room to room without moving oxygen cylinder.

Oximeter may be used to assess oxygenation instead of requiring blood samples for blood gases.

Geriatric

Monitor for signs of chronic lung disease and take appropriate precautions.

 Transcultural

- Prior to touching the client's head, note ethnic/cultural background. Acknowledge related cultural taboos, and discuss alternatives (eg, have client or family member apply cannula/mask).

- With clients of African or Mediterranean descent, exercise caution when assessing for cyanosis, particularly around the mouth, as this area may be dark blue normally. Coloration varies from client to client and should be carefully evaluated on an individual basis.*

*Boyle and Andrews. Transcultural Concepts in Nursing Care. p 80. Scott, Foresman/Little, Brown, 1989.

IMPLEMENTATION

Action	Rationale
1. Wash hands and organize equipment.	*Decreases microorganism transfer* *Promotes efficiency*
2. Explain equipment and procedure to client.	*Decreases anxiety and facilitates cooperation*
3. Insert flow meter into outlet on wall, or place oxygen cylinder near client.	
4. Prepare humidifier: Add distilled water if needed, or remove prefilled bottle from package and screw enclosed spiked cap to bottle (Fig. 4.6.1*A*).	*Delivers moistened oxygen to mucous membranes of airway*
5. Connect humidifier to flow meter (Fig. 4.6.1*B*).	*Controls flow of oxygen*
6. Connect humidifier to tubing attached to cannula or mask (Fig. 4.6.1C).	*Connects humidification to delivery mechanism*
7. Turn on oxygen flow meter until bubbling is noted in humidifier. If no bubbling is noted, check that flow meter is securely inserted, ports of humidifier are patent, and connections are tight. Contact respiratory therapist or supervisor if unable to correct problem.	*Determines if oxygen flow is adequate and connections are intact*
8. Regulate flow meter as ordered (with Venturi masks, attach oxygen percentage regulator to oxygen mask). Regulate flow as indicated.	*Regulates oxygen delivery*
9. Instruct family to check oxygen flow rate every 8 hours.	*Assures correct level of oxygen administration*
10. Don gloves.	
11. Place oxygen cannula or mask on client.	

Action	Rationale

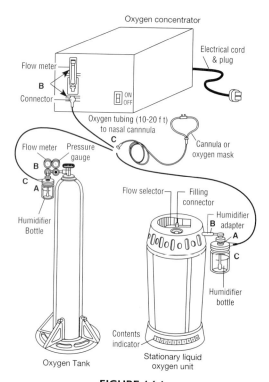

FIGURE 4.6.1

Cannula

- Clear nares of secretions with moist cotton balls.

    Removes secretions

- Place cannula prongs into client's nares.

- Slip attached tubing around client's ears and under chin (Fig. 4.6.2).

    Holds tubing in place

Action	Rationale

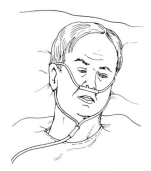

FIGURE 4.6.2

Cotton between tubing
and ear may add
comfort.
- Tighten tubing to secure
cannula, but make sure
client is comfortable.

Mask
- Place mask over nose,
mouth, and chin.

Places mask correctly

- Adjust metal strip at
nose bridge of mask to
fit securely over bridge
of client's nose.

Individualizes fit

- Pull elastic band
around back of head or
neck.

Secures mask

- Pull band at sides of
mask to tighten (Fig.
4.6.3). Cotton under
bridge of face mask
may decrease pressure
on nose.

Ensures secure fit

12. Instruct family to remove
cannula every 4–8 hours
to assess skin and apply
lubricating jelly to nares,

*Provides opportunity to
assess skin condition*
Promotes comfort
Prevents infection

Action	Rationale

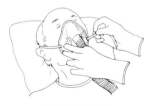

FIGURE 4.6.3

and clean away accumulated secretions.
Remove mask every 2 to 4 hours, wipe away accumulated mist, and assess underlying skin.

13. Position client for comfort with head of bed elevated.

Facilitates lung expansion for gas exchange

14. Dispose of or store equipment appropriately.

Decreases spread of microorganisms

15. Place "NO SMOKING" signs on door and over bed.

Prevents contact of fire with combustible oxygen

Evaluation

Were desired outcomes achieved?

DOCUMENTATION

The following should be noted on the visit note:

- Time of initiation of oxygen therapy
- Amount of oxygen and delivery method
- Respiratory status prior to and after initiation
- Color of skin and mucous membranes
- Client teaching performed regarding therapy and client/caregiver understanding of teaching
- Blood gas results

Sample Documentation

DATE	TIME	
1/12/98	1200	Client complained of chest pain and shortness of breath. Three liters of O_2 begun per nasal cannula. Respiratory rate, 32/minute prior to oxygen administration, decreased to 24/minute within 10 minutes. Resting comfortably, states pain decreased.

Nursing **P**rocedure 4.7

🖐 *Oral Airway Insertion*

✖ EQUIPMENT

- Oral airway
- Equipment for suctioning
- Tape strips—one approximately 20 inches, one 16 inches (may use commercially manufactured airway holder)
- Tongue depressor
- Lubricating jelly
- Mouth moistener or swabs with mouthwash
- Nonsterile gloves

Purpose

Holds tongue forward and maintains open airway
Facilitates easy removal of secretions

Desired Outcomes (sample)

Airway is patent and free of secretions.
Skin and mucous membranes of lips and oral area are intact without dryness or irritation.

Assessment

Assessment should focus on the following:

Level of consciousness, agitation, and ability to push airway from mouth
Respiratory status (respiratory rate, congestion in upper airways), blood pressure, pulse
Color, amount, and consistency of secretions
Alternative methods of maintaining airway

Outcome Identification and Planning

Key Goals and Sample Goal Criteria
The client will:

Attain and maintain clear airway passage, evidenced by nonlabored respirations and clear breath sounds

Maintain skin integrity of lips and moist, intact oral mucous membranes

Special Considerations

If client is alert and agitated enough to push airway out or resist it, DO NOT INSERT. Airway could stimulate gag reflex and cause client to vomit and to aspirate. Use another method of maintaining airway, if needed.

IMPLEMENTATION

Action	Rationale
1. Explain procedure to client and family.	*Decreases anxiety and facilitates cooperation*
2. Wash hands and organize equipment.	*Reduces microorganism transfer* *Promotes efficiency*
3. Lay long strip of tape down with sticky side up, and place short strip of tape over it with sticky side down, leaving equal length of sticky tape exposed on each end of long strip. Split each end of tape 2 inches (See Figure 4.12.1 and Procedure 4.12) May substitute commercial holder.	*Prepares tape as holder for oral airway*
4. Don gloves.	*Avoids contact with secretions*
5. Rinse airway in cool water.	*Facilitates insertion*
6. Open mouth and place tongue blade on front half of tongue.	*Flattens tongue and opens mouth, facilitating airway insertion*
7. Turn airway on side and insert tip on top of tongue (Fig. 4.7.1).	*Promotes deeper insertion of airway without stimulating gag*
8. Slide airway in until tip is at lower half of tongue.	*Assures accurate placement*
9. Remove tongue blade.	
10. Turn airway so that tip points toward tongue, (outer ends of airway should be vertical).	*Places tongue under curve of airway, thus holding tongue forward and away from pharynx*

Action   **Rationale**

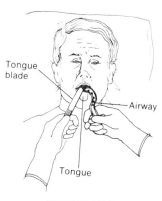

FIGURE 4.7.1

Action	Rationale
11. Place tape under client's neck with ends lying on either side.	*Places nonsticky portion under neck*
12. Pull one end of tape across client's mouth with splits taped across upper and lower ends of airway (Fig. 4.7.2).	*Secures airway in mouth*
13. Repeat with other end of tape.	
14. Suction mouth and throat, if needed.	*Removes pooled secretions*
15. Swab mouth with moisturizer and mouthwash.	*Freshens mouth and removes microoganisms*
16. Apply lubricating jelly to lips.	*Decreases dryness of lips*
17. Assist client to position that is in good alignment and comfortable.	
18. Remove gloves and wash hands.	*Removes microorganisms*

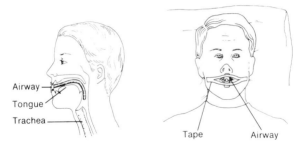

FIGURE 4.7.2

Evaluation

Were desired outcomes achieved?

DOCUMENTATION

The following should be noted on the visit note:

- Respiratory rate, quality, degree of congestion
- Status of lips and mucous membranes
- Time of airway insertion
- Suctioning and mouth care performed
- Tolerance of procedure

Sample Documentation

DATE	TIME	
3/4/98	0830	Client semicomatose, moves arms to painful stimuli. Upper airway congestion noted with tongue at back of throat. Oral airway inserted with no resistance. Suctioned clear secretions from mouth. Lemon-glycerin swabs to oral area, lubricating jelly to lips. No broken skin noted on lips or in oral area.

Nursing **P**rocedure *4.8*

🖐 *Nasal Airway Insertion*

❎ EQUIPMENT

- Nasal airway
- Equipment for suctioning
- Lubricating jelly
- Moist tissue/cotton balls
- Cotton-tip swabs
- Nonsterile gloves
- Washcloth

Purpose

Facilitates easy removal of secretions

Desired Outcomes (sample)

Client's airway is patent and free of secretions.
Skin and mucous membranes of nasal area are intact, without dryness or irritation.

Assessment

Assessment should focus on the following:

Level of consciousness, agitation, and inability to tolerate oral airway
Available alternative methods of maintaining airway
Respiratory status (respiratory rate, congestion in upper airways)
Blood pressure, pulse
Color, amount, and consistency of secretions

Outcome Identification and Planning

Key Goals and Sample Goal Criteria

The client will:

Attain and maintain clear airway passage, evidenced by smooth, nonlabored respirations, and clear breath sounds

Maintain good skin integrity of nose and intact nasal mucous
   membranes

Special Considerations

The decision to use continuous or intermittent nasal airway
   should be based on client's needs and the status of circulation
   to the underlying tissue. If circulation is poor, the nasal airway may need to be alternated between nares frequently or an
   alternate method of airway maintenance should be considered.

If airway is difficult to insert, it may be maintained continu-
   ously, but it will require frequent checks and care.

Teach family to insert airway and perform maintenance for care
   between nurse's visits.

Geriatric

Tissue is often thin and fragile, requiring frequent checks and
   skin care.

IMPLEMENTATION

Action	Rationale
1. Explain procedure to client and family.	*Decreases anxiety* *Facilitates cooperation*
2. Wash hands and organize equipment.	*Reduces microorganism transfer* *Promotes efficiency*
3. Don gloves.	*Avoids contact with secretions*
4. Ask client to breathe through one naris while the other is occluded.	*Determines patency of nasal passage*
5. Repeat step 4 with other naris.	*Determines patency of nasal passage*
6. Have client blow nose with both nares open (if client is comatose pro-ceed to next step).	*Facilitates removal of excess mucus and dried secretions*
7. Clean mucus and dried secretions from nares with wet tissue or cotton-tip swab.	*Clears nasal passage*
8. Lubricate airway.	*Facilitates insertion*
9. Insert airway into naris in a smooth downward arch Fig. 4.8).	*Decreases trauma to nasal tissue*
10. Roll airway side to side while gently pushing downward.	*Promotes deeper insertion of airway without tissue damage*

Action	Rationale
11. Slide airway in until horn of airway fits against outer naris.	*Ensures accurate placement*
12. Remove excess lubricant.	
13. Suction pharynx and mouth, if needed (see Procedure 4.9).	*Removes pooled secretions*
14. Apply lubricating jelly to nares.	*Decreases dryness of nares*
15. Assist client to position of comfort. Evaluate respirations of client.	
16. Discard gloves.	*Decreases spread of organisms*
17. Raise side rails and place call light within reach.	*Facilitates client safety and permits communication*

Maintenance Techniques

18. Instruct caregiver at least once each day, to don gloves, slide airway slightly outward, and inspect underlying tissue.	
19. Lubricate naris with lubricating jelly and massage gently.	*Keeps tissue moist* *Promotes skin circulation*

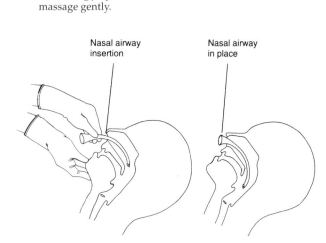

Nasal airway insertion

Nasal airway in place

FIGURE 4.8

Action	Rationale

20. Alternate nares (if both are unobstructed) if airway is to be maintained for extended periods or inserted and removed for each suctioning episode.

Cleaning and Storage
21. Remove tube by:
    - Donning gloves
    - Gently pulling airway out using a side-to-side twisting motion
    - Covering tube with washcloth as it is withdrawn

    Prevents client witness of dirty tube

22. Clean nares with moist cotton ball and apply lubricating jelly to nares.

    Decreases dryness of nares

23. Place tube in warm, soapy water and soak for 5 to 10 minutes; pass water through tube several times.

    Loosens thick and dried secretions

24. Use cotton and cotton-tip swabs to clean lumen of tube.

    Removes secretions

25. Rinse tube with clear water.

    Removes soap and secretions

26. Dry lumen with cotton-tip swabs.

    Removes remaining water

27. Cover in clean, dry cloth and store at bedside.

    Keeps airway clean and dry for future use

28. Remove gloves and discard soiled equipment appropriately.

    Removes microorganisms

Evaluation

Were desired outcomes achieved?

DOCUMENTATION

The following should be noted on the visit note:

- Time of airway insertion
- Client's tolerance of procedure
- Suctioning and skin care performed
- Respiratory rate, quality, degree of congestion
- Status of nares

Sample Documentation

DATE	TIME	
3/4/98	0830	Client alert, restless, moves arms to painful stimuli. Upper airway congestion noted with tongue at back of throat. Nasal airway inserted with no resistance. Suctioned clear secretions from pharynx. Lemon-glycerin swabs to oral area, lubricating jelly to nasal entrance. No broken skin on nares.

*N*ursing *P*rocedure **4.9**

🖐 *Oral Airway Suctioning*

☒ EQUIPMENT

- Suction source
- Large towel
- Nonsterile gloves
- Irrigation saline or sterile water
- Oral moisturizer swabs
- Mouthwash (optional)
- Lubricating jelly
- Suction catheter (adult, size 14 to 16 French; pediatric, 8 to 12 Fr), or oral suction (Yankauer).

Purpose

Clears oral airway of secretions
Facilitates breathing
Decreases halitosis and anorexia

Desired Outcomes (sample)

Respirations are 14 to 20 breaths per minute, the oral airway is clear, and oral intake is adequate.

Assessment

Assessment should focus on the following:

Respiratory status (respirations, breath sounds)
Lips and mucous membranes (dryness, color, amount and consistency of secretions)
Ability or desire of client or caregiver to perform suctioning

Outcome Identification and Planning

Key Goals and Sample Goal Criterion
The client will:

Attain and maintain a patent upper airway, evidenced by respiratory rate of 14 to 20 breaths per minute (or within normal limits for client), with clear upper airway and no pooling of oral secretions

Special Considerations

If a client is capable and wishes to manage suctioning independently, provide instruction in the use of the suction catheter or Yankauer.

Suctioning of disoriented clients may require two people. Family or significant others may be particularly helpful in assisting and in allaying the client's fears.

A bulb syringe may be purchased at pharmacy and used.

IMPLEMENTATION

Action	Rationale
1. Explain procedure to client.	*Reduces anxiety*
2. Wash hands and organize equipment.	*Reduces microorganism transfer* *Promotes efficiency*
3. Check suction apparatus for appropriate functioning.	*Maintains safety*
4. Position client in semi-Fowler's or Fowler's position.	*Facilitates forward draining of secretions in mouth*
5. Turn suction source on and place finger over end of attached tubing.	*Tests suction apparatus (use 50 to 120 mmHg pressure)*
6. Open sterile irrigation solution and pour into sterile cup.	*Allows for sterile rinsing of catheter*
7. Open mouthwash and dilute with water (optional).	*Freshens mouth and decreases oral microorganisms*
8. Don gloves.	*Prevents contact with secretions*
9. Open suction catheter package.	*Facilitates organization*
10. Place towel under client's chin.	*Prevents soiling of clothing*
11. Attach suction control port of suction catheter to tubing of suction source.	*Ensures correct attachment of catheter to suction source*
12. Lubricate 3 to 4 inches of	*Prevents mucosal trauma when*

Action	Rationale
catheter tip with irrigating solution.	*catheter is inserted*
13. Ask client to push secretions to front of mouth.	*Facilitates secretion removal*
14. Insert catheter into mouth along jawline and slide to oropharynx until client coughs or resistance is felt. BE SURE FINGER IS NOT COVERING OPENING OF SUCTION PORT.	*Promotes removal of pooled secretions* *Prevents application of suction as catheter is inserted*
15. Withdraw catheter slowly while applying suction and rotating catheter between fingers. AVOID DIRECT CONTACT OF CATHETER WITH IRRITATED OR TORN MUCOUS MEMBRANES.	*Facilitates removal of secretions from oropharynx* *Prevents additional trauma to oral tissue*
16. Place tip of suction catheter in sterile solution and apply suction for 1 to 2 seconds.	*Clears secretions from tubing*
17. Ask client to take three to four breaths while you auscultate for bronchial breath sounds and assess status of secretions.	*Permits reoxygenation* *Determines need for repeat suctioning*
18. Repeat steps 13 to 17 once or twice if secretions are still present.	*Promotes adequate clearing of airway*
19. When secretions are adequately removed, irrigate mouth with 5 to 10 mL of mouthwash and ask client to rinse out mouth.	*Removes microorganisms and thick secretions* *Freshens breath and improves taste sensation*
20. Suction mouth; repeat irrigation and suctioning.	*Removes secretions and residual mouthwash*
21. Disconnect suction catheter from machine tubing, turn off suction source and discard catheter.	
22. Apply lubricating jelly to	*Prevents cracking of lips and*

Action	Rationale
lips, and mouth moistener to inner lips and tongue, if desired.	*maintains moist membranes*
23. Dispose of or store equipment properly.	*Decreases spread of microorganisms*
24. Assist client to position of comfort with head of bed elevated 45 degrees.	*Lowers diaphragm and promotes lung expansion*

Evaluation

Were desired outcomes achieved?

DOCUMENTATION

The following should be noted on the visit note:

- Breath sounds after suctioning
- Character of respirations after suctioning
- Color, amount, and consistency of secretions
- Tolerance to treatment
- Replacement of oxygen equipment on client after treatment

Sample Documentation

DATE	TIME	
2/30/98	1400	Suctioned moderate amount of thick cream-colored secretions from mouth and oropharynx. Mouth care given. Upper airway clear; respirations non-labored. Continues on O_2 per nasal cannula at 3 liters.

*N*ursing *P*rocedure 4.10

Nasopharyngeal/ Nasotracheal Suctioning

✖ EQUIPMENT

- Suction source
- Large towel or linen saver
- Sterile irrigation saline or water
- Suction catheter (adults, size 14 to 16 French)
- Sterile gloves
- Cotton-tip swabs
- Moist tissue/cotton swabs

Purpose

Clears airway of secretions
Facilitates breathing

Desired Outcomes (sample)

Respirations are 14 to 20 breaths per minute, of normal depth, smooth, and symmetrical.
Upper lung fields are clear; no cyanosis.

Assessment

Assessment should focus on the following:

Doctor's order
Respiratory status (respiratory character, breath sounds)
Circulatory indicators (skin color and temperature, capillary refill, blood pressure, pulse)
Nasal skin and mucous membranes
Color, amount, and consistency of secretions
Client's and caregiver's ability to perform the suctioning procedure

Outcome Identification and Planning

Key Goals and Sample Goal Criterion

The client will:

Attain or maintain a patent upper airway, indicated by respiratory rate of 14 to 20 breaths per minute, normal depth, smooth
symmetrical, lungs clear, no cyanosis

Special Considerations

Clients sensitive to decreased oxygen levels should be suctioned for shorter durations, but more frequently, to ensure
adequate airway clearance without hypoxia.

Two people may be required for the suction procedure to minimize trauma. Whenever possible, an assistant should be secured to minimize unnecessary tube manipulation and to facilitate bagging with less risk of contamination.

IMPLEMENTATION

Action	Rationale
1. Explain procedure to client and caregiver.	*Reduces anxiety*
2. Wash hands and organize equipment.	*Reduces microorganism transfer Promotes efficiency*
3. Apply nonsterile gloves.	*Prevents contact with secretions*
4. Assist client into a sitting or reclining position.	*Facilitates maximal breathing during procedure*
5. Turn suction machine on and place finger over end of tubing attached to suction machine.	*Tests suction pressure (use 60 mmHg for children and up to 120 mmHg for adults for normal secretions)*
6. Open sterile irrigation solution and pour into sterile cup.	*Allows for sterile rinsing of catheter*
7. Open sterile gloves and suction catheter package.	*Maintains aseptic procedure*
8. Place towel under client's chin.	*Prevents soiling of clothing*
9. Ask client to breathe through one nostril while the other is occluded.	*Determines patency of nasal passage*
10. Repeat step 9 with other naris.	*Determines patency of nasal passage*
11. Have client blow nose with both nares open.	*Clears nasal passage without pushing microorganisms into inner ear*
12. Clean mucus and dried secretions from nares with moist tissues or cotton-tip swabs.	*Clears nasal passage*

Action	Rationale
13. Don sterile glove on dominant hand.	*Maintains sterile technique*
14. Holding suction catheter in sterile hand, attach suction control port to tubing of suction source (held in nonsterile hand).	*Maintains sterility while establishing suction*
15. Slide sterile hand from control port to suction catheter tubing (wrap tubing partially around hand).	*Facilitates control of tubing*
16. Lubricate 3 to 4 inches of catheter tip with irrigating solution.	*Prevents mucosal trauma when catheter is inserted*
17. Ask client to take several deep breaths—with oxygen source near.	*Provides additional oxygen to body tissues before suctioning*
18. Insert catheter into an unobstructed naris, using a slanted, downward motion. BE SURE FINGER IS NOT COVERING OPENING OF SUCTION PORT.	*Facilitates unrestricted insertion of catheter* *Prevents trauma to membranes due to suction from catheter*
19. As catheter is being inserted, ask client to open mouth.	*Allows for visibility of tip of catheter once inserted*
20. Proceed to step 21 for pharyngeal suctioning or to step 26 for nasotracheal suctioning.	

Nasopharyngeal Suctioning

Action	Rationale
21. Once catheter is visible in back of throat or resistance is felt, place thumb over suction port (Fig. 4.10).	*Applies suction*
22. Withdraw catheter in a circular motion, rotating it between thumb and finger. SUCTION SHOULD NOT BE APPLIED FOR MORE THAN 10 to 12 SECONDS.	*Promotes cleaning of large area and sides of lumen* *Prevents unnecessary hypoxia*
23. Place tip of suction cath-	*Clears secretions from tubing*

Action	Rationale

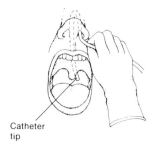

Catheter
tip

FIGURE 4.10

eter in sterile solution and apply suction for 1 to 2 seconds.

24. Allow client to take about five breaths while you listen to bronchial breath sounds and assess status of secretions.

Determines if repeat suctioning is needed

25. Repeat steps 21 to 24 once or twice if assessment indicates that secretions have not cleared well. Proceed to step 34 for completion of procedure.

Promotes adequate clearing of airway

Nasotracheal Suctioning

26. Once catheter is visible in back of throat or resistance is felt, ask client to pant or cough.

Opens trachea and facilitates entrance into trachea

27. With each pant or cough, attempt to insert the catheter deeper.

Decreases resistance to catheter insertion

28. Place thumb over suction port.

Initiates suction of secretions

29. Encourage client to cough.

Facilitates loosening and removal of secretions

30. Withdraw catheter in a circular motion, rotating

Minimizes adherence of catheter to the sides of the airway

Action	Rationale
it between thumb and finger. SUCTION SHOULD NOT BE APPLIED FOR MORE THAN 10 to 12 SECONDS.	*Prevents unnecessary hypoxia*
31. Place tip of suction catheter in sterile solution and apply suction for 1 to 2 seconds.	*Clears clogged tubing*
32. Allow client to take about five breaths while you listen to bronchial breath sounds and assess status of secretions.	*Determines if repeat suctioning is needed*
33. Repeat steps 26 to 32 once or twice if assessment indicates that secretions have not cleared well.	*Promotes adequate clearing of airway*
34. To complete the suctioning procedure:	
- Perform oral airway suctioning	*Clears secretions from oral airway*
- Disconnect suction catheter from suction tubing and turn off suction machine	
- Properly dispose of or store all equipment	*Prevents spread of microorganisms*
35. Assess incisions and wounds for drainage and approximation.	*Detects complications, such as bleeding or weakened incisions, from coughing and straining*
36. Assist client into a position of comfort.	*Facilitates slow, deep breathing* *Promotes safety* *Permits communication*
37. Wash hands.	*Removes microorganisms*

Evaluation

Were desired outcomes achieved?

DOCUMENTATION

The following should be noted on the visit note:

- Breath sounds after suctioning
- Character of respirations
- Significant changes in vital signs
- Color, amount, and consistency of secretions
- Tolerance to treatment (eg, state of incisions, drains)
- Replacement of oxygen equipment on patient after treatment

Sample Documentation

DATE	TIME	
12/3/98	0400	Suctioned moderate amount of thick, cream-colored secretions via nasopharynx (nasotrachea). Lungs clear in all fields after suctioning. Client slightly short of breath after procedure. Deep breaths with 100% O_2 taken. Respirations are 22, smooth and nonlabored. O_2 per nasal cannula reapplied at 3 liters/minute. Chest dressing dry and intact.

Nursing **P**rocedures   **4.11, 4.12, 4.13**

Tracheostomy Suctioning (4.11)

Tracheostomy Cleaning (4.12)

Tracheostomy Dressing and Tie Change (4.13)

⊠ EQUIPMENT

- Tracheostomy care kit:
  - sterile bowls or trays (two)
  - cotton-tip swabs
  - pipe cleaners
  - nonabrasive cleaning brush
  - tracheostomy ties
  - gauze pads
- Normal saline (500-mL bottle)
- Hydrogen peroxide
- Equipment for suctioning:
  - suction machine
  - suction catheter (size should be ½ lumen of trachea; adult, 14 to 16 French)
- Pair of nonsterile gloves
- Pair of sterile gloves (often in suction catheter kit)
- Towel or waterproof drape
- Goggles or protective glasses or face shield
- Face mask
- Gown or protective apron (optional)
- Irrigation saline (prefilled tubes or filled 3-, 5-, or 10-mL syringe)
- Hemostat
- Obturator (have available in case tube is dislodged)

Purpose

Clears airway of secretions
Facilitates tracheostomy healing
Minimizes tracheal trauma or necrosis

Desired Outcomes (sample)

Respirations are 14 to 20 breaths/minute, of normal depth, smooth, and symmetrical.

Upper lung fields are clear; no cyanosis.

Tracheostomy site remains intact without redness or signs of infection.

Assessment

Assessment should focus on the following:

Agency policy regarding tracheostomy care

Status of tracheostomy (ie, time since immediate postoperative period)

Type of tracheostomy tube (ie, metal, plastic, cuffed)

Respiratory status (respiratory character, breath sounds)

Color, amount, and consistency of secretions

Skin around tracheostomy site

Outcome Identification and Planning

Key Goals and Sample Goal Criterion

The client will:

Attain and maintain a patent airway, indicated by respiratory rate of 14 to 20 breaths/minute, smooth, symmetrical, normal depth; breath sounds clear, and no cyanosis

Special Considerations

For maximum client safety and oxygenation during suctioning and tracheostomy care, an assistant should be secured before beginning procedure.

Clients sensitive to decreased oxygen levels should be suctioned for shorter durations but more frequently to ensure adequate airway clearance without hypoxia or carbon dioxide buildup.

If client has nasogastric (NG) tube and cuffed tracheostomy, monitor closely for signs of pharyngeal trauma.

Client participation in tracheostomy care provides opportunity to teach home care.

Clean technique may be substituted for sterile technique in home health care, extended care, and care in other facilities.

Family members should be taught to perform care and assist nurse in care.

Tape hemostat to head of bed or wall above bed for emergency use if tracheostomy tube becomes dislodged.

IMPLEMENTATION

Action	Rationale
1. Explain procedure to client and caregiver.	*Reduces anxiety*
2. Wash hands and organize equipment.	*Reduces microorganism transfer* *Promotes efficiency*
3. Perform any procedure that loosens secretions (eg, postural drainage, percussion, nebulization).	*Facilitates removal of secretions from all lobes of lungs*

Procedure 4.11 Tracheostomy Suctioning

Action	Rationale
4. Don nonsterile gloves, goggles, gown, and mask.	*Protects nurse from contact with secretions*
5. Assist client into position on side or back with head of bed elevated.	*Facilitates maximal breathing during procedure*
6. Turn suction machine on and place finger over end of tubing attached to suction machine.	*Tests suction pressure (should not exceed 120 mmHg)*
7. Open sterile irrigation solution and pour into sterile cup.	*Allows for sterile rinsing of catheter*
8. Draw 10 mL sterile saline into syringe and place back into sterile holder (or place 3-mL saline containers on table).	*Provides fluid for irrigation of lungs to loosen secretions by stimulating cough during suctioning*
9. If performing tracheostomy care, set up tracheostomy care equipment (see Fig. 4.12.1 and Procedure 4.12). If not, proceed to step 10.	
10. Increase oxygen concentration to tracheostomy collar to 100% if O_2 being used.	*Increases oxygen level inspired before suctioning*
11. Open sterile gloves and suction catheter package.	*Ensures aseptic procedure*
12. Place towel or drape on client's chest under tracheostomy.	*Prevents soiling of clothing*
13. Don sterile glove on dominant hand.	*Maintains sterile technique*

Action	Rationale
14. Pick up suction catheter with sterile hand and attach suction control port to tubing of suction source (held with non-sterile hand).	*Maintains sterility* *Ensures correct attachment of catheter*
15. Slide sterile hand from control port to suction catheter tubing (may wrap tubing around hand).	*Facilitates control of tubing*
16. Lubricate 3 to 4 inches of catheter tip with irrigating solution.	*Prevents mucosal trauma when catheter is inserted*
17. Ask client to take several deep breaths with tracheostomy collar intact (Fig. 4.11) at tracheostomy tube entrance.	*Provides additional oxygen to body tissues before suctioning*
18. Remove tracheostomy collar.	*Allows entrance into tracheostomy*
19. Insert catheter approximately 6 inches into inner cannula (or until resistance is met or cough re-	*Places catheter in upper airway and facilitates clearance* *Prevents trauma to membranes due to suction from catheter*

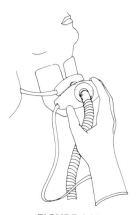

FIGURE 4.11

Action	Rationale
flex is stimulated). BE SURE FINGER IS NOT COVERING OPENING OF SUCTION PORT.	
20. Encourage client to cough.	*Facilitates loosening and removal of secretions*
21. Place thumb over suction port.	*Initiates suction of secretions (often catheter stimulates cough)*
22. Withdraw catheter in a circular motion, rotating catheter between thumb and finger. Intermittent release and application of suction during withdrawal is recommended. APPLY SUCTION FOR NO MORE THAN 10 TO 15 SECONDS.	*Facilitates removal of secretions from sides of the airway* *Prevents unnecessary hypoxia* *Minimizes trauma to mucosa*
23. Place tip of suction catheter in sterile solution and apply suction for 1 to 2 seconds.	*Clears clogged tubing*
24. Encourage client to take about five breaths while you auscultate bronchial breath sounds and assess status of secretions.	*Assesses if repeat suctioning is needed* *Permits reoxygenation*
25. Repeat steps 19 to 24 once or twice if secretions are still present.	*Promotes adequate clearing of airway*
26. If performing tracheostomy cleaning, wrap catheter around sterile hand (do not touch suction port), and proceed to step 4 of Procedure 4.12, Tracheostomy Cleaning.	*Maintains sterility and control*
27. If not performing tracheostomy cleaning or dressing/tie change, discard materials.	*Completes procedure*
28. Assist client to position of comfort.	*Provides for client safety and communication*
29. Wash hands.	*Prevents spread of microorganisms*

Action	Rationale

Procedure 4.12 Tracheostomy Cleaning

1. If tracheostomy cleaning is to follow tracheostomy suctioning, leave suction catheter around sterile hand (see Procedure 4.11), and proceed to step 4.

Clears secretions
Maintains sterility

2. If suctioning is not required, set up tracheostomy care equipment (Fig. 4.12.1):
   - Open tracheostomy care kit and spread package on bedside table.

   Provides sterile field

   - Maintaining sterility, place bowls and tray with supplies in separate locations on paper.

   Arranges equipment for easy access without contamination

   - Open sterile saline and peroxide bottles and fill first bowl with equal parts of peroxide and saline (do not touch container to bowl).

   Provides ½ strength peroxide mixture for tracheostomy cannula cleaning
   Maintains sterility of supplies

   - Fill second bowl with saline.

   Provides rinse for cannula

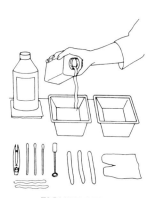

FIGURE 4.12.1

Action	Rationale
- Don sterile gloves.	
3. Place four cotton-tip swabs in peroxide mixture, then place across tracheal care tray.	*Provides moist swabs for cleaning skin*
4. Pick up one sterile gauze with fingers of sterile hand.	*Allows nurse to touch nonsterile items while maintaining sterility*
5. Stabilize neck plate with nonsterile hand (or have assistant do so).	*Decreases discomfort and trauma during removal of cannula*
6. With sterile hand, use gauze to turn inner cannula counterclockwise until catch is released (unlocked).	*Separates inner and outer cannula*
7. Gently slide cannula out using an outward and downward arch (Fig. 4.12.2).	*Follows curve of tracheostomy tube*
8. Place cannula in bowl of half-strength peroxide.	*Softens secretions*
9. Discard gauze.	*Avoids contaminating sterile items*
10. Unwrap catheter and suction outer cannula of tracheostomy.	*Removes remaining secretions*
11. Have client take deep breaths from trach collar	*Provides oxygenation after suctioning*

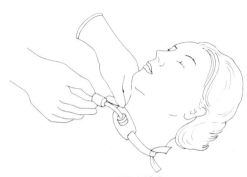

FIGURE 4.12.2

Action	Rationale
to deliver 100% oxygen.	
12. Disconnect suction catheter from suction tubing and discard sterile glove and catheter.	*Prevents spread of microorganisms*
13. Remove tracheostomy dressing.	*Exposes skin for cleaning*
14. Using gauze pads, wipe secretions and crustation from around tracheostomy tube.	*Removes possible airway obstruction and medium for infection*
15. Use moist swabs to clean area under neck plate at insertion site.	*Decreases possible infection*
16. Discard gloves.	*Prevents spread of microorganisms*
17. Don sterile gloves.	
18. Pick up inner cannula and scrub gently with cleaning brush.	*Removes crustation and secretions from outside and inside of cannula*
19. Use pipe cleaners to clean lumen of inner cannula thoroughly.	*Decreases accumulation of mucus in lumen*
20. Run inner cannula through peroxide mixture.	*Removes remaining debris*
21. Rinse cannula in bowl containing sterile saline.	*Rinses away peroxide mixture and residual debris*
22. Place cannula in sterile gauze and dry thoroughly; use dry pipe cleaner to remove residual moisture from lumen.	*Prevents introducing fluid into trachea*
23. Slide inner cannula into outer cannula (keeping inner cannula sterile), using smooth inward and downward arch, and rolling inner cannula side to side with fingers.	*Facilitates insertion and reduces resistance*
24. Hold neck plate stable with other hand and turn inner cannula clockwise until catch (lock) is felt and dots are in alignment.	*Assures inner cannula is securely attached to outer cannula*
25. If performing tracheostomy	

Action	**Rationale**

dressing or tie change, proceed to Procedure 4.13.

26. If not performing dressing or tie change, discard materials, wash hands and assist client to position of comfort.

Completes procedure and prevents spread of microorganisms

Procedure 4.13 Tracheostomy Dressing and Tie Change

1. Have assistant hold tracheostomy by neck plate while you clip old tracheostomy ties and remove them.

Prevents accidental dislodgment of tracheostomy during tie replacement

2. Slip end of new tie through tie holder on neck plate and tie a square knot 2 to 3 inches from neck plate (Fig. 4.13.1).

Facilitates removal of tie while holding tracheostomy tube firm

3. Place tie around back of client's neck and repeat above step with other end of tie, cutting away excess tie.

4. Apply tracheostomy dressing:

Places dressing in position to catch secretions from tra-

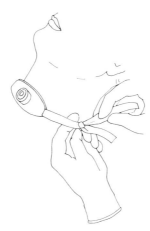

FIGURE 4.13.1

Action	Rationale
- Hold ends of tracheostomy dressing (or open gauze and fold into V shape).	*cheostomy or surrounding insertion site*
- Gently lift neck plate and slide end of dressing under plate and tie.	
- Pull other end of dressing under neck plate and tie.	
- Slide both ends up toward neck, using a gentle rocking motion, until middle of dressing (or gauze) rests under neck plate (Fig. 4.13.2).	
5. Assist client to position of comfort.	
6. Discard materials and wash hands.	*Reduces spread of infection*

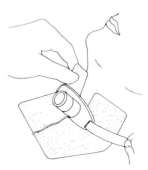

FIGURE 4.13.2

Evaluation

Were desired outcomes achieved?

DOCUMENTATION

The following should be noted on the visit note:

- Breath sounds after suctioning

- Character of respirations
- Status of tracheostomy site
- Significant changes in vital signs
- Color, amount, and consistency of secretions
- Tolerance to treatment (ie, state of incisions, drains)
- Replacement of oxygen equipment after treatment

Sample Documentation

DATE	TIME	
7/3/98	0400	Suctioned moderate amount of thick, cream-colored secretions via trachea. Lungs clear in all fields after suctioning. Tracheostomy care done. Stoma site dry with no redness or swelling. Client slightly short of breath after procedure. Respirations smooth and nonlabored after deep breaths with 100% O$_2$ taken. O$_2$ per tracheostomy collar reapplied. Client tolerated procedure with no pain or excess gagging. Client observed procedure with mirror to learn care procedure.

Nursing Procedures 4.14, 4.15

Tracheostomy Tube Cuff Management (4.14)

Tracheostomy Tube Removal and Reinsertion (4.15)

EQUIPMENT

- 10-mL syringe
- Blood pressure manometer
- Three-way stopcock
- Mouth-care swabs, moistener, and mouthwash
- Suctioning equipment
- Nonsterile gloves
- Sterile gloves
- Sterile 4 × 4 gauze
- Obturator

Purpose

Maintains minimum amount of air in cuff to ensure adequate ventilation without trauma to trachea

Desired Outcomes (sample)

Respirations are 14 to 20 breaths/minute, of normal depth, smooth, and symmetrical.

Lung fields are clear; no cyanosis.

Minimum occlusive pressure is maintained while cuff is inflated.

Tracheostomy tube is reinserted quickly without contamination or impaired oxygenation.

Assessment

Assessment should focus on the following:

Size of cuff

Maximum cuff inflation pressure (check cuff box)
Bronchial breath sounds
Respiratory rate and character
Agency policy or doctor's orders regarding cuff care

Outcome Identification and Planning

Key Goals and Sample Goal Criteria

The client will:

Maintain adequate ventilation, evidenced by pink mucous
   membranes, smooth nonlabored respirations, and respiratory
   rate of 12 to 16 breaths/minute
Experience no undetected tracheal damage

Special Considerations

Some cuffs are low-pressure cuffs and require minimum manipulation; however, client should still be monitored periodically
   to ensure proper cuff function.

IMPLEMENTATION

Action	Rationale

Cuff Pressure Check (for long-term cuff inflation)

Action	Rationale
1. Wash hands and organize equipment.	*Reduces microorganism transfer* *Promotes efficiency*
2. Check cuff balloon for in-flation by compressing be-tween thumb and finger (should feel resistance).	*Indicates cuff is inflated*
3. Attach 10-mL syringe to one end of 3-way stopcock. Attach manometer to an-other stopcock port. Close remaining stopcock port.	*Establishes connection between syringe and manometer*
4. Attach pilot balloon port to closed port of three-way stopcock (Fig. 4.14).	
5. Instill air from syringe into manometer until 10-mmHg reading is obtained.	*Prevents rapid loss of air from cuff*
6. Auscultate tracheal breath sounds, noting presence of smooth breath sounds or gurgling (cuff leak).	*Determines if cuff leak is present*

Action	Rationale

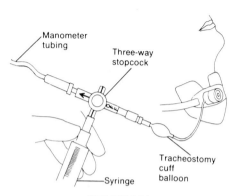

Manometer tubing

Three-way stopcock

Tracheostomy cuff balloon

Syringe

FIGURE 4.14

7. If smooth breath sounds are noted:
   - Turn stopcock off to manometer.
   - Withdraw air from cuff until gurgling is noted with respirations.
8. Once gurgling breath sounds are noted, insert air into cuff until gurgling is noted only on inspiration.

Provides minimum leak and minimizes pressure on trachea (airway is larger on inspiration)

9. Turn stopcock off to syringe.

Allows reading of pressure in cuff

10. Note manometer reading as client exhales. Record reading (note if pressure exceeds recommended volume. Do not exceed 20 mmHg). Notify physician if excessive leak persists or if excess pressure is needed to inflate cuff.

Expiratory cuff pressure indicates minimum occlusive volume (cuff pressure on tracheal wall)

11. Turn stopcock off to pilot balloon and disconnect.

Action	Rationale

Intermittent Cuff Inflation

12. Auscultate tracheal breath sounds noting presence of smooth breath sounds (cuff inflated), or vocalization/hiss (cuff deflated).

Determines if cuff leak is present

13. If smooth breath sounds are noted, withdraw air from cuff until faint gurgling is noted with respirations. If vocalization or hiss is noted, insert air into cuff until faint gurgling is noted with respirations.

14. Once gurgling breath sounds are noted, insert air into cuff until gurgling is noted only on inspiration.

Provides minimum leak and minimizes pressure on trachea (airway is larger on inspiration)

15. Instruct caregiver to monitor breath sounds every 2 hours until cuff is deflated.

Determines that minimum leak remains present

Cuff Maintenance Principles

16. Instruct caregiver to check tracheal breath sounds every 4 to 8 hours (more frequently if indicated) and note pressure of pilot balloon between fingers.

Determines if minimum or excessive cuff leak is present

17. Every 8 to 12 hours or per agency policy, caregiver should check cuff pressure and note if minimum occlusive volume increases or decreases.

Indicates if tracheal tissue damage or softening is occurring or if tracheal swelling is present

18. If oral or tube feedings are being received, assess secretions for tube feeding or food particles.

Indicates possible tracheo-esophageal fistula

19. To perform cuff deflation:

Prepares for removal of secre-

Action	Rationale
- Obtain and set up suctioning equipment.	*tions pooled on top of cuff* *Facilitates oxygenation*
- Enlist assistance and perform oral or naso-pharyngeal suctioning.	*Removes secretions pooled in pharyngeal area*
- Set up Ambu bag (if client is not on ventilator and long-term cuff inflation has been used).	*Provides for deep ventilations to move secretions*
- Have assistant initiate deep sigh with ventilator or administer deep ventilation with Ambu bag as you remove air from cuff with syringe.	*Pushes pooled secretions into oral cavity as cuff is deflated*
- Suction pharynx and oral cavity again.	*Removes remaining secretions*
20. Perform mouth care with swabs and mouthwash.	*Freshens mouth and moistens mucous membranes*
21. Apply lubricant to lips.	
22. Dispose of supplies appropriately.	
23. Assist client to position of comfort.	*Promotes comfort and safety* *Permits communication*

Procedure 4.15 Tracheostomy Tube Removal and Reinsertion

Removal

1. Explain procedure to the client/caregiver.	
2. Don unsterile gloves. Open several packets of sterile gauze. Prepare suction and cleaning materials if applicable (see Procedure 4.12).	*Permits manipulation of tracheostomy tube without contamination* *Prepares for cleaning of tube*
3. Untie or cut tracheostomy ties, remove and discard.	*Prepares tracheostomy for removal*
4. If cuffed tube and cuff is inflated, attach 10 mL-syringe to tracheostomy cuff balloon port and aspirate air from the cuff until the pilot balloon is flat.	*Deflates the tracheostomy cuff fully to prevent tissue trauma during tube removal*
5. Using a sterile gauze grasp	*Prevents contamination of the*

Action	Rationale

the tracheostomy neck plate, being careful not to obstruct the opening of the inner cannula. Gently, in an outward and downward curving motion, slide the neck plate and the inner and outer tracheostomy cannulas out of the tracheostomy opening in the neck. *Touch the outer cannula with sterile gauze only.*

tracheostomy tube
Promotes removal of the tube with minimal trauma to the tissues

6. Remove and clean the inner cannula (see Procedure 4.12). Use similar techniques to clean mucous plugs, and secretions from the lumen and external surfaces of the outer cannula as needed. Place inner cannula aside in cleansing soak or on sterile gauze and reinsert outer cannula (see steps below).

Reinsertion

1. If tube was accidentally removed or coughed out, and a cuffed tube is present, check tracheostomy tube cuff and deflate.

2. Don sterile gloves and clean the inner and outer cannulas as indicated. Replace ties as indicated. Place inner cannula on sterile 4 × 4 or let it remain in the cleansing soak.

Prepares outer cannula for reinsertion and stabilization
Maintains outer cannula lumen for insertion of obturator

3. Place the obturator into the outer cannula (Fig. 4.15.1A). Use the obturator to reinsert the trache-

Action	Rationale

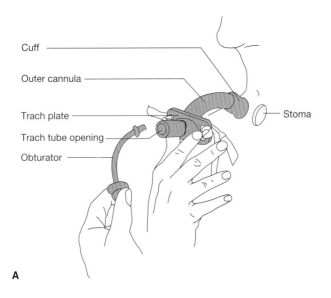

A

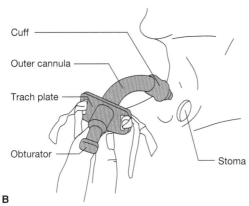

B

FIGURE 4.15.1

Action	Rationale

ostomy tube into the stoma in the client's neck (Fig. 4.15.1B).

4. Hold the trach plate in place and quickly remove the obturator (Fig. 4.15.2).

Prevents hypoxia from prolonged obstruction of airway by obturator
Prevents dislodgment of tracheostomy tube due to cough or gag stimulated by tube manipulation

5. Inflate cuff, if cuffed tube present, using a 10-mL syringe. Secure trach ties and tuck gauze pad under trach plate.

Prevents accidental dislodgement of tube

6. Using a sterile gauze or sterile gloves, dry and in-

Maintains sterility of inner cannula and reinserts with

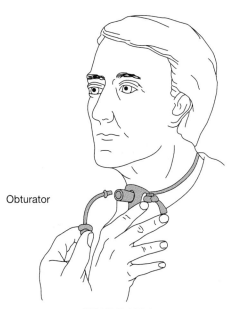

Obturator

FIGURE 4.15.2

Action	Rationale
sert the inner cannula in an inward and downward motion. Holding neckplate secure with one hand, turn cannula hub clockwise until it locks in place.	*minimal stimulation of cough or gag due to manipulation*
7. Discard gloves and used supplies. Wash your hands and assist the client to a position of comfort.	

Evaluation

Were desired outcomes achieved?

DOCUMENTATION

The following should be noted on the client's visit note:

- Cuff pressures noted and tracheal breath sounds
- Suctioning performed and nature of secretions
- Tolerance to procedure (changes in respiratory status and vital signs)
- Condition of the stoma
- Client/caregiver instructions and compliance with the procedure

Sample Documentation

DATE	TIME	
1/2/98	1800	Tracheal tube dislodged accidentally while client coughing. Inner and outer tube cannulas cleaned and tube reinserted without discomfort. Tracheal tube cuff checked with 15-mmHg minimum occlusive pressure noted. Suctioned scant thin secretions via nasopharynx, then cuff deflated fully. Client remains in bed with head of bed elevated. Respirations even and nonlabored.

Nursing **P**rocedure **4.16**

Suctioned Sputum Specimen Collection

EQUIPMENT

- Gown and mask
- Goggles
- Sterile sputum trap
- Suctioning equipment (see procedure for specific type of suctioning)
- Sterile saline in sterile container and prefilled tubes for irrigation
- Specimen bag and labels
- Sterile gloves
- Nonsterile gloves

Purpose

Obtain sputum specimen for analysis while minimizing risk of contamination

Desired Outcomes (sample)

Airway is clear of secretions.
Uncontaminated sputum specimen is obtained.

Assessment

Assessment should focus on the following:

Doctor's orders for test to be done and method of obtaining specimen
Breath sounds indicating congestion and need for suction
Previous notes of nurses and respiratory therapists to determine if secretions are thick or if catheter insertion (nasotracheal or nasopharyngeal) was difficult

Outcome Identification and Planning

Key Goals and Sample Goal Criteria
The client will:

Maintain clear airway
Receive proper treatment based on noncontaminated sputum
  specimen

Special Considerations

Time home visits to coincide with scheduled suctioning and
  specimen collection. Deliver specimen to laboratory immediately.

IMPLEMENTATION

Action	Rationale
1. Explain procedure to client.	*Reduces anxiety*
2. Wash hands and organize equipment.	*Reduces microorganism transfer* *Promotes efficiency*
3. Don clean gloves, goggles, gown, and mask.	*Protects nurse from contact with secretions*
4. Prepare suction equipment for type of suction to be performed (see appropriate procedure in this chapter).	*Promotes efficiency*
5. Open sputum trap package.	
6. Remove sputum trap from package cover and attach suction tubing to short spout of trap.	*Establishes suction for secretion aspiration*
7. Don sterile glove on dominant hand.	*Maintains sterility of process*
8. Wrap suction catheter around sterile hand.	*Maintains control of catheter*
9. Holding catheter suction port in sterile hand and rubber tube of sputum trap with nonsterile hand, connect suction to sputum trap (Fig. 4.16.1).	*Maintains sterility of procedure*
10. Suction client until secretions are collected in tubing and sputum trap. (If secretions are thick and need to be removed from catheter, suction small amount of sterile saline	*Obtains specimen* *Facilitates collection of thick sputum specimen*

Action	Rationale

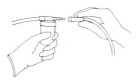

FIGURE 4.16.1

until specimen is cleared from tubing.)	
11. If insufficient amount of sputum is collected, repeat suction process.	*Ensures adequate specimen*
12. Using nonsterile hand, disconnect suction from sputum trap.	
13. Disconnect suction catheter and sputum trap, maintaining sterility of suction catheter control port, trap tubing, and sterile glove.	*Maintains catheter sterility for further suctioning, if needed*
14. Reconnect suction tubing to catheter and continue suction process, if needed.	*Clears remaining secretions from airway*
15. Discard suction catheter and sterile glove when suctioning is complete.	*Prevents spread of microorganisms*
16. Connect rubber tubing to sputum trap suction port (Fig. 4.16.2).	*Seals specimen closed*
17. Place specimen in plastic bag (if agency policy) and label with client's name, date, time, and nurse's initials.	*Ensures proper identification of specimen*
18. Discard equipment	*Prevents spread of microorganisms*
19. Assist client to position of comfort.	*Facilitates client comfort*
20. Wash hands.	*Reduces spread of infection*

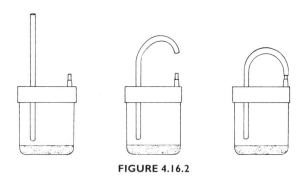

FIGURE 4.16.2

Evaluation

Were desired outcomes achieved?

DOCUMENTATION

The following should be noted on the visit note:

- Date, time, and type of specimen collection
- Type of suction done
- Amount and character of secretions
- Client tolerance of process

Sample Documentation

DATE	TIME	
1/6/98	1415	Sputum specimen obtained by naso-tracheal suctioning. Large amounts of thick, white mucus obtained; cough reflex stimulated with strong cough noted. Respirations even and nonla-bored, breath sounds clear. Specimen sent to lab.

Nursing **P**rocedure **4.17**

Pulse Oximetry

⊠ EQUIPMENT

- Pulse oximeter
- Sensor (permanent or disposable)
- Alcohol wipe(s)
- Nail polish remover

Purpose

Noninvasive monitoring of the oxygen saturation of arterial blood

Desired Outcomes (sample)
Client's SaO_2 remains between 90% and 100%.
Client has no undetected signs or symptoms of hypoxemia.

Assessment

Assessment should focus on the following:

Other signs and symptoms of hypoxemia (restlessness; confusion; dusky skin, nailbeds, or mucous membranes)
Quality of pulse and capillary refill proximal to potential sensor application site
Respiratory rate and character
Amount and type of oxygen administration, if applicable

Outcome Identification and Planning

Key Goals and Sample Goal Criteria
The client will:

Maintain an SaO_2 (arterial oxygen saturation) between 90% and 100%
Demonstrate knowledge of exogenous factors affecting pulse oximeter readings (ie, movement-restrictive probe placement, outside light, and anemia)

Special Considerations

Geriatric

Be sensitive to probe placement. This includes tension on probe site as well as tape applied to dry, thin skin.

 Transcultural

When choosing the earlobe as a site for pulse oximetry in clients of African descent, be sensitive to the presence of keloids. These ropelike scars, which are the result of an exaggerated wound healing process, may occur as a result of ear piercing. These scars may not allow accurate SaO_2 readings.

IMPLEMENTATION

Action	Rationale
1. Wash hands. Organize equipment.	*Reduces microorganism transfer* *Promotes efficiency*
2. Explain procedure to conscious client.	*Decreases anxiety and facilitates cooperation*
3. Choose sensor.	*Sensor types may vary according to weight of client and site considerations*
4. Prepare site. Use alcohol wipe to cleanse site gently. Remove nail polish or acrylic nails if needed when using finger as monitoring site.	*Alcohol wipes aid in ensuring that site is clean and dry.* *Frosted or colored nail polish and acrylic nails may interfere with pulse oximetry reading*
5. Check capillary refill and pulse proximal to the chosen site.	*Compromised peripheral circulation, caused by restriction (probe applied too tightly) or poor circulation due to medications or other conditions, may yield false readings*
6. Ascertain the alignment of the light-emitting diodes (LEDs) and the photo detector (light-receiving sensor). These sensors should be directly opposite each other (Fig. 4.17).	*Sensors that are not properly aligned will not yield an accurate SaO_2 reading via the pulse oximeter*
7. Turn the pulse oximeter to the ON position. REMEMBER: DISPOSABLE	*The emitting sensors (LEDs) will transmit red and infrared light through the*

Action	Rationale

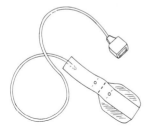 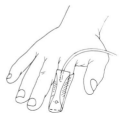

FIGURE 4.17

SENSORS NEED TO BE ATTACHED TO THE PATIENT CABLE BEFORE TURNING THE PULSE OXIMETER ON.	*tissue* *The receiving sensor (photo-detector) will measure the amount of oxygenated hemoglobin (which absorbs more infrared light) and deoxygenated hemoglobin (which absorbs more red light)* *SaO_2 will be computed by the pulse oximeter using these data*
8. Listen for a beep and note waveform or bar of light on front of pulse oximeter.	*Each beep indicates a pulse detected by the pulse oximeter. The light or waveform changes and indicates the strenth of the pulse. A weak pulse may not yield accurate SaO_2.*
9. Note reading and remove sensor and equipment. If continuous monitoring, check alarm limits. Reset if necessary. Always make certain that both high and low alarms are on before leaving the client.	*Alarm limits for both high and low SaO_2 and high and low pulse rate are preset by the manufacturer, but can be easily reset in response to doctor's orders*
10. Teach client common position changes that may trigger the alarm, such as bending the elbow and gripping the	*Patient participates in care, thus decreasing anxiety*

Action	Rationale
side rails or other objects.	
11. Instruct client or caregiver to relocate finger sensor at least every 4 hours. Relocate spring tension sensor at least every 2 hours.	*Prevents tissue necrosis*
Check adhesive sensors at least every 8 hours.	*Irritation may occur because of the adhesive*

Evaluation

Were desired outcomes achieved?

DOCUMENTATION

The following should be noted on the visit note:

- Type and location of sensor
- Presence of pulse proximal to sensor and status of capillary refill
- Percentage of oxygen saturated in arterial blood (SaO_2)
- Rotation of sensor site according to guidelines
- Percentage of oxygen client receiving or room air
- Interventions as a result of deviations from the norm

Sample Documentation		
DATE	**TIME**	
7/26/98	1800	Finger sensor (probe) applied to left index finger, capillary refill brisk, radial pulse present. Pulse oximeter yielding SaO_2 of 96% on room air.
	2200	Finger probe applied to right index finger, capillary refill brisk, radial pulse present. Pulse oximeter yielding SaO_2 of 97% of room air.

Chapter 5

Nutrition—Fluid and Nutrient Balance

OVERVIEW

▶ Initiation of intake and output measurement is an appropriate nursing decision any time potential for fluid imbalance is present.

▶ Malnourished clients have a high susceptibility to infection, and nutrition support substances provide a medium for possible microorganism growth; thus, good asepsis is a crucial concern.

▶ Careful monitoring and regulation of fluid administration are essential to prevent a potentially lethal fluid overload.

▶ Intake and output and daily weights are crucial in assessing nutritional support and fluid balance.

▶ Infusion of hyperosmotic solutions into the thoracic cavity or aspiration into the pulmonary tree could result in major respiratory compromise; thus, verification of feeding tube or central line placement is a primary concern in nutritional support.

▶ To prevent possible exposure to infectious organisms, nurses should wear gloves when contact with body fluids is probable.

Nursing **P**rocedure **5.1**

🖐 *Intake and Output Measurement*

⊠ EQUIPMENT

- Graduated 1000-mL measuring container
- Graduated water pitcher
- Graduated cups
- Scale
- Nonsterile gloves
- Felt pen or fine-tip marker

Purpose

Facilitates control of fluid balance
Provides data to indicate effects of diuretic or rehydration therapy

Desired Outcomes (sample)

Skin turgor is normal (ie, pinched skin returns to position immediately).
Edema is reduced from pitting to nonpitting type.
Indications of fluid excess or deficit are detected, if present.

Assessment

Assessment should focus on the following:

Doctor's orders for frequency of intake and output (I & O; hourly, every shift, 24-hourly)
Client status indicating need for I & O: edema, poor skin turgor, severely low or high blood pressure, congestive heart failure, dyspnea, reduced urinary output, intravenous infusion
Medications being taken that alter fluid status

Outcome Identification and Planning

Key Goals and Sample Goal Criteria

The client will:

Demonstrate an output equal to intake (plus or minus insensible loss)

Demonstrate a reduction in ankle edema, evidenced by a decrease in ankle measurement from 6.0 to 5.5 inches within 48 hours

Special Considerations

Strict I & O involves accounting for incontinent urine, emesis and diaphoresis, if possible. Weigh soiled linens to determine fluid loss, or estimate it.

Family members could be important allies in obtaining accurate I & O measurement. Explain procedure and enlist their assistance.

When measuring output, gloves should be worn to protect the caregiver from exposure to contaminated body fluids.

If the homebound client has difficulty understanding units of measure or seeing calibration lines, make an I & O sheet including columns of drinking glasses, cups of ice, bowls of jello and soup, and so forth, to represent intake and for client to cross off. Have client measure output by number of voidings.

IMPLEMENTATION

Action	Rationale
1. Wash hands and organize equipment.	*Reduces microorganism transfer* *Promotes efficiency*
2. Post pad on refrigerator; instruct client and family on use of intake and output record, with return demonstration. (If calorie count is in progress, list type of food and fluid consumed as well.)	*Ensures complete, accurate record of intake and output*

Intake

3. Place graduated cups in room and request that all fluids be measured in the cups prior to consumption.	*Ensures common units of measurement* *Minimizes error of measurement* *Facilitates accurate calculation of intake*
4. Semisolid substance intake should be recorded in percentage or fraction amount.	
5. Measure all oral intake: - Water: note volume in pitcher at the beginning	*Takes into account the wide variety of fluids consumed orally*

Action	Rationale
of the day, plus any fluid added, and substract fluid remaining in pitcher at the end of the day.	
- Ice chips: multiply volume by 0.5	*When melted, the volume of ice is approximately half its previous volume*
- All liquids (juice, beverage, broth) should be measured in graduated container.	
- Soup: indicate kind; measure volume.	
- Jello, ice cream, sherbet: use volume on container.	
6. Measure nasogastric (NG) or gastric tube feedings:	*Maintains accurate record by including gastrointestinal (GI) intake besides oral*
- Note volume in bottle hanging at beginning of the day (amount left from previous 24 hours) plus any feeding added during the day. (Allow prior feeding to infuse almost totally before adding new solution.)	*Indicates volume infusing during current period*
- Subtract fluid remaining in bag at end of the day (or read infusion total from pump).	
- Liquid—oral or NG— medications should be mixed with a measured volume of water.	*Maintains complete I & O measurement*
7. Measure all intravenous intake using same methodology as step 6. Volume of each type of intake is often designated on flowsheet (eg, colloids, blood products).	*Maintains complete I & O measurement*
8. If NG irrigation is performed and irrigant is left to drain out with other gastric contents, enter irrigant in intake section of	

Action	Rationale

flowsheet (or subtract
irrigant amount from
total output; see step 13).

Output

9. Place one or more (de-
pending on amount of
drainage) large graduated
containers in room. For
small amounts of drain-
age (wound drains or
scant NG drainage),
place graduated cups in
room with clearly marked
labels:
"*For Drainage Measure-
ment*"
Designate if urine mea-
surement from urinals
will be used or if urine
should be poured into
graduated containers.

*Maintains accurate output
measurement*
*Standardizes measurement
units (some containers vary
slightly)*

*Prevents inadvertent use of cup
for use of intake*

10. At end of each 24 hour
period, *don gloves* and
empty drainage into
graduated container. An
alternate method of
measuring output drain-
ing into a graduated con-
tainer is to mark the level
of drainage on a tape
strip on the container.
Mark drainage level with
date and time of each
measurement—or cali-
brate in intervals of
desired number of hours
(Fig. 5.1). When container
is nearly full, empty or
dispose of container and
replace with new con-
tainer.

*Minimizes exposure to body
fluids*
*Allows monitoring on a more
frequent basis*

11. Record amount and
source of drainage, particularly with drains from
different sites.

*Identifies abnormal drainage and
source*

Action	Rationale

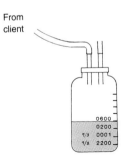

From
client

0600
0200
9/3 0001
9/2 2200

FIGURE 5.1

12. Measure output from:
    - NG or gastrostomy tubes
    - Ostomy drainage
    - Wound drains
    - Chest tube drainage
    - Urinary drainage or voidings
    - Emesis
    - Liquid stool
    - Blood or serous drainage and extreme diaphoresis (weigh soiled pads or linens and subtract dry weight to estimate output)

    Takes into account output from all sources

13. If intermittent or ongoing irrigation is performed, calculate true output (urinary or NG) by measuring total output and subtracting total irrigant infused (record only true output or indicate calculations on forms).

    Eliminates errors of double counting output

14. At end of 24-hour period, usually at end of the night, add total intake and total output. Report

    Indicates I & O status over 24-hour period

Action	Rationale
extreme input/output discrepancy to doctor (eg, if input is 1 to 2 liters more than output). Correlate weight gains with fluid intake excesses.	
15. Clean containers and store in client's room. Discard gloves, and wash hands.	*Prevents spread of infection*

Evaluation

Were desired outcomes achieved?

DOCUMENTATION

The following should be noted on the visit note:

- Intake from all sources on appropriate graphic sheet
- Output from all sources on appropriate graphic sheet
- Medication or fluid given to improve fluid balance and immediate response noted (eg, diuresis, blood pressure increase)
- Vital signs and skin status indicating fluid balance or imbalance

---

Sample Documentation

DATE	TIME	
6/9/98	0600	Client excreted 1200 mL urine after Lasix administration. Ankle diameter measurement remains 6 inches with 2+ pitting edema. D_5W infusing into right wrist angiocath at 10 mL/ hour by infusion pump.

*N*ursing *P*rocedures **5.2, 5.3, 5.4**

Intravenous Therapy: Vein Selection (5.2)

Intravenous Therapy: Solution Preparation (5.3)

Intravenous Therapy: Catheter/Infusion Plug Insertion (5.4)

☒ EQUIPMENT

- Nonsterile gloves
- Over-the-needle catheter or butterfly catheter/needle
- IV fluid (if continuous infusion) *or* infusion plug and heparin flush solution (if IV lock)
- Armboard (optional)
- Infusion tubing (vented for IV-fluid bag, unvented for IV bottles)
- IV pole (bed or rolling) *or* IV pump/controller
- IV insertion kit or supplies:
  - tourniquet (or blood pressure cuff)
  - tape—1 inch wide (or 2-inch tape, cut)
  - alcohol pads
  - Povidone pad (optional)
  - ointment (optional)
  - dressing—2 × 2-inch gauze, transparent semipermeable dressing
  - adhesive bandage
  - adhesive labels
- Scissors to clip hair (optional)
- Towel or linen saver

Purpose

Provides safe venous route for administration of fluids, medications, blood, or nutrients

Desired Outcomes (sample)

Skin is warm with good capillary refill and no edema.

IV intake is consistent with ordered rate.

Electrolytes are within normal limits.

Client performs self-care activities without disruption of IV assembly.

IV insertion site is clean and dry with no pain, redness, or swelling.

Assessment

Assessment should focus on the following:

Reason for initiation of IV therapy for particular client

Orders for type and rate of fluid and/or specified IV site

Status of skin on hand and arms; presence of hair or abrasions; previous IV sites

Client's ability to avoid movement of arms or hands for duration of procedure

Allergy to tape, iodine, antibiotic pads, or ointment

Client knowledge of IV therapy

Client's ability to care for IV site

Outcome Identification and Planning

Key Goals and Sample Goal Criteria

The client will:

Be able to verbalize and demonstrate safe management of IV site

Obtain and maintain fluid and electrolyte balance, as evidenced by good skin turgor, brisk capillary refill, no edema

Maintain intact skin integrity and absence of infection at insertion site, as evidenced by lack of pain, redness, or swelling at site

Verbalize understanding of movement limitations related to IV infusions and complications to be reported to the nurse

Demonstrate no extreme anxiety during or after IV insertion procedure

Special Considerations

Gloves should be worn since contact with blood is likely.

Maintenance of aseptic technique is a prime concern for the nurse performing IV therapy.

Choose tubing and needle appropriate for solution to provide optimal fluid flow: viscous solutions require larger needles.

Small catheters cause less vein wall irritation than large ones: choose the smallest gauge needle that will meet the need.

When working with confused clients, or other clients who are restless, obtain an assistant to help hold extremities still.

Because venous blood runs upward toward the heart, attempt to enter a vein at its lower (distal) end so that the same vein can be used later without leakage.

If it is difficult to insert catheter fully, wait until fluid infusion is initiated and then gently insert catheter.

To facilitate accurate 24-hour management, the client or care provider should record the amount of fluid infused each day.

Microdrip tubing with volume control chambers should be used for strict volume control. Infusion devices are often used for additional safety.

Clear explanations should be given with a demonstration of the equipment (except needles). Explain need for a helper to "assist" client in holding extremity stable during needle insertion.

Armboards may be used for stabilization of IV in an extremity.

If nursing visits are intermittent and IV therapy is continuous, instruct client and family on rate regulation, signs and symptoms of infiltration, and method for discontinuing IV catheter.

Geriatric

Veins are often fragile. When veins are elevated and clearly visible, needle insertion may be performed without tourniquet.

IMPLEMENTATION

Action	Rationale
Procedure 5.2 Intravenous Therapy: Vein Selection	
1. Wash hands and organize equipment.	*Reduces microorganisms* *Promotes efficiency*
2. Explain procedure, including client assistance needed during and after therapy initiation.	*Decreases anxiety and ensures cooperation*
3. Encourage client to use bedpan or commode before beginning.	*Avoids interruption during IV insertion process*
4. Help client into loose-fitting gown or clothing.	*Promotes ease of gown changes during IV therapy*
5. Ask client which is dominant hand.	*Facilitates placement of needle in nondominant hand or arm*
6. Tie tourniquet on arm 3 to 5 inches below elbow.	*Facilitates assessment of distal arm veins and hand veins*

Action	Rationale
7. Ask client to open and close hand or hang arm at side of bed.	*Pumps blood to extremity* *Dilates vein*
8. Look for vein with fewest curves or junctions and largest diameter (puffiness).	*Allows more complete insertion of catheter and use of large-gauge catheters*
9. Find vein on lower arm, if possible. Check anterior and posterior surfaces.	*Lower arm has natural splint of radial and ulnar bones*
10. If lower arm veins are unsuitable, look at hand and wrist veins.	
11. Look for site with 2 inches of skin surface below it (Fig. 5.2). If a large vein is needed, tie tourniquet just above antecubital area and search upper arm for suitable vein. A doctor's order is usually required before a vein in the lower extremities can be used. For PICC catheter the basilic or cephalic veins are most appropriate.	*Permits taping with greater stability* *Upper arm veins are large and support large needle gauges (18 or 16) often needed for blood or blood products* *Lower extremities are more prone to thrombophlebitis and other peripheral vascular problems*
12. Release tourniquet.	*Re-establishes blood flow*
13. Obtain supplies.	
14. Select smallest catheter size that meets infusion needs and is appropriate for vein size.	*Prevents irritation of vein lining, which causes phlebitis and infiltration*
15. Include two appropriately sized catheters and one smaller gauge catheter with other supplies.	*Prevents delay if second attempt is needed or smaller vein must be used*

Procedure 5.3 Intravenous Therapy: Solution Preparation

1. Select vein (see Procedure 5.2).	
2. Open tubing package and check tubing for cracks or flaws. Check ends for covers and verify that regulator clamp is closed (rolled	*Ensures that no defective materials are used and that tubing remains sterile* *Allows better fluid control, minimizing air in tubing*

Action	Rationale

Note: A doctor's order is usually needed for lower extremity IV.

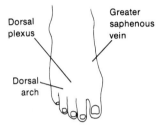

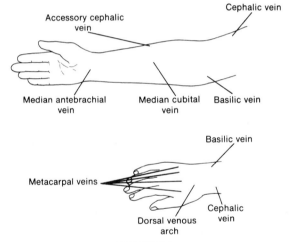

FIGURE 5.2

down, clamped off, or screwed closed).

3. Open IV fluid container:
   - **Bottles:** With one hand, hold bottle firmly on counter; with other hand, lift, then pull metal tab down, outward, and

Prevents injury or bottle breakage

Action	Rationale

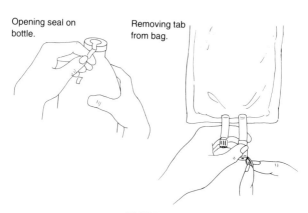

Opening seal on bottle.

Removing tab from bag.

FIGURE 5.3

around until entire ring is removed (Fig. 5.3); lift metal cap and pull flat rubber pad up and off. MAINTAIN STERILITY OF BOTTLE TOP.

Avoids introducing micro-organisms into client's vein

- **Bags:** Remove outer bag covering; hold bag by neck in one hand; pull down on plastic tab with other hand and remove (Fig. 5.3).

Prevents squeezing of fluid or air from bag when spike is inserted, increasing accuracy of fluid measurement

4. To attach tubing, first re-move cap from tubing spikes:
   - **Bottles:** Wipe top with alcohol; push spike into bottle port that is *not* attached to white tube.

Prevents blockage of tube that provides air vent

   - **Bags:** Push spike into port until flat end of tub-ing and bag meet.

Ensures complete connection of bag and tubing

5. Prime the tubing (remove air):
   - Hang bottle or bag on IV pole or wall hook;

Action	Rationale
squeeze and release drip chamber until fluid level reaches ring mark.	*Eliminates introduction of air into tubing*
- Remove cap from end of tubing.	
- Open roller clamp and flush tubing until air is removed.	*Removes air from tubing*
- Hold rubber medication plugs and in-line filter (if present) upside down and tap while fluid is running.	*Forces air bubbles from plugs and filter*
- Close roller clamp.	
6. Replace cap on end of tubing.	*Maintains sterility*
7. Apply time strip (see Procedure 5.8).	*Identifies when fluid should be replaced* *Facilitates monitoring of in- fusion rate*
8. Proceed to client with equipment. Drape tubing over pole.	*Maintains sterility of tubing*

Procedure 5.4 Intravenous Therapy: Catheter/ IV Lock Insertion

For Primary Infusion Line and IV Lock

1. Select vein (see Procedure 5.2) and prepare solution (see Procedure 5.3). Place IV tubing beside client.	*Selects most appropriate vein* *Provides fluid for infusion* *Places tubing at easy access*
2. Assist client into a supine or sitting position. Sit along side of bed or chair.	*Provides easier access to veins* *Promotes comfort during proce- dure* *Promotes use of good body mechanics*
3. Tear (3 one-inch) tape strips. Cut one piece down center.	*Narrow strip will secure cathe- ter without covering insertion site*
4. Prepare needle/catheter for insertion: **Over-the-needle catheter:** Examine the catheter for cracks or flaws. Rotate the catheter on needle. **Butterfly:** Check needle	*Ensures that catheter and needle are intact and plastic sheath will thread smoothly into vein* *Prevents shearing of vein by*

Action	Rationale
tip for straight edge without bends or chips.	*jagged needle*
5. Open antimicrobial solution or alcohol pad.	*Provides fast access to cleaning supplies*
6. Place towel under extremity.	*Prevents soiling of linens*
7. Place tourniquet on extremity.	*Restricts blood flow, distending vein*
8. Locate largest, most distal vein.	*Permits entrance of vein at higher point on future attempts without leakage*
9. Don gloves.	*Prevents contact with blood*
10. With alcohol or antimicrobial solution, clean vein area, beginning at the vein and circling outward in a 2-inch diameter. Repeat with povidone solution. Allow to air dry completely.	*Maintains asepsis* *Complete air drying is necessary to achieve maximum antimicrobial effectiveness*
11. Encourage client to take slow, deep breaths as you begin.	*Facilitates relaxation*
12. Hold skin taut with one hand while holding catheter with other (Fig. 5.4.1).	*Stabilizes vein and prevents skin movement during insertion*
Over-the-needle catheter: Hold the catheter by holding fingers on opposite sides of needle housing, *not* over catheter hub.	*Facilitates viewing of initial blood flashback in catheter and reduces potential for contamination*
Butterfly: Pinch "wings" of butterfly together to	*Decreases pain during needle insertion*

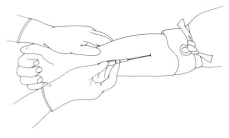

FIGURE 5.4.1

Action	Rationale

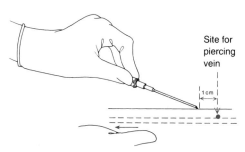

Site for
piercing
vein

|1 cm|

FIGURE 5.4.2

insert needle.
13. Maintaining sterility,
    insert catheter into vein
    with bevel of needle up.
    Insert needle parallel to   *Allows for full insertion of*
    straightest section of vein.   *catheter*
    Puncture skin at a 30-de-   *Ensures catheter stability*
    gree angle, 1 cm below
    site where the vein will be
    entered (Fig. 5.4.2).
14. When needle has entered   *Prevents penetration of both*
    skin, lower it until it is al-   *walls of the vein*
    most flush with the skin
    (Fig. 5.4.3).
15. Following path of vein,
    insert catheter into side
    of vein wall (*If using a*
    needle-stick protective over-

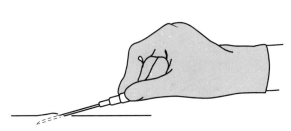

FIGURE 5.4.3

Action	Rationale
the-needle catheter system, insert needle at a 30-degree angle with bevel and push-off tabs in the up position. Place index finger on the push-off tab and thread the catheter to the desired length.)	
16. Watch for first backflow of blood, then push needle gently into vein.	*Indicates needle has pierced vein wall*
Over-the-needle catheter: Push needle into vein about ¼ inch after blood is noted. Slide catheter over needle and into vein. Apply digital pressure distal to catheter tip before pulling needle out of vein and skin (Fig. 5.4.4). IF UNABLE TO INSERT CATHETER FULLY, DO NOT FORCE; WAIT UNTIL FLUID FLOW IS INITIATED.	*Prevents piercing both walls of vein with needle* *Permits insertion of catheter without needle to prevent puncture of other vein wall* *Prevents excessive bleeding from the hub* *Fluid infusion facilitates dilatation of vein*
17. Holding catheter securely, remove cap from IV tubing and insert into hub of catheter; with **IV LOCK**	*Prevents dislodging of catheter*

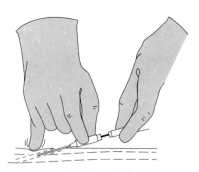

FIGURE 5.4.4

Action	Rationale

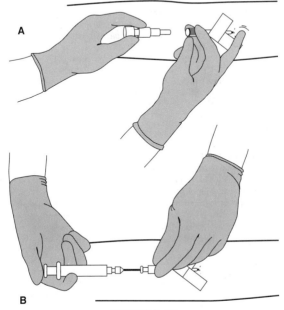

FIGURE 5.4.5

twist on infusion plug
(Fig. 5.4.5*A*).
18. Remove tourniquet.

    Prevents vein rupture from infusion of fluid against closed vessel

19. Open roller clamp and allow fluid to flow freely for a few seconds; with **heparin lock,** wipe plug with alcohol and flush with saline (Fig. 5.4.5*B*).

    Determines if catheter is in vein or wedged against vessel wall

    Fluid infusion prevents clot formation

20. Monitor for swelling or pain.

    Indicates infiltration

21. Tape catheter in position that allows free flow of the fluid. Tape catheter

    Eliminates positional flow of IV fluids

Action	**Rationale**
in one of the following methods:	
Over-the-needle catheter: Put small piece of tape under hub of catheter and fold ends straight down towards the insertion site, place a tape strip across the top of the hub to secure hub to skin. DO NOT PLACE TAPE OVER INSERTION SITE.	*Maintains sterility of insertion site by covering with sterile material only*
Butterfly: Put smallest pieces of tape across "wings" of butterfly; put another tape piece across middle to form an H (see Fig. 5.8 for an example).	*Provides catheter stabilization without tape covering insertion site*
22. Slow IV fluids to a moderate drip.	*Prevents accidental fluid bolus while completing site care*
23. Place ointment over insertion site, if desired, and cover with adhesive bandage, 2 × 2-inch dressing, or transparent dressing (omit ointment with this dressing type).	*Decreased exposure to and growth of microorganism*
24. Remove gloves and secure tubing:	
Over-the-needle catheter: Place tape across top of tubing, just below catheter. Loop tubing and tape to dressing. Secure length of tubing to arm with short piece of tape. Tape the tubing/catheter hub junction.	*Prevents disconnection of tubing*
Butterfly: Coil needle tubing around and on top of IV site.	*Prevents weight of tubing or movement from dislodging needle*
- Tape across coil and hub of needle.	
IV lock: Flush with dilute heparin solution (1:10 or	*Prevents clot formation* *Secures needle/catheter*

Action	Rationale
1:100) or saline. Tape across infusion plug.	
25. On a piece of tape or label, record: needle size, type, date, and time of insertion and your initials. Place label over top of dressing.	*Provides information needed for follow-up care*
26. Apply armboard if needed.	*Stabilizes sites of frequent movement*
27. Discard gloves and dispose of equipment properly.	*Prevents spread of microorganisms and accidental contaminated needle exposures*
28. Regulate IV flow manually or set infusion device at appropriate rate (see Procedure 5.7).	
29. Review limitations in range of motion with client. Instruct client to notify nurse of problems or discomfort.	*Enlists client's assistance in maintenance of catheter*
30. Remove towel and assist client to a comfortable position.	*Promotes comfort and safety*
31. Check infusion accuracy after 5 minutes and again after 15 minutes. Teach client how to check volume every 1 to 2 hours for infusion rate accuracy.	*Determines if rate needs to be adjusted.* *Promotes client autonomy and infusion safety*

Evaluation

Were desired outcomes achieved?

DOCUMENTATION

The following should be noted on the visit note:

- Client's tolerance of insertion procedure and fluid infusion
- Status of IV site, dressing, fluids, and tubing
- Size and type of catheter/needle
- Type and rate of infusion (if continuous infusion)

- Client teaching accomplished
- Follow-up assessments of the infusion
- Accuracy of return demonstration observed
- Type and amount of flush solution used if IV lock device is in place

Sample Documentation
DATE   TIME

12/3/98   1200   Client has 20-gauge Jelco inserted in right lower arm. One liter D_5W infusing at 125 mL/hr. Site intact. Client tolerated insertion procedure and fluid infusion without significant changes in vital signs. Teaching done regarding mobility limitations and IV maintenance procedures. Client voiced understanding and accurately demonstrated IV care.

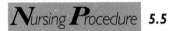

*N*ursing *P*rocedure 5.5

Intravenous (IV) Therapy: Midline Catheter Insertion

☒ EQUIPMENT

- Midline venous access device
- Sterile drapes
- 70% Isopropyl alcohol swab sticks ×3
- Povidone–iodine swab sticks ×3
- Tourniquet
- Sterile gloves, 2 pair
- Face mask ×2 (optional)
- Steri strips
- Flush solutions; normal saline and heparin
- Towel roll
- 10-mL syringes ×2
- Extension set and needleless cap

Purpose

To provide safe and cost-effective vascular access for the intermediate term IV therapy administration in the home environment.

Desired Outcomes (sample)

Provide peripheral IV vascular access that remains intact without complication or problems throughout the entire course of therapy

Completion of vascular access for intermediate term therapies with one IV access stick

Assessment

Assessment should focus on the following:

Client's vascular access condition and client allergies
Anticipated type and duration of therapy
Ability of the client or caregiver to understand and perform appropriate catheter maintenance procedures
Client lifestyle and preference

Outcome Identification and Planning

Key Goals and Sample Goal Criteria

The client or significant other will:

Demonstrate the care and maintenance activities required to keep the midline patent

Verbalize an understanding of the purpose of the catheter

Remain as comfortable as possible throughout the procedure

Verbalize and demonstrate emergency interventions

Special Considerations

Each client must be measured from the anticipated site of insertion to desired tip location.

Optimal tip location on the chest is level with the axilla

Midline catheters are intended to be threaded from three (3) to eight (8) inches into the peripheral vascular system. These catheters have various length and gauge sizes and are available in both single and dual lumen catheters.

Midline catheters are compatible with any peripheral IV therapies, ie, antibiotics, pain medication and should be used when therapy is anticipated to last from 1 week to 1 month.

Midline catheters are inserted by RNs who have been specially trained and are qualified in the insertion technique. Some agencies require a physician's order for insertion of these lines. Other agencies do not.

Some agencies require sterile procedure for insertion, other agencies require that a clean technique be used. Regardless, aseptic technique is used throughout this procedure. If the client is allergic to iodine solutions or preparations, the prepping agent is 70% isopropyl alcohol applied with friction for a minimum of 30 seconds per swab, until the final swab comes away visually clean.

Before using any catheter, visually inspect it for product integrity. If the package is opened or has an irregularity, do not use this device.

If there is resistance during catheter advancement, rotating the wrist, moving the arm to a different angle, or flushing the catheter with normal saline may assist progression.

Geriatric

These clients may have sclerotic or fragile vascular systems with a loss of vessel elasticity. Midline catheters may be a good choice for this population as the frequency of IV sticks is greatly decreased.

Economic

Midline catheters are initially more expensive than the standard IV catheter but the length of dwell is increased. The client could save health care dollars and visiting nurse time with this device. Inform the client of insurance coverage for home care transfusion services before insertion is done. Discuss the cost–benefit ratio with the client/caregiver.

HINTS

Specific insertion techniques varies from one manufacturer to another. Check the specific product directions for use before starting.

Ask the patient which hand is dominant as that hand will be needed for preparing home IV infusions. If possible, place the catheter in the nondominate arm.

IMPLEMENTATION

Action	Rationale
1. Cleanse hands and working area, and assemble equipment.	*Reduces transfer of microorganisms*
2. Assist the client to a comfortable supine position.	
3. Position the arm at a 45° angle abducted from the body. The arm should be fully extended with the elbow supported with a rolled towel.	*Assists with vessel visualization and helps to keep the ante cubital area prominent*
4. Position protective drape under the client's arm.	*Maintains clean field and keeps linens free from preparation solutions and blood*
5. Apply the tourniquet and perform a final assessment of the condition of the veins in the antecubital area. The insertion site should be 2 to 3 finger widths above or 1 to 2 finger widths below the antecubital space.	*Proper placement ensures catheter function throughout the length of dwell*
6. Release the tourniquet.	

Action	Rationale
7. Apply face mask and assist the client or caregiver with applying a mask also.	*Decreases potential for site contamination.*
8. Apply sterile gloves.	
9. Prep the insertion area 3 times with alcohol in a concentric motion working from the planned insertion site outward to a diameter of 3 to 4 inches. Allow to dry.	*Drying is very important for the antiseptic effects on the skin and as wet alcohol negates the effect of iodophor preparations.*
10. Repeat the above step– with the povidine iodine swabs. Allow to dry.	*Antibacterial effects are enhanced over time as the Betadine solution remains on the skin.*
11. Remove gloves and reapply tourniquet.	
12. Apply the second pair of sterile gloves.	
13. Drape with sterile towel or fenestrated drape, keeping the venipuncture site visible.	*Removes potential for contaminating sterile field*
14. Perform the venipuncture and observe for flashback before threading the catheter. Insert the catheter according to the specific manufacturer's directions.	*Safeguards vascular access*
15. Thread the catheter into the vein using slow, small increments. If resistance is felt, stop advancement and troubleshoot the line.	*Prevents damage to vein by forcing the catheter through the vein wall*
16. Remove tourniquet.	
17. Attach appropriate IV equipment.	
18. Infuse fluids or flush the line with normal saline and observe the upper arm for any signs of infiltration.	*Visual inspection of upper arm helps to affirm correct tip location*
19. Apply sterile dressing.	
20. Explain emergency pro-	

Action	Rationale
cedures to client. Client should be instructed to notify the doctor or nurse immediately if: - you are unable to infuse any of the solution - resistance is met when flushing the catheter - if you have a hole or break the line - you have any pain in the neck or shoulder - any symptoms of infection (fever sweats or drainage at the insertion site) are present - There is redness or swelling in the arm	*Reinforces safe practice in the home*

Evaluation

Were desired outcomes achieved?

DOCUMENTATION

The following should be noted on the visit note:

- Date and time of insertion
- Catheter type, length, and gauge
- Location of insertion site
- Type of dressing applied
- Brief description of the procedure and client's tolerance

SAMPLE DOCUMENTATION

A 6-inch, 20-g, midline catheter inserted into the left basilic vein. Insertion procedure followed according to policy. Client tolerated 45-minute supine position well. Occlusive semipermeable transparent applied. Catheter easily flushed with 0.9% NS. Potential problems and warning signs of complications explained to client and caregiver. Understanding of emergency procedures verbalized.

*N*ursing *P*rocedure 5.6

Intravenous (IV) Therapy: Peripherally Inserted Central Catheter (PICC) Insertion

☒ EQUIPMENT

- PICC and insertion kit or individually collect: PICC
- Sterile drapes: polylined, fenestrated and nonfenestrated
- Sterile 2 × 2 and 4 × 4 gauze squares
- Sterile nontoothed forceps and scissors
- Sterile nonpowdered gloves, 2 pair
- 70% isopropyl alcohol swab sticks × 3
- Povidone–iodine swab sticks × 3
- Flush solutions; normal saline and heparin
- Local Anesthetics—Optional
  1. Intradermal injection xylocaine (without epinephrine)
  2. Topical cream
- Tourniquet
- Face mask × 2
- Eye protection (goggles)
- Steri strips (½ inch)
- 10-mL syringes with 21 g needle × 2
- 1-mL syringe with 25 g needle
- Luer-Lok extension set and needle less cap
- Protective gown (optional)
- Measuring tape

Purpose

To provide safe, efficacious means of providing long-term vascular access for intravenous therapy administration in the home environment.

Desired Outcomes (sample)

Provide central vascular access that remains without complications or problems throughout the entire course of therapy

Completion of vascular access for long term therapies with one IV access puncture

Assessment

Assessment should focus on the following:

Physician order for PICC insertion
Consent form: signed or verbal
Client's vascular access condition and client allergies
Anticipated type and duration of therapy
Ability of the client or caregiver to understand and perform appropriate catheter maintenance procedures and emergency interventions
Client lifestyle and preference

Outcome Identification and Planning

Key Goals and Sample Goal Criteria
The client or significant other will:

Demonstrate the care and maintenance activities required to keep the PICC patent and free from potential complications
Verbalize an understanding of the purpose of the catheter
Remain as comfortable as possible throughout the insertion procedure
Verbalize and demonstrate emergency interventions

Special Considerations
PICCs are to be inserted by nurses who possess advanced IV skills, have completed a formal theoretical and clinical education program for PICC insertion and have demonstrated competency for safe insertion. The Nurse Practice Act of some states may not allow nurses to insert PICCs.
Portable radiographic confirmation of catheter tip location must be obtained before initiation of prescribed IV therapy.
PICCs are available in both single and dual lumen designs. The line may be inserted through a variety of methods, including break-away needle or a peel-away sheath introducer.
Aseptic technique is used throughout this procedure. If the client is allergic to iodine solutions or preparations, the prepping agent is 70% isopropyl alcohol applied with friction for a minimum of 30 seconds per swab, until the final swab comes away visually clean.
Before using any catheter, visually inspect it for product integrity. If the package is opened or has an irregularity, do not use this device.

Geriatric

These clients may have sclerotic or fragile vascular systems with a loss of vessel elasticity. The large introducing device of the PICC may be especially painful for this population. The PICC is a good choice for this generation as the frequency of IV sticks is greatly decreased and the daily care and maintenance procedures are minimal.

Economic

PICC catheters are initially more expensive than the standard IV catheter but the length of dwell is greatly increased. Health care dollars and visiting nurse time are saved with this device. Inform the client of insurance coverage for home care infusion services before insertion is done. Discuss the cost–benefit ratio with the client/caregiver.

HINT

Ask the patient which hand is dominant as that hand will be needed for preparing home IV infusions. If possible, place the catheter in the nondominate arm. Specific insertion techniques varies from one manufacturer to another. Check the specific product directions for use before starting.

IMPLEMENTATION

Action	Rationale
1. Assist the client to a comfortable supine or semi-reclining position.	*Assists in decreasing client anxiety*
2. Using a tourniquet, assess the clients antecubital fossa for appropriate vein selection.	*Basilic, medium cubital, and cephalic veins are the vessels of choice*
3. Remove tourniquet.	
4. Thoroughly wash hands using an approved antiseptic soap.	*Reduces transfer of microorganisms*
5. Gather all necessary supplies.	*Improves procedure efficiency*
6. Measure the client for the final tip. The junction of the SVC and the right location (SVC) with the arm abducted at atrium	*The junction of the SVC and right atrium is in this area*

Action	Rationale

is in this area, 45° angle from the body. Carefully measure from 1 cm below the anticipated site of insertion, across the clavicle to the sternum down to the third intercostal space (Fig. 5.6).

7. Put mask, protective eye wear, and gown on.

Maintains universal precautions

8. If necessary, clip hair from antecubital fossa.

Clipping decreases potential for microscopic skin abrasions that occur with shaving

9. Place a moisture-proof drape under client's arm.

Maintains clean field and keeps linens free from preparation solutions and blood

10. Position arm at a 90° angle. It should be fully

Assists with vessel visualization and helps to keep the ante-

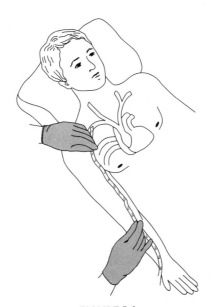

FIGURE 5.6

Action	Rationale
extended with the elbow supported with a rolled towel.	*cubital area prominent*
11. Open the insertion kit, creating a sterile field, dropping additional supplies onto the field.	
12. Apply sterile gloves.	*Decreases potential for site contamination*
13. Carefully place a sterile towel under the client's arm.	
14. Cleanse the selected insertion area three times with alcohol swabs in a concentric motion working from the planned insertion site outward to a diameter of 5–6 inches in diameter. Allow to air dry.	*Drying is very important for the antiseptic effects on the skin and as wet alcohol negates the effect of iodophor preparations*
15. Repeat the above step with the povidone–iodine swabs. Allow to air dry.	*Antibacterial effects are enhanced over time as the Betadine solutions remains on the skin*
16. Trim the catheter to the appropriate premeasured length and flush the line if necessary.	*Some manufacturers suggest trimming to ensure correct tip placement*
17. Anesthetize insertion site with 0.2–0.4 mL 1% lidocaine intradermally or apply topical cream.	*Assists in decreasing pain from needle or sheath introducer.*
18. Remove gloves and reapply tourniquet.	
19. Apply the second pair of sterile nonpowdered gloves.	*Removes potential for contaminating sterile field*
20. Drape the area with sterile towel or fenestrated drape, keeping the venipuncture site visible, creating a sterile field.	*Decreases risk of contaminating equipment and assists in diminishing the potential for post-insertion infection*
21. Perform the venipunc-	*Ensures that entire bevel of the*

Action	Rationale
ture. When blood return is obtained, advance the introducer 1–2 millimeters.	*introducer is inserted into the vessel*
(a.) If using a sheath introducer, remove the stylet.	*Prevents trauma to the vascular intima*
22. Remove the tourniquet.	
23. Using a nontoothed forceps, grasp catheter ½ inch from tip and thread through the introducer.	
24. Slowly advance the line into the vessel in ½-inch increments until 10–20 cm of length is reached.	*Prevents damage to the vein and safeguards vascular access*
25. Carefully pull introducer back along the catheter, almost to hub. Cautiously peel or break away introducer from the catheter.	*Using caution protects against catheter damage or shearing*
26. Ask the client to turn toward the cannulated arm and drop their chin to the shoulder.	*Keeps the entrance into the internal jugular restricted and assists in guiding the catheter towards the SVC*
27. Thread the catheter into the vein using slow, small increments. If resistance is felt, stop advancement and troubleshoot the line.	*If resistance continues after various advancement techniques are implemented the procedure must be discontinued*
28. Continue to advance catheter to the premeasured length.	
29. If present, remove guidewire.	
30. Securely attach Luer-Lok extension set and injection cap.	
31. Stabilize the catheter with a steristrip.	
32. Confirm patency by aspirating for blood return and flush with 5–10 mL NS then,	

Action	Rationale
33. Flush with 2–3 mL (100 u/cc) heparin solution.	
34. If necessary, apply a folded 2 × 2 to the insertion site for 24 hours.	*To absorb any excess blood from insertion site*
35. Apply a sterile, occlusive semipermeable transparent dressing.	
36. Obtain chest x-ray confirmation of catheter tip placement.	*Tip should be in the SVC*
37. Explain emergency procedures to client instructing him/her to notify the doctor or the nurse immediately if: - you are unable to infuse any of the solution - resistance is met when flushing the catheter - if you have a hole or break the line - you have any pain in the neck or shoulder - any symptoms of infection (fever sweats or drainage at the insertion site) are present - There is redness or swelling in the arm	*Reinforces safe practice in the home*

Evaluation

Were desired outcomes achieved?

DOCUMENTATION

The following should be noted on the visit note:

- Date and time of insertion
- Catheter type, manufacturer name
- Catheter length and gauge
- Location of insertion site with measured internal and external lengths

- Type of dressing applied
- Brief description of the procedure and client's tolerance
- Upper arm circumference and designation of measurement
- Radiographic confirmation of tip location

Sample Documentation

DATE	TIME	
2/6/98	1100	Insertion of a 50-cm, 4.0 Fr., dual lumen PICC in the left basilic vein. Inserted 52 cm with 6 cm left on patient's skin. Insertion procedure followed according to policy. Client tolerated the 60-minute supine position well. Occlusive, semipermeable transparent applied. No bleeding at insertion site post insertion noted. Catheter easily flushed with 0.9% N.S. and 2.5 mL heparin. Tip location in SVC confirmed by chest x-ray. Potential problems and warning signs of complications explained to client and caregiver. Understanding of emergency procedures verbalized.

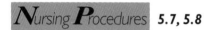
5.7, 5.8

Flow Rate Calculation (5.7)

Intravenous Fluid Regulation (5.8)

☒ EQUIPMENT

- IV pole (bed or rolling) *or* IV pump/controller
- Calculator (or pencil and pad)
- Watch with second hand

Purpose

Ensures delivery of correct amount of IV fluids

Desired Outcome (sample)

Correct volume of fluid is infused within designated time frame.

Client/caregiver verbalizes understanding of, and purpose of, infusion equipment used.

Assessment

Assessment should focus on the following:

- Orders for type and rate of fluid
- Type of infusion control devices available or ordered
- Viscosity of ordered fluids
- Client's knowledge of infusion therapy
- Client or caregiver's ability to use infusion equipment

Outcome Identification and Planning

Key Goals and Sample Goal Criterion

The client or caregiver will:

Infuse the correct fluid volume

Demonstrate the ability to perform the procedures necessary for completing infusions

Special Considerations

Viscous solutions may require rate adjustments throughout infusion process based on actual flow due to accumulation in filter or on sides of tubing.

Manual Flow Control Devices

Add-on manual flow regulating devices are available from many manufacturers; consult package directions for precise instruction. These add-on devices may provide a greater accuracy than regular in-line roller clamps. Some also compensate for client head height. This is important for the ambulatory patient. These devices can provide an extra measure of safety for the gravity infusions but **are not** intended to replace electronic infusion devices.

Geriatric

These clients are often volume sensitive and prone to fluid overload, particularly with rapid infusion of large volumes. Infusions must be regulated carefully and checked frequently, and clients must be watched closely for tolerance.

Economic

The cost for home infusion therapy may be expensive for the client. Many items are not covered by insurance nor are they reimbursed to the provider. The use of infusion equipment and devices must be examined for real versus perceived need.

HINT

Simple, lightweight or programmable ambulatory infusion devices assist the nurse in ensuring patient/caregiver compliance with infusion therapy.

IMPLEMENTATION

Action	Rationale

Procedure 5.5 Flow Rate Calculation

Action	Rationale
1. Check tubing package to determine drop factor of tubing.	*Indicates drops per mL for drip rate calculation*
2. Determine the infusion *volume in milliliters* (mL) per hour using the following formula:	*Simplifies calculations by limiting time to 60 minutes* *Facilitates monitoring of fluid and time taping container*

Action	Rationale

$$\frac{\text{TOTAL VOLUME}}{\text{TOTAL NUMBER OF HOURS}} = \boxed{\begin{array}{c}\text{Hourly infusion rate}\\ \text{(volume to infuse each hour)}\end{array}}$$

Example: 1000 mL to be infused over 6 hours

$$1000/6 = 167 \text{ mL/hr}$$

3. Determine *flow rate* by using the following formula:

$$\frac{\text{TOTAL FLUID VOLUME}}{\text{TOTAL TIME (minutes)}} \times \begin{array}{c}\text{DROP FACTOR} \\ \text{(drops/mL)}\end{array} = \boxed{\begin{array}{c}\text{INFUSION}\\ \text{RATE}\\ \text{(drops/min)}\end{array}}$$

Example: Volume ordered is 1000 mL of D_5W over 6 hours; tubing drop factor is 15 drops/mL

$$\frac{1000 \text{ mL}}{6 (60) \text{ min}} \times 15 \text{ drops/mL} = \frac{15,000 \text{ drops}}{360 \text{ min}} = \begin{array}{c}41.7 \text{ or}\\ 42 \text{ drops/min}\end{array}$$

Or use hourly infusion rate (see above):

$$\frac{167 \text{ mL} \times 15 \text{ drops}}{60 \text{ min/mL}} = \begin{array}{c}41.7 \text{ or}\\ 42 \text{ drops/min}\end{array}$$

Total fluid volume equals the amount of fluid, expressed in mL, to infuse over the ordered period of time (if order is 1 liter of D_5W over 12 hours, the total volume is 1 liter [1000 mL]).

Total time is the number of minutes (hours $\times$ 60) over which the fluid should infuse. IF FLUID IS ORDERED PER HOUR OR YOU CALCULATE VOLUME PER HOUR, THE TOTAL TIME WILL EQUAL 60 MINUTES. Total volume will equal hourly infusion rate.

The drop factor is the number of drops from the chosen tubing that will equal 1 mL. This amount is found on the tubing package and is expressed in drops per mL.

4. *If available, use precalculated infusion chart by:*
   - Looking across chart for drop factor of tubing
   - Coming down chart to line indicating amount of

Indicates drops per minute at point of intersection

TABLE 5.7 Flow Rates for Intravenous Infusions

Drop Factor of Tubing (drops/mL)	1000 mL/6 hr (drops/min)	1000 mL/8 hr (drops/min)	1000 mL/10 hr (drops/min)	1000 mL/12 hr (drops/min)	1000 mL/24 hr (drops/min)
10	28	21	17	14	7
15	42	31	25	21	10
20	56	42	34	28	14
60	167	125	100	84	42

Action	Rationale

fluid infusing per hour
(see Table 5.7)
5. Regulate fluid or set drop
rate on fluid regulator (see
Procedure 5.5).

Procedure 5.8 Intravenous Fluid Regulation

1. Calculate or determine appropriate volume per hour
and drip rate (drops per
minute; see Procedure 5.7).
2. Prepare time tape for fluid   *Facilitates close monitoring of*
based on volume of fluid   *fluid infusion*
to infuse over 1 hour (Fig.   *Prevents puncture of container*
5.8.1). Use felt pen to mark.
- Tear an 11-inch strip of
1-inch tape.
- Place tape on IV fluid
container beside fluid-
level indicators.
- Mark tape at intervals in-   *Simplifies marking of fluid*
dicating fluid level after   *amounts (ie, instead of 75*
each hour of infusion (for   *mL/hr mark 150 mL at 2-hour*
small hourly volumes,   *intervals)*
mark the volume for a 2-

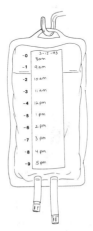

FIGURE 5.8.1

Action	Rationale

or 3-hour interval instead).

3. Attach appropriate tubing (for electronic infusion device, with chamber, or infusion flow regulator) and clear tubing of air. Proceed to appropriate section for step 4.

Manual Rate Regulation

4. Open all clamps except roller/screw clamp. — *Limits fluid rate control to regulator*

5. Open clamp fully; then slowly close clamp while observing drip chamber—fluid should initially run in a stream (Table 5.8 lists troubleshooting tips). — *Determines catheter patency*

6. Close roller/screw clamp until fluid is dropping at slow but steady pace.

7. Count the number of drops falling within 15 seconds and multiply by 4 (see Procedure 5.7). — *Determines drops falling per minute*

8. Open clamp to increase drop flow if drops-per-minute rate is less than calculated drip rate; close clamp if drops-per-minute rate is more than needed.

9. Count drops again and continue to adjust flow until desired drip rate is obtained. — *Produces correct drip rate*

10. Recheck drip rate after 5 minutes and again after 15 minutes. Proceed to Finishing Steps 11 to 15. — *Detects changes in rate due to expansion/contraction of tubing*

Manual Flow Control Device Regulation

See steps 1 to 3 for initial preparation.

Action	Rationale

TABLE 5.8	**Troubleshooting Tips for Intravenous Infusion Management**

Problem	Actions
1. Drip chamber is overfilled.	Close regulator clamp, turn fluid container upside down, and squeeze fluid from drip chamber until half full or slightly below.
2. Air is in tubing.	Check adequacy of fluid level in drip chamber and security of tubing connections. Insert needle and syringe into rubber port distal to air and aspirate to remove air.
3. Blood is backing up into tubing.	Be sure fluid is above the level of the IV catheter site and the level of the heart. Check security of tubing connections. Check that infusing fluid has not run out and that catheter is in a vein, not an artery (note pulsation of blood in tubing).
4. Infusion pump alarms indicate flow problem.	Check drip chamber for excess or inadequate fluid level. Check that clamps and regulators are open, air vent is open (if applicable), and tubing is free of kinks. Check IV catheter site for infiltration, blood clot, kinks, and positional obstruction (open fluid regulator fully and change position of arm to see if fluid flows better in various positions). Insert needle and syringe into medication port and gently flush fluid through catheter. If resistance is met, try to aspirate blood/clot into tubing; if unsuccessful, discontinue IV and restart.
5. IV is positional (ie, runs well only when arm or hand is in a certain position).	Stabilize IV site with armboard or handboard and have caregiver or client monitor infusion and IV site closely.
6. Fluid is dripping but is also leaking into tissue surrounding puncture site.	Discontinue IV and restart in another site. Place warm soak over infiltrated site, and elevate extremity. Reassess frequently.

Action	Rationale

4. At end of IV tubing attach manual flow control device (Ex: Dial-A-Flo tubing) (Fig. 5.8.2).
5. Open all clamps and regulator on IV tubing.
6. Adjust flow control device to open position and clear tubing of air (remove cap if needed).

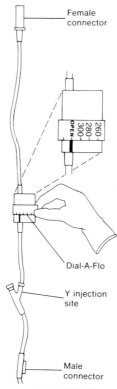

Female connector

Dial-A-Flo

Y injection site

Male connector

FIGURE 5.8.2

Action	Rationale
7. Close fluid regulator roller/screw.	*Prevents fluid flow during connection to IV catheter*
8. Attach flow control device to catheter hub (following initial insertion or during tubing change) and open fluid regulator.	
9. Turn flow control device regulator until arrow is aligned with desired volume of fluid to infuse over 1 hour.	*Regulates fluid to infuse at desired rate*
10. Check drip rate over 15 seconds and multiply by 4 (should coincide with calculated drip rate).	*Verifies fluid infusion rate*
- Adjust height of pole if necessary.	*Gravity facilitates flow*
- Recheck drip rate after 5 minutes and again after 15 minutes.	*Detects changes in rate due to expansion/contraction of tubing*
- Proceed to finishing steps 11 to 15.	

Electronic Infusion Regulation

See steps 1 to 3 for initial preparation. (See manufacturer's instructions for equipment unlike the example provided.)

Action	Rationale
4. Insert tubing into infusion pump/regulator according to pump manual.	*Ensures proper functioning of infusion regulator*
5. Close door to pump/controller and open all tubing clamps and regulator roller/screw.	*Allows pump/controller to regulate fluids*
6. Set volume dials for appropriate volume per hour *or* drops per minute (check type of pump *carefully*).	*Determines amount of fluid pump/controller will deliver*
7. Place electronic eye clamp over drip chamber (optional in some in-	*Allows pump/controller to monitor fluid flow*

Action	Rationale

fusion regulators; consult
manual; Fig. 5.8.3).

8. Push ON or START
button.

9. Check drip rate (if
present) over 15 seconds
and multiply by 4 (should
coincide with calculated
drip rate).

10. Set volume infusion
alarm. If tubing does not

Initiates fluid flow and regulation

Verifies fluid infusion rate

*Notifies nurse/client when set
volume has been infused*

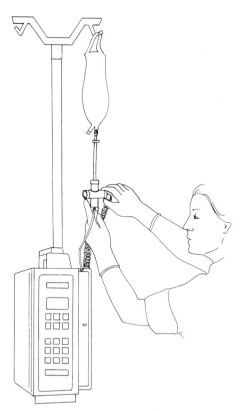

FIGURE 5.8.3

Action	Rationale
contain a regulator cassette, periodically change the sections of tubing placed inside infusion clamp. Proceed to finishing steps 11 to 15.	*Prevents tubing collapse due to constant squeezing by pump*

Volume Control Chamber (Buretrol) Regulation

See steps 1 and 2 for initial preparation.

Action	Rationale
3. Close off roller clamp 1 (above chamber) and roller clamp 2 (below chamber).	*Controls fluids more precisely*
4. Open roller clamp 1. Fill chamber with 10 mL fluid, prime drip chamber, and clear tubing of air (Fig. 5.8.4A).	*Facilitates clearing of air from tubing*
5. Fill chamber with volume of fluid to infuse in one hour (or 2 or 3 hours' worth, if volume is small).	*Allows for close monitoring of fluid volume (needed for volume-sensitive or pediatric clients)*
6. Close roller clamp 1. Make sure air vent is open (Fig. 5.8.4B).	*Stops flow from bottle. Allows fluid to flow from buretrol*
7. Open roller clamp 2 and regulate drops to calculated rate (drip rate should equal volume per hour if minidrip tubing system is used [check drop factor]), *or:* - Attach flow control device to tubing and leave roller clamp 2 open, *or* - Use an electronic infusion pump or controller and leave clamp 2 open.	*Sets volume to infuse over an hour* *Allows infusion pump/ controller to regulate fluid*
8. Check drip rate over 15 seconds and multiply by 4 (should coincide with calculated drip rate).	*Verifies fluid infusion rate*
9. Put a time tape on the chamber (if pump/ controller is not used).	*Allows for quick, easy check of fluid infusion progress and the need to add fluid to chamber.*

Action	Rationale

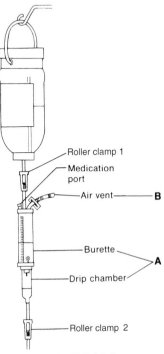

Roller clamp 1
Medication port
Air vent — **B**
Burette —
— **A**
Drip chamber
Roller clamp 2

FIGURE 5.8.4

10. Check chamber each hour or two, and add 1 to 2 hours' more fluid volume as needed. IF CLOSE FLUID MONITORING IS NOT NEEDED, CLAMP AIR VENT AND OPEN CLAMP 1.
Proceed to finishing steps 11 to 15.

Maintains fluid infusion and catheter patency
Prevents air entrance into tubing
Allows fluid to flow directly from bottle/bag into chamber and to client

Finishing Steps
11. Mark beginning hour of

Sets times for subsequent checks

Action	Rationale
fluid infusion on time tape.	
12. Teach client to check volume every 1 to 2 hours and compare with time tape.	*Determines actual volume infusion*
13. If volume depleted does not coincide with time mark:	
- Check time tape for accuracy.	
- Check settings on infusion device or flow control device and readjust if indicated.	
- Elevate fluid container on pole.	*Facilitates flow by gravity*
- Check catheter site and position for obstruction (see Table 5.8).	
14. Review limitations in ambulating with equipment and range of motion with client. Instruct client to notify nurse of problems or discomfort.	*Facilitates early detection of problems with catheter or fluid flow*

Evaluation

Were desired outcomes achieved?

DOCUMENTATION

The following should be noted on the visit note:

- Time of initiation of fluid infusion
- Type and volume of fluid infusing
- Infusion device used, if applicable
- Status of catheter insertion site
- Problems with infusion procedure and solutions applied (eg, armboard used, catheter repositioned)
- Client tolerance to fluid infusion
- Client teaching and response

Sample Documentation

DATE	TIME	
2/9/98	1400	Client receiving D_5W; 1000-mL bag infusing at 125 mL/hour per ambulatory pump. Tolerating fluid infusion well. Catheter site clean and dry without signs of infiltration or infection. Return demonstration noted arm positions to be avoided during IV fluid infusion.

Nursing Procedures **5.9, 5.10**

Intravenous Tubing Change/Conversion to IV Lock (5.9)

Intravenous Dressing Change (5.10)

EQUIPMENT

- Alcohol pads, povidone pad, 1%–2% tincture of iodine, or chlorhexidine
- Infusion tubing (vented for IV fluid bag, unvented for IV bottles)
- IV infusion plug
- Towel
- Tape 1 inch wide (may cut 2-inch tape)
- Saline or heparin flush solution
- Dressing: 2 × 2-inch gauze, adhesive bandage or transparent IV dressing
- IV pole (bed or rolling) *or* IV pump/controller
- Ointment (optional)
- Scissors to clip hair (optional)
- Armboard (optional)
- Adhesive labels
- Nonsterile gloves

Purpose

Decreases opportunity for growth of microorganisms by removing possible medium for infection

Desired Outcomes (sample)

No evidence of infection exists around insertion site, and skin integrity is intact. Client verbalizes understanding of movement limitations related to intravenous infusions and of complications to be reported to the nurse.

Assessment

Assessment should focus on the following:

Doctor's orders for type and rate of fluid
Status of skin on hand and arms, presence of hair or abrasions
Ability to hold arm and hand without movement or resistance
    for duration of procedure
Allergy to tape, iodine, antibiotic pads, or ointment

Outcome Identification and Planning

Key Goals and Sample Goal Criteria
The client will:

Maintain skin integrity and absence of infection around inser-
    tion site, as evidenced by lack of pain, redness, or swelling at
    site
Verbalize understanding of movement limitations related to in-
    travenous infusions and complications to be reported to the
    nurse

Special Considerations
If possible, replace IV fluid and tubing and change dressing at
    the same time. This reduces risk of introducing microorgan-
    isms. *Many agencies have specified procedures and times for dress-
    ing and tubing change. If unsure, consult policy manual.*

Geriatric
If the client is resistant, confused, or frightened, obtain an assis-
    tant to immobilize arm to ensure that IV line is not acciden-
    tally dislodged during dressing change.
Be constantly alert for subtle signs and symptoms of infection
    associated with long-term IV therapy.

IMPLEMENTATION

Action	Rationale
Procedure 5.9 Intravenous Tubing Change/Conversion to IV Lock	
1. Wash hands and organize equipment.	*Reduces microorganism transfer* *Promotes efficiency*
2. Open package and check tubing for cracks or flaws. Be sure caps are on all	*Ensures that no defective ma-terials are used and that tub-ing remains sterile*

Action	Rationale
ports and that the regulator clamp is closed (rolled down, clamped off, or screwed closed).	*Allows better fluid control minimizing air in tubing*
3. Check infusing fluid against doctor's orders.	*Validates correct fluid infusion*
4. Tape old tubing to IV pole or pump pole with strip of tape and fill drip chamber full (Fig. 5.9.1).	*Allows fluid in tubing to infuse into vein while new tubing is being prepared*
5. Remove infusing fluid bag/bottle from IV pole or pump (put pump on hold) and disconnect from old tubing.	*Provides fluid for new tubing*
6. Attach new tubing to bag/bottle and prime tubing (remove air): - Hang bottle or bag on IV	*Forces air to bottle/bag top and*

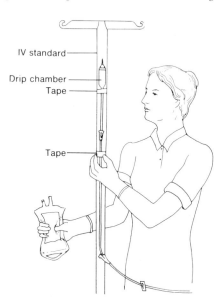

IV standard

Drip chamber

Tape

Tape

FIGURE 5.9.1

Action	Rationale

pole or infusion pump hook).

- Squeeze and release drip chamber until fluid level reaches ring mark on chamber.

- Remove cap from end of tubing.

- Open roller clamp and flush tubing until air is removed.

- Hold rubber medication plugs and in-line filter (if present) upside down and tap while fluid is running; close clamp.

7. Loosely cover end of tubing with cap and lay on bed near IV dressing.
Place towel under extremity.

8. Don gloves.
9. Close off flow from old tubing.

10. a. Exchange old tubing for new at IV catheter hub:

- Place alcohol swab under the catheter hub–tubing junction.

- Loosen connection at junction of IV catheter and old tubing.

- Holding catheter firm with one hand, apply digital pressure above IV insertion site with one finger, remove old tubing; *and*

- Quickly insert new tubing into catheter hub (Fig. 5.9.2*A*), maintaining sterility of catheter and tip of new tubing.

places fluid at entrance to tubing

Fills drip chamber and prevents introduction of air into tubing

Allows total removal of air from tubing

Forces air bubbles from plugs and filters

Maintains sterility

Prevents soiling of linen

Prevents exposure to blood
Prevents wetting dressing and bed

Removes medium for micro-organism growth

Decreases blood soiling of dressing or bed

Prevents dislodgment of catheter and bleeding from the hub when changing tubing

Action	Rationale

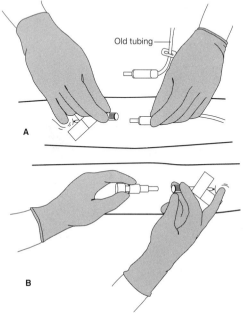

FIGURE 5.9.2

Action	Rationale
- Secure the junction with tape or Leur-Lok connections.	*Minimizes risk of tubing disconnection*
b. Begin flow from new tubing.	*Prevents clot formation in catheter*
c. Regulate fluid flow or place tubing into pump.	*Promotes accurate infusion rate*
d. Tape tubing to dressing and arm unless dressing is to be changed.	*Decreases accidental pull on catheter*
e. Tag tubing with date, time hung, and own initials.	*Indicates when tubing replacement is due (every 48 hours or per agency policy)*

Action	Rationale

11. **Conversion to IV lock**
    a. Perform steps 1 to 9. Remove old tubing and apply infusion plug/heparin lock (Fig. 5.9.2*B*).
    b. Flush catheter with saline or heparin flush.
    c. Tape infusion plug and catheter securely in place or perform dressing change if indicated.
    d. Tag site with date, time, and initials.
12. Discard old tubing and other trash. — *Promotes clean environment*
13. If performing dressing change, see Procedure 5.10, Intravenous Dressing Change. If not, place tape across junction of tubing and catheter. — *Prevents dislodging of tubing from catheter*
14. Discard gloves and wash hands. — *Reduces microorganism transfer*

Procedure 5.10 Intravenous Dressing Change

1. Wash hands and organize equipment. — *Reduces microorganism transfer* / *Promotes efficiency*
2. Explain procedure to client. — *Decreases anxiety*
3. Tear tape strips 3 inches in length, 1 inch wide. Cut one strip down the center. Hang tape pieces from edge of table. — *Secures catheter without covering insertion site* / *Places tape in available position without disrupting adhesive*
4. Open antimicrobial solution (alcohol/povidone, etc), dressing and adhesive bandage, and ointment. — *Provides fast access to supplies*
5. Assist client into sitting or supine position. — *Provides easy access to IV site* / *Promotes comfort during procedure*
6. Place towel under extremity. — *Prevents soiling of linens*

Action	Rationale
7. Don gloves	*Protects from potential contamination*
8. Remove dressing and all tape except tape holding catheter.	*Prevents dislodging of catheter while cleaning site*
9. Using alcohol first and then Betadine swabs, clean catheter-insertion site beginning at catheter and cleaning outward in a 2-inch diameter circle.	*Removes blood and drainage from site and surrounding area*
10. Allow to dry completely.	*Achieves maximum antimicrobial effectiveness*
11. Holding catheter secure with one hand, remove remaining tape and clean under catheter.	*Prevents catheter dislodgment*
12. Allow area to dry and secure catheter in position:	
- **Over-the-needle catheter:** With tape edges sticking to thumb and fingertip, slide small strip of tape under catheter hub with adhesive side up (Fig. 5.10*A*). Fold ends straight down toward insertion site. DO NOT place tape over insertion site; put other small strip of tape across catheter hub (Fig. 5.10*B*).	*Provides greater control of tape* *Insertion site should be covered with sterile material only* *Adds stability to catheter and decreases tension on IV insertion site*
- **Butterfly:** Put smallest pieces of tape across wings of butterfly and another tape piece across middle to form an H.	*Eliminates positional flow of IV fluids* *Allows for catheter stabilization without tape covering insertion site*
13. Place ointment over insertion site, if desired, and cover site with adhesive bandage, 2 × 2-inch dressing, or transparent IV dressing (if	

Action	Rationale

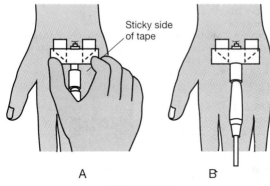

Sticky side of tape

A   B

FIGURE 5.10

client is allergic to iodine, use Neosporin ointment).
14. Remove gloves and secure tubing:
- **Over-the-needle catheter:** Place tape across top of tubing just below catheter, loop tubing and tape to dressing, and secure tubing to arm with short piece of tape (taping the tubing/catheter hub junction is optional). | *Prevents disconnection of tubing*
- **Butterfly:** Coil catheter tubing around on top of IV site; tape across coil and catheter hub. | *Prevents weight of tubing or movement from dislodging catheter*
- **IV lock:** Flush with with heparin or saline flush solution and tape across infusion plug. | *Prevents clot formation and secures catheter*
15. Apply armboard if needed. | *Stabilizes sites of frequent movement*
16. On a piece of tape or label, record needle size, | *Provides information needed for follow-up care*

Action	Rationale
type, date and time of site care and your initials; place label over top of dressing.	
17. Explain limitations of movement to client with return demonstrations, as well as need to report pain or swelling at site.	*Decreases client anxiety regarding proper maintenance of IV needle* *Promotes early detection of infiltration or other complications*
18. Discard or restore supplies; wash hands.	*Decreases the spread of organisms*

Evaluation

Were desired outcomes achieved?

DOCUMENTATION

The following should be noted on the visit note:

- Location and status of IV site, dressing, fluids, and tubing
- Size and type of catheter/needle
- Reports of pain at site
- IV site care rendered and client tolerance to care
- Client teaching
- Client subjective comments

Sample Documentation

DATE	TIME	
4/9/98	1200	Tubing changed to IV of D_5W infusing at 125 mL/hr in right lower arm. Site care done, #20 Jelco present, site clean without swelling or pain. Client tolerated procedure well. Reinforced teaching regarding mobility limitations; client verbalized understanding.

Nursing **P**rocedure **5.11**

🖐 Centrally Inserted IV Catheter Maintenance

⊠ EQUIPMENT

- Sterile gloves
- Sterile gauze pads (4 × 4 inches) or transparent dressing
- 2 Face masks
- 2-inch tape
- Alcohol pads
- Betadine swabs (optional)
- IV fluids and tubing or heparin flush or saline flush
- Prep razor
- Suture with needle holder
- CVP insertion kit containing:
  - sterile gloves (multiple sizes)
  - Betadine swabs or solution and gauze
  - sterile towels/drapes
  - 10-mL syringe (slip-tip)
  - ⅜, 1-, and 1½-inch needles
- Lidocaine/Xylocaine (without epinephrine) 1% or 2%
- Central line with introducer (eg, single-lumen or multilumen catheter, Hickman catheter, angiocath)

Purpose

Permits administration of medications and nutritional support that should not be given via a peripheral route or when peripheral routes cannot be obtained

Desired Outcomes (sample)

Client remains free of embolism, pleural effusion, and infection, both systemic and at catheter site.
Central line remains patent.

Assessment

Assessment should focus on the following:

Type of catheter

Location of catheter
Type of infusion(s)
Agency policy regarding central line care

Outcome Identification and Planning

Key Goals and Sample Goal Criteria
The client will:

Maintain skin turgor during parenteral nutrition (PN) administration
Gain ½ to 1 kg per week

Special Considerations
If central line was inserted for infusion of PN, infuse only $D_{10}W$ or D_5W until PN is available.
If multilumen catheter is used, select and mark a catheter port for PN only.
Policy varies greatly regarding use of saline or Heparin solution for flushing catheter; consult agency policy manual.
A central line is likely to be in place for a long time. Therefore, be constantly alert for early signs and symptoms of infection.

HINTS

Heparin/saline flush solutions may range from 10 µ/mL to 100 µ/mL concentrations; some agencies use saline flush.
   Internal volume of each device and extension volumes must be considered when preparing flush solutions.
   Check the manufacturer's guidelines for specific catheter internal volumes.

Safety
Use a 10-mL syringe for all flushing and administration of medications for these devices. This assists in keeping the PSI syringe pressures below most manufacturers's recommendations.
Use the lowest possible concentration of heparin locking solution. This helps to prevent untoward bleeding complications that have been associated with frequent flushing of these lines.
It is best to use Luer locking tubing on all connections.

IMPLEMENTATION

Action	Rationale
1. Wash hands and organize equipment.	*Reduces microorganism transfer* *Promotes efficiency*
2. Arrange supplies on tray, using appropriate-size gloves.	
3. Reinforce explanation of procedure to client.	*Reduces client anxiety*
4. Mark each lumen of multilumen catheter with name of fluid/medication infusing.	*Prevents mixing of medications*
5. Lumens without continuing infusion of fluids are capped with infusion plug and flushed every day (or as ordered) with heparin solution (usually 1:100 dilution) or saline.	*Prevents obstruction of catheter lumen with blood clot*
The amount depends on length of tubing and size of catheter (see Table 5.11).	*Minimizes leakage of plug or damage to catheter*
6. Flush tubings, between infusion of medications and drawing of blood first using saline, and then heparin.	*Prevents medication interaction or lumen obstruction with blood*
7. ALWAYS ASPIRATE BEFORE INFUSING MEDICATIONS OR FLUSHING TUBINGS.	*Assures patency of line and validates presence in vessel*
8. Monitor for clot formation in lumen: If resistance is met when flushing tubing, DO NOT FORCE; aspirate and remove clot if possible; if not, notify doctor.	*Prevents clot from reaching client and causing emboli*
9. Monitor respirations and breath sounds every visit.	*Promotes early detection of fluid entering chest cavity or of pulmonary embolism*
10. Maintain IV fluids above the level of the heart. Do not allow fluid to run out and air to enter tubing	*Prevents blood reflux into tubing* *Prevents infusion of air*

Action	Rationale
(see Table 5.6 and Procedure 5.6).	

Tubing Change

1. Review Procedure 5.9. Prepare fluid and tubing (see Procedure 5.3). — *Minimizes exposure to microorganisms*
2. Don gloves. — *Protects from potential contamination*
3. Expose catheter hub or rubber port of multilumen catheter. — *Precedes connection of tubing*
4. Ask client to take a deep breath and bear down (Valsalva's maneuver). — *Increases intrathoracic pressure* *Prevents air from entering vein*
5. Disconnect old tubing and quickly connect new tubing. Instruct client to breathe normally after tubing is connected.
6. Open fluid and adjust to appropriate infusion rate.
7. Proceed to dressing change, if needed.

Dressing Change (see Table 5.11 for various catheter types)

1. Explain procedure to client. — *Reduces anxiety*
2. Wash hands and gather equipment. — *Reduces microorganism transfer* *Promotes efficiency*
3. Open packages, keeping supplies sterile. — *Prevents contamination of catheter site*
4. Apply clean gloves and mask. Assist client in applying mask also.
5. Remove tape.
6. Don sterile gloves.
7. Beginning at catheter and wiping outward to the surrounding skin, clean insertion site with alcohol and Povidone. — *Decreases contamination* *Removes microorganisms from site*
8. Place ointment over insertion site (optional) and cover with sterile gauze

TABLE 5.11 — Central Line Equipment

Catheter Type	Definition	Examples	Flushing Frequency (intermittent)	Dressing Change Frequency (may vary per agency)
Non-tunneled	Short-term lines that are percutaneously introduced	Subclavian lines Hohn catheter	q24 hr; 3 mL hep-lock flush	1. Sterile gauze, occlusive; q3 days 2. Transparent semi-permeable membrane (TSM) set at specific intervals (q3–7 days) 3. When dressing integrity compromised
Tunneled	Long term catheters, surgically implanted through a subcutaneous tunnel	Hickman Broviac	q24 hr; 3 mL hep-lock flush	1. Airstrip—q3 days 2. Sterile gauze, occlusive; q3 days 3. TSM at specific intervals (ie q3–7 days) 4. When dressing integrity compromised
		Groshong	q7 days; vigorous 5 mL NS flush	
Implanted venous access ports	Surgically placed drug reservoir	Intravenous port Peripheral port	monthly; 3 mL hep-lock flush	When accessed, TSM at specific intervals
PICC	Peripherally inserted central catheter	Break-away needle Peelable sheath introducer	q24 hr; 3 mL hep-lock flush	1. TSM at specific intervals (ie q3–7 days) 2. When dressing integrity compromised

Action	Rationale
or transparent IV dressing.	
9. Frame gauze with tape or transparent IV dressing. Wrap tubing on top of tape, and cover tubing with tape.	*Secures dressing* *Prevents pull on catheter*
10. Remove gloves and mask.	
11. On a piece of tape or label, record date and time of site care and your initials. Place label over top of dressing.	*Determines next site care (required every 48 to 72 hours)*
12. Assist client to position of comfort.	*Promotes client comfort*

Evaluation

Were desired outcomes achieved?

DOCUMENTATION

The following should be noted on the visit note:

- Date and time of catheter insertion
- Type and location of catheter
- Care and maintenance procedures performed
- Equipment used with catheter
- Client tolerance to procedures

Sample Documentation

DATE	TIME	
1/9/98	0400	Dressing changed at right subclavian triple-lumen catheter site. No redness, edema, or drainage at site. Povidone ointment applied. IV fluid bag and tubing changed. D_5W infusing via IVAC pump at 50 mL/hr.

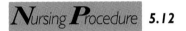

*N*ursing *P*rocedure **5.12**

Peripherally Inserted Central Catheter (PICC) Maintenance

⊠ EQUIPMENT

- PICC dressing change kit

Purpose

To provide a safe, antiseptic routine dressing change for a PICC

Desired Outcomes (sample)

Completion of IV therapy without catheter or insertion site infection.

Client and care giver will provide continual PICC maintenance without interruption of therapy.

Assessment

Assessment should focus on the following:

Insertion site
Catheter tract
Integrity of the surrounding tissue
Use of the device
Catheter integrity and patency

Outcome Identification and Planning

Key Goals and Sample Goal Criteria

The client or significant other will:

Demonstrate the catheter dressing change procedure
Verbalize an understanding of the rationale for changing a PICC dressing
Demonstrate the ability to self-assess for any potential complications associated with PICC IV access

Special Considerations

The frequency of in-home monitoring of the venous access device is determined by the client's condition, the type of therapy, and the type of access. The nurse is responsible for monitoring for local and systemic complications. Appropriate catheter care is essential in the prevention of complications associated with IV therapy. Recommended dwell time for a PICC is a topic of controversy. There is no one answer that fits every client. Factors related to the environment, the infusate, the client, and all care givers must be evaluated.

The frequency of dressing changes also varies from agency to agency. Routine changes range from every 72 hours to once per week or prn. Check for specific policy expectations.

Techniques and methods used in the maintenance of these catheters can have a significant effect on the incidence of complications. There are ongoing debates about the best methods for use in the scope of care. Check for specific agency policy.

Transparent semipermeable membrane (TSM) may be used on PICCs. Sterile, occlusive gauze and tape dressings also may be used.

HINTS

> *When a PICC is indwelling, no blood draws, tourniquet, or blood pressures are to be taken on the accessed arm.*
> *When used intermittently, heparin lock flush (100 units : 1 mL) is administered after each medication administration and daily. Use only 10-mL syringes for flushing the lumen(s).*

Economic

The PICC is an invasive device that may predispose the client to complications that can be financially expensive and physically debilitating. It is essential that the home care nurse is knowledgeable about these and other vascular access devices that are available for the home-based client.

IMPLEMENTATION

Action	Rationale
1. Explain the dressing change procedure to the client.	*Enhances nurse–client trust and assists to establish a comfortable environment for education*
2. Assist the client to a comfortable supine position	*Decreases client and care provider anxiety. Reinforces pre-*

Action	Rationale
or to a chair. If there is a care provider present, have them perform the dressing change with your guidance.	*viously taught material.*
3. Instruct the client to keep their head turned away from the insertion site or have them wear a mask.	*Decreases the chance of airborne pathogen contamination*
4. Establish a clean working area.	*Reduces transfer of micro-organisms*
5. Wash hands and assemble supplies.	
6. Apply a mask and a pair of sterile gloves.	*Decreases the potential for site contamination*
7. Secure the extension tubing to the arm with tape.	*Stabilizes the PICC during the procedure*
8. Carefully remove the old dressing. Pull the dressing away from the hub toward the insertion site, keeping the old dressings parallel to the skin.	*Helps to keep the catheter from migrating out of the insertion site*
9. Inspect the insertion site and surrounding skin.	*Assess for signs of inflammation, infection, phlebitis, irritation, or drainage*
10. Remove dirty gloves and rewash hands.	
11. Put on second pair of sterile gloves.	
12. Cleanse the insertion area three times with 70% isopropyl alcohol swabs in a concentric motion working from the insertion site outward to a diameter of 3–4 inches. With last swab clean the catheter and any sutures. Allow to air dry.	*Drying is very important for antiseptic effects on the skin and as wet alcohol negates the effect of iodophor preparations*
13. Repeat the cleansing procedure with three iodophor swabs. Allow to air dry.	*Antibacterial effects are enhanced over time as the Betadine solutions remains on the skin*
14. Cover the insertion site and catheter with the	*A semipermeable transparent or sterile gauze dressing with tape*

Action	Rationale
sterile dressing. Secure all edges.	*over the entire gauze provides an occlusive seal*
15. If used, replace the extension set(s), maintaining sterile technique.	*Reduces transfer of microorganisms and assists in keeping potential infectious complications minimal*
16. Flush catheter to maintain patency.	*When used intermittently heparin lock after each IV administration and daily*
17. Write date, time and sign the dressing label.	

Evaluation

Were desired outcomes achieved?

DOCUMENTATION

The following should be noted on the visit note:

- Date and time of the dressing change
- Condition of the insertion site
- Approximate length of catheter on the skin
- Type of dressing applied
- Any patient or care giver education with outcomes observed

Sample Documentation

DATE	TIME	
9/15/97	1430	PICC dressing procedure completed without complication. Client tolerated procedure well. Insertion site without redness or swelling. No problems verbalized. Five cm of catheter external. Semipermeable transparent, occlusive dressing applied. Client able to verbalize signs and symptoms of infection.

*N*ursing *P*rocedure 5.13

Parenteral Nutrition (PN) Management

EQUIPMENT

- IV tubing with filter (for total parenteral nutrition; PN)
- IV tubing without filter for lipids, if ordered
- Infusion pumps, if available
- Appropriate labels
- Sterile gloves

Purpose

Permits administration of nutritional support when gastrointestinal tract is traumatized or nonfunctional

Desired Outcomes (sample)

Skin turgor is good; no edema is present.
Albumin and potassium levels are within normal range; glucose level is within acceptable range.
Delivery of adequate calories and protein to meet the client's daily nutritional requirements.

Assessment

Assessment should focus on the following:

Doctor's orders for PN type (central or peripheral), contents, and rate
Doctor's orders for lipid infusion frequency and rate
Current nutritional status (weight, height, skin turgor, edema)
Laboratory values, particularly albumin level, glucose, and potassium

Outcome Identification and Planning

Key Goals and Sample Goal Criteria

The client will:

Maintain skin turgor during PN administration
Gain ½ to 1 kg per week

Special Considerations

Cyclic PN, infusing 12 hours while asleep, is the most common form of home PN.

High glucose levels in PN provide a good medium for bacterial growth; thus, strict asepsis is needed to prevent septicemia.

3 in 1 PN solutions eliminate the need for separate lipid infusion.

Geriatric

The elderly tend to be very sensitive to volume changes; thus, volume should be infused cautiously.

They are also susceptible to infection; therefore, instruct client and caregiver to check client's temperature frequently.

IMPLEMENTATION

Action	Rationale

Central Parenteral Nutrition

Action	Rationale
1. Wash hands and organize equipment.	*Reduces microorganism transfer* *Promotes efficiency*
2. Assess central line (see Procedure 5.11) and monitor client appropriately.	*Provides venous access for PN*
3. Don gloves.	*Reduces contamination*
4. Mark port intended for PN and close it with infusion plug; or prepare infusion of $D_{10}W$ or D_5W to be used until PN solution is available.	*Preserves sterility of port for PN* *Maintains tubing for PN* *Minimizes contamination of tubing*
5. DO NOT INFUSE MEDICATIONS OR OTHER SOLUTIONS THROUGH PORT.	
6. Compare PN label with doctor's orders.	*Verifies correct dosage of nutrients*
7. Prepare PN: - If refrigerated, allow bag/bottle to stand at room temperature 15 to 30 minutes or have client	*Prevents infusion of cold fluid with resulting discomfort and chilling*

Action	Rationale
remove from refrigerator 30 minutes before visit.	
- Put time tape on bag/bottle.	
- Close drip regulator on filtered tubing.	
- Remove cap from filtered IV tubing to expose spike.	
- Remove tab/cover from PN bag/bottle.	
- Insert tubing spike.	
- Prime drip chamber.	
- Open drip regulator.	
- Clear air from tubing.	
- Close drip regulator.	
- Place tubing at bedside.	
8. Prepare lipids (if lipids and PN are to infuse simultaneously):	
- Put time tape on bottle (every 2 hours if small hourly infusion).	*Facilitates correct infusion rate*
- Insert vented, nonfiltered tubing spike into lipid container.	
- Prime drip chamber and clear air from tubing.	*Prevents infusion of air into chest*
- Place needle (21 gauge) on end of tubing and plug into medication plug at distal end of PN tubing (Fig. 5.13).	
9. Attach PN tubing to central line port (see Fig. 5.13).	
10. Discard gloves and disposable materials; position client for comfort.	*Promotes clean environment Facilitates comfort*
11. Set pumps to deliver appropriate volumes per hour.	
12. Calculate and check drip rate. Instruct client to	*Verifies correct infusion rate*

Action	Rationale

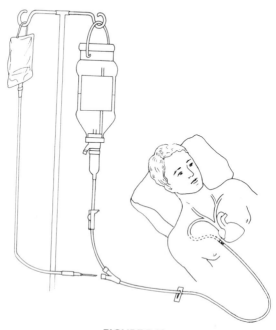

FIGURE 5.13

monitor infusion the first 1 to 2 hours. (If infusion is behind schedule, DO NOT SPEED UP IN-FUSION RATE. Correct infusion rate and resume proper administration.)	*Prevents volume overload or glucose bolus*
13. Perform client teaching regarding:	
- Need to keep solution higher than chest, avoid manipulating catheter	*Facilitates proper flow of solution*
- Need to report any pain,	*Indicates possible catheter*

Action	Rationale
respiratory distress, warmth, or flushing	*dislodgment or infection*
14. Emphasize need for client to monitor:	
- Temperature check every 8 hours (depending on orders)	*Facilitates early detection of infection or complications*
- For the diabetic client, check blood glucose level every 12 to 24 hours or as ordered	*Detects glucose intolerance*
- Central line site every 12 hours; provide care every 48 to 72 hours (see Procedure 5.11)	
- For dyspnea (ie, rales in lung bases)	*Indicates possible fluid overload*
15. Instruct client to weigh daily.	*Indicates benefits of nutritional intake*
16. Place PN and lipids on rolling infusion pumps and encourage client ambulation, if allowed.	*Facilitates pulmonary toilet Facilitates muscle development Promotes sense of well-being*

Evaluation

Were desired outcomes achieved?

DOCUMENTATION

The following should be noted on the visit note:

- Time of PN bottle/bag is hung, number of bottles/bags, and rate of infusion
- Time lipid bottle is hung and rate of infusion
- Site of IV catheter and verification of patency
- Status of dressing and site, if visible
- Laboratory results of electrolytes
- Client tolerance to PN

Sample Documentation

DATE	TIME	
3/9/98	2400	2-L bag of 3 in 1 PN infusing into the proximal port of the Hickman catheter. Infusion pump programmed to run 80 mL/hour for 2 hours then increase rate to 225 mL per hour for 7.5 hours, then to decrease rate to 80 mL per hour for the final 2 hours of the cyclic infusion. Catheter insertion site intact with good blood return. Fingerstick blood sugar 110.

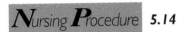

*N*ursing *P*rocedure 5.14

🖐 *Blood Transfusion Management*

☒ EQUIPMENT

- Blood transfusion tubing (Blood Y set with in-line filter)
- 250- to 500-mL bag/bottle normal saline
- Packed cells or whole blood, as ordered
- Blood warmer or coiled tubing and pan of warm water (optional)
- Order slips for blood
- Flow sheet for documentation
- Nonsterile gloves
- Materials for IV start (see Procedures 5.3 and 5.4)

Purpose

Increases client's hemoglobin and hematocrit for improved circulation and oxygen distribution

Desired Outcomes (sample)

Blood pressure, pulse, respirations, and temperature are within normal range for client.

Client's activity tolerance has increased to ambulation in home without dyspnea.

Transfusion therapy is completed with no untoward physical reactions.

Assessment

Assessment should focus on the following:

Indications infusion can be completed safely: Client is noncombative with no signs of heart or renal failure

Baseline vital signs; circulatory and respiratory status

Skin status (eg, rash)

Doctor's orders for type, amount, and rate of blood administration

Size of IV catheter or need for catheter insertion

Documentation that client has had at least one prior transfusion of the ordered product without experiencing adverse reactions

Religious or other personal objections to client's receipt of blood

Compatibility of client to blood (matching blood sheet numbers to name band; see page 222).

Access to a working phone and available physician

The presence of a signed consent form

Outcome Identification and Planning

Key Goals and Sample Goal Criteria

The client will:

Demonstrate adequate circulation evidenced by capillary refill time of 2 to 3 seconds, pink mucous membranes, and warm, dry skin

Understand the medical necessity for transfusion

Tolerate the transfusion without complication

Verbalize the signs and symptoms of transfusion reactions both during and post infusion

Special Considerations

Clients with a history of previous transfusions must be watched carefully for a transfusion reaction.

The maximum transfusion time for packed cells or whole blood is 4 hours.

The RN must stay with the client throughout the entire infusion and for a minimum of 30 minutes after completion.

Have the client sign an informed consent stating that they were provided the information regarding treatment, goals, and potential complications of transfusion therapy.

Geriatric

Fluid sensitive clients may not tolerate a rapid change in blood volume; they must receive the product as slowly as possible.

 Transcultural

Some clients have religious or personal objections to receipt of blood and blood products.

Economic

Inform the client of insurance coverage for home care transfusion services before all preparations are done.

HINTS

In the event of an emergency, have an anaphylaxis kit available.

Schedule a pretransfusion home visit to educate the client, gather the necessary information, and schedule a time for the infusion visit.

IMPLEMENTATION

Action	Rationale

Obtaining the Blood or Blood Components (Units)

1. Obtain the unit(s) from the blood bank immediately before transfusion.

   Promotes infusion of blood within limited time prior to loss of product integrity

2. Inspect the unit for general appearance, clots, and coloration. Do not accept it if it appears abnormal.

   Prevents infusion of ruined blood product

3. Check each unit against the transfusion requisition. The client's name and ID number, ABO, Rh type, product unit number, and expiration date must be the same on both slips.

   Prevents infusion of incompatible blood

   - The units must be checked by the blood bank representative and RN.
   - The double check forms are to be signed by the persons checking each unit.
   - If there are discrepancies in any area, do not use the product unit until compatibility is confirmed.

4. Secure unit in cool container.

   Prevents spoilage of blood product

   Fasten with seat belt or in trunk. The blood bank will

Action	Rationale
provide coolers and ice packs for transportation of the blood/components. Internal temperature of blood should remain below 10°C.	
5. Remove blood from cooler 20 minutes before administration.	*Allows blood to warm to room temperature, prevents chilling of client*

Blood Administration

Action	Rationale
1. Before administration, ask the client to state name. Have the caregiver double check each unit with the RN again.	*Verifies correct client identification*
2. Cleanse hands with approved antiseptic for 2 minutes and clean the working area.	*Reduces transfer of microorganisms*
3. Assemble equipment (including the anaphylaxis kit).	*Promotes organization and efficiency*
4. Explain procedure to client, particularly the need for frequent vital sign checks.	*Decreases client anxiety*
5. **Prepare tubing:**	
- Open tubing package and close drip regulator (which may be a clamp, roller, or screw). Note red and white caps over tubing spikes.	*Prepares for infusion of saline before and after transfusion*
- Remove white cap to reveal spike on one side of blood tubing (Fig. 5.14A).	
- Remove tab from normal saline bag/bottle and insert tubing spike.	
- Remove cap from end of tubing, open saline roller clamp 1, prime drip chamber with saline, and flush tubing to end.	*Prevents air entering tubing* *Clears air from tubing*
- Close fluid roller clamp.	
- Replace cap on tubing	*Retains sterility*

Action	Rationale

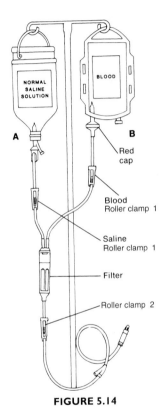

A

NORMAL
SALINE
SOLUTION

B

Red
cap

Blood
Roller clamp 1

Saline
Roller clamp 1

Filter

Roller clamp 2

FIGURE 5.14

end and place on bed
near IV catheter. (If infusing blood rapidly, con-
nect to warming-coil
tubing and flush tubing
to end. Place coil in
warm water bath.)
6. Don gloves and insert IV
catheter, if needed (see

*Prepares medium for warming
blood before infusing*
*Prevents infusion of cold blood
and lowering of body temperature*
*Permits access for connection
of blood tubing*

Action	Rationale
Procedure 5.4); or if IV catheter is present and is of adequate size (catheter should be 20 gauge or larger). Remove dressing enough to expose catheter hub.	*Decreases hemolysis* *Allows free flow of blood*
7. Connect blood tubing to catheter hub (discard infusion plug or place needle cap over previous infusion-tubing tip).	*Connects blood directly to catheter* *Preserves previous infusion for future use*
8. Open fluid regulator regulate to a rate that will keep vein open (15 to 30 mL/hour).	*Verifies and maintains patency of catheter*
9. Check and record pulse, respirations, blood pressure, and temperature.	*Provides baseline vital signs prior to blood transfusion*
10. Remove red cap to reveal spike on other side of blood tubing and, using a twisting motion, push spike into port on blood bag (Fig. 5.14B).	
11. Close roller clamp 1 on normal saline side of tubing and open roller clamp 1 on blood side of tubing.	*Prevents saline infusing into blood bag* *Allows blood tubing to fill with blood*
12. Regulate drip rate to deliver:	*Most reactions occur within the first 15 minutes*
a. A maximum of 30 mL of blood within the first 15 minutes.	*Delivers blood volume in 2 to 4 hours*
b. ½ to ¼ of the volume of blood each hour (62 to 125 mL per hour)—depending on client tolerance to volume change and volume of blood to be infused; if client has poor tolerance to volume change, some blood banks will divide units in half so that 8 hours may be used to	*Allows slower infusion of total unit without violating 4-hour transfusion time limit*

Action	Rationale
infuse one unit of packed cells.	
13. Check vital signs and temperature again 15 minutes after beginning the transfusion, then half an hour or hourly until transfusion is completed (refer to agency policy); check at the completion of delivery of each unit of blood.	*Detects transfusion reaction (Most reactions occur within the first 15 minutes.)*
14. When blood transfusion is complete:	
- Clamp off roller clamp 1.	*Clears bloodline for infusion of other fluids*
- Turn on normal saline.	
- Remove empty blood bag/bottle. Recap spike.	*Maintains sterility for future transfusions*
- Fill in time of completion on blood bank slip and place copy of slip with empty bag.	*Complies with agency regulations for confirmation of blood administration*
- Place all used tubing and blood bag into cooler and return to the blood bank. If a second transfusion is to be given, use new tubing.	*Complies with Standards of the American Association of Blood Banks*
- Instruct client on signs/ symptoms of delayed transfusion reactions.	*Reinforces previously learned material and decreases client anxiety*
- Remove peripheral line or flush access device per policy.	
- Remove gloves and cleanse hands.	*Reduces transfer of microorganisms*
15. During and after transfusion, monitor client closely and instruct client and caregiver to observe for signs of a transfusion reaction, which include the following:	*Prevents severe complications from undetected reaction*

Action	Rationale
- **Allergic reaction,** evidenced by rash, chills, fever, nausea, or severe hypotension (shock)	*Indicates incompatibility between transfused red cells and the host cells*
- **Pyrogenic reaction** (usually noted toward end or after transfusion), evidenced by nausea, chilling, fever, and headache	*Indicates sepsis and subsequent renal shutdown*
- **Circulatory overload,** evidenced by cough, dyspnea, distended neck veins, and rales in lung bases	*Indicates acute pulmonary edema or congestive failure*
16. *If allergic or pyrogenic reaction is noted:*	
- Turn off blood transfusion.	*Decreases further infusion of incompatible or contaminated blood*
- Remove blood tubing and replace with tubing primed with normal saline.	*Maintains catheter patency*
- Turn on normal saline at slow rate.	
- Contact doctor immediately.	
17. *If fluid overload is noted:*	
- Slow blood transfusion rate and contact doctor.	*Decreases workload of the heart and avoids further overload*
- Take vital signs frequently (every 10 to 15 minutes until stable), and perform emergency treatment as needed or ordered.	*Detects and treats resulting shock or cardiac insufficiency*
- Remove and send remaining blood and blood tubing to blood bank with completed blood transfusion forms.	
- Send first voided urine specimen to laboratory.	*Confirms hemolytic reaction, if red blood cells present*
- Monitor input and out-	*Detects renal shutdown sec-*

Action	Rationale
put (particularly urinary output).	*ondary to reaction*
- Instruct client/caregiver to check vital signs every 4 hours for 24 hours (or per agency policy).	*Facilitates early detection of complications*

Evaluation

Were desired outcomes achieved?

DOCUMENTATION

The following should be noted on the visit note:

- Date and initiation and completion time for each unit of blood transfused
- Initial and subsequent vital signs
- Presence or absence of transfusion reaction and actions taken
- Home transfusion care plan
- Name of primary provider with phone and pager numbers
- Primary and secondary diagnosis
- Copies of the order form, pretransfusion assessment, transfusion flow sheet, reaction
- Signed informed consent
- Type of access device and maintenance information
- Type of product infused
- Progress notes stating client's status before, during, and after transfusion

Sample Documentation

DATE	TIME	
1/9/98	1000	Transfused 1 unit of packed red blood cells (unit #R46862, O positive) through an 18-g, 1½ inch teflon catheter without problem. Transfusion started at 10:30 AM and completed at 13:00 Signs and symptoms of posttransfusion reaction reinforced. Emergency phone numbers given to client. See transfusion flow sheet for specific information.

*N*ursing *P*rocedure 5.15

🖐 *Nasogastric/Nasointestinal Tube Insertion*

☒ EQUIPMENT

- Nasogastric (NG) tube (14 to 18 French sump tube) or nasointestinal (8 to 12 French, small-bore feeding tube)
- Lubricant
- Ice chips or glass of water
- Appropriate-sized syringe:
  - *NG:* 30- or 60-mL syringe with catheter tip
  - *Small bore:* 20- to 30-mL Luer-Lok syringe
- Nonsterile gloves
- Stethoscope
- 1-inch tape (two 3-inch strips and one 1-inch strip)
- Washcloth, gauze, cotton balls, cotton-tip swab
- Petroleum jelly
- Emesis basin
- Tissues
- Tongue blade
- Moisture-resistant drape
- Flashlight or penlight
- Safety pin and rubber band

Purpose

Permits nutritional support through gastrointestinal tract
Allows evacuation of gastric contents
Relieves nausea

Desired Outcomes (sample)

Client gains ½ to 1 kg per week.
Client has no complaints of nausea or vomiting.

Assessment

Assessment should focus on the following:

Doctor's order for type of tube and use of tube
Size of previous tube used, if any

History of nasal or sinus problems
Abdominal distension, pain, or nausea

Outcome Identification and Planning

Key Goals and Sample Goal Criteria
The client will:

Gain ½ to 1 kg per week after initiation of tube feeding
Experience no episodes of nausea and vomiting within 1 hour
of NG suction initiation

Special Considerations
Be prepared to restrain client to prevent pulling on NG tube.
The tube should be taped to side of client's face rather than nostril to prevent nasal ulceration.

IMPLEMENTATION

Action	Rationale
1. Wash hands and organize equipment.	*Reduces microorganism transfer* *Promotes efficiency*
2. Explain procedure to client.	*Reduces anxiety* *Promotes cooperation and participation*
3. Assist client into semi-Fowler's position.	*Facilitates passage of tube into esophagus instead of trachea*
4. Check and improve nasal patency:	
- Ask client to breathe through one naris while the other is occluded. (Assess nares of an unconscious client with a penlight)	*Determines patency of nasal passage*
- Repeat with other naris	*Determines patency of nasal passage*
- Have client blow nose with both nares open.	*Clears nasal passage without pushing microorganisms into inner ear*
- Clean mucus and secretions from nares with moist tissues or cotton-tip swabs	*Clears nasal passage*
5. Measure length of tubing	

Action	Rationale
needed by using tube itself as a tape measure:	
- Measure distance from tip of nose to earlobe, placing the rounded end of the tubing at earlobe (Fig. 5.15.1*A*).	*Indicates distance from nasal entrance to pharyngeal area*
- Continue measurement from earlobe to sternal notch (Fig. 5.15.1*B*).	*Indicates distance from pharyngeal area to stomach*
- Mark location of sternal notch along the tubing with small strip of tape.	*Indicates depth to which tube should be inserted*
- Place tube in ice-water bath (optional).	*Makes tube less pliable*
(If a feeding tube with weighted tip is used [small-bore feeding tube], insert guide wire and prepare the tube as instructed on package insert [usually by flushing with 10 to 20 mL of irrigation saline]).	*Facilitates insertion of tube*
6. Don gloves and dip feeding tube in water or water-soluble jelly to lubricate tip.	*Reduces contamination* *Promotes smooth insertion of tube*
7. Ask client to tilt head	*Facilitates smooth entrance of*

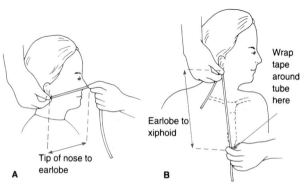

Wrap tape around tube here

Earlobe to xiphoid

Tip of nose to earlobe

A

B

FIGURE 5.15.1

Action	Rationale
backward; insert tube into clearest naris.	*tube into naris*
8. As you insert tube deeper into naris have client hold head and neck straight and open mouth.	*Decreases possibility of insertion into trachea* *Allows nurse to see when tube is in pharynx*
9. When tube is seen and client can feel tube in pharynx, instruct client to flex head forward and swallow (offer ice chips or sips of water).	*Facilitates passage of tube into esophagus*
10. Insert tube further into esophagus applying gentle pressure without force as client swallows (if client coughs or tube curls in throat, withdraw tube to pharynx and repeat attempts); between attempts, encourage client to take deep breaths.	*Prevents trauma from forcing tube and prevents tube entering trachea* *Maintains good oxygenation*
11. When tape mark on tube reaches entrance to naris, stop tube insertion and check placement: - Have client open mouth for tube visualization. - Aspirate with syringe and monitor for gastric drainage (or old tube feeding if insertion). - Connect syringe with 10 to 20 mL (10 mL for peditric clients) air to tube and push air in while listening to stomach with stethoscope (see Fig. 5.16); if gurgling is heard, secure tube. (If tube is a feeding tube, remove the stylet from small bore feeding tube and store it.)	*Indicates tube is in stomach and not curled in mouth or in tracheobronchial tree* *Preserves guide wire for reinsertion of tube, if needed*

Action	Rationale
12. To secure tube: - Split 2 inches of long tape strip, leaving 1 inch of strip intact. - Apply 1-inch base of tape on bridge of nose. - Wrap first one, then the other, side of split tape around tube (Fig. 5.15.2).	*Maintains tube placement with client activity*
13. Tape loop of tube to side of client's face (if feeding tube) or pin to client's gown (if sump tube). May use rubber band to secure tube.	*Decreases pull on client's nose and possible dislodgment*
14. Store stylet from small-bore feeding tube in a plastic bag at the bedside.	
15. Begin suction or tube feeding as ordered.	

Evaluation

Were desired outcomes achieved?

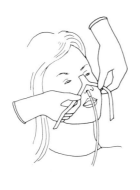 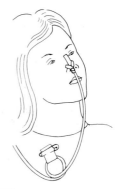

FIGURE 5.15.2

DOCUMENTATION

The following should be noted on the visit note:

- Date and time of tube insertion
- Color and amount of drainage return
- Size and type of tube
- Client tolerance to procedure
- Confirmation of tube placement by radiograph
- Suction applied or tube feeding started and rate

Sample Documentation		
DATE	**TIME**	
3/9/98	1230	Sump tube (#18) inserted via left naris with no obstruction or difficulty, tolerated with no visible clinical problems. Gurgling audible with insertion of air.

Nursing Procedures **5.16, 5.17**

Nasogastric Tube Maintenance (5.16)

Nasogastric Tube Discontinuation (5.17)

✖ EQUIPMENT

- Syringe and container with saline
- Tape or tube holder
- Washcloth, gauze, cotton balls, cotton-tip swabs
- Petroleum jelly or ointment
- Towel or linen saver
- 500- or 1000-mL bottle saline or ordered irrigant
- Stethoscope
- Mouth moistener
- Nonsterile gloves

Purpose

Minimizes damage and irrigation to naris from tube
Maintains proper tube placement
Promotes proper gastric suctioning or tube feeding
Terminates nasogastric (NG) therapy properly

Desired Outcomes (sample)

Tubing patency is maintained.
Client experiences no nausea or vomiting.

Assessment

Assessment should focus on the following:

Size and type of tube
Purpose of tube
Doctor's orders regarding type and frequency
Type and rate of tube feeding

Outcome Identification and Planning

Key Goals and Sample Goal Criterion

The client will:

Have no episodes of nausea or vomiting
NG tube will remain patent.

Special Considerations

General

Aspiration is a primary problem with nasogastric tubes. Clients at risk for aspiration are those with decreased levels of consciousness, absent or diminished cough reflex, and those who are noncommunicative and recumbent most of the time (Young and White, 1992)

When NG therapy is long term, include in plan of care replacement of tube at specified intervals to avoid complications.

Home caregivers should be taught signs of and ways to avoid aspiration.

IMPLEMENTATION

Action	Rationale

Procedure 5.16 Nasogastric Tube Maintenance

Action	Rationale
1. Question client regarding discomfort from tube and determine need for adjustments.	*Facilitates client comfort*
2. Observe tube insertion site for signs of irritation or pressure.	*Indicates need to adjust or remove tube from current site*
3. Apply gloves.	*Reduces contamination*
4. Check tube placement before irrigation or medication administration and instruct client caregiver to check placement every 4 to 8 hours of tube feeding:	
- Have client open mouth for tube visualization.	*Indicates tube is in stomach and not curled in mouth or in tracheobronchial tree*
- Aspirate and check for gastric contents (or old tube feeding if reinsertion).	
- Connect syringe with 15 to 20 mL air to NG tube	

Action	Rationale

and push air in while listening to stomach with stethoscope; if gurgling is heard, secure tube (Fig. 5.16).

5. Cleanse nares with moist gauze or cloth and apply ointment or oil to site.

Maintains skin integrity and patency of nares

6. Every 4 hours, caregiver should perform mouth care: apply moistener to oral cavity and ointment to lips.

Maintains integrity of oral mucous membranes

7. Irrigate tube (if permitted by doctor) with 20 to 30 mL of saline every 3 hours:
   - Connect saline-filled syringe to tube.

Maintains patency of tube

   - Slowly and gently push fluid into tube.

Prevents rupture of tube

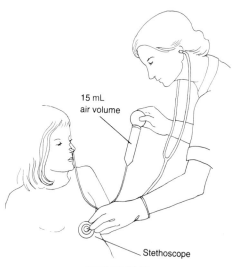

15 mL
air volume

Stethoscope

FIGURE 5.16

Action	Rationale
- Aspirate fluid gently; note appearance and discard. - Repeat irrigation and aspiration. - Reconnect tube to suction or tube feeding.	*Removes irrigant and detects possible gastric bleeding*
8. Remove and reapply tape if loose or soiled. Cleanse skin prior to reapplication of tape.	*Prevents dislodgment of tube* *Promotes cleanliness*
9. If entrance to naris is irritated, place tube in other naris, if clear.	*Prevents additional skin breakdown*
10. Reconnect to tube feeding (see Procedure 5.15) or suction.	

Gastric Suction

Teach client or caregiver to:

Action	Rationale
11. Every 2 hours, check suction for appropriate suction pressure (usually 80 to 120 mmHg = low suction) and frequency (ie, constant or intermittent).	
12. Monitor drainage in tubing and bag for color, consistency, and odor.	*Indicates presence of bleeding or infection or need for irrigation*
13. Every 8 hours, mark drainage level (if bottle or canister is used) or empty and measure amount of drainage.	*Monitors amounts of drainage*
14. To empty drainage bag (if 75% to 100% full), first turn off suction and wait until suction meter returns to 0. Measure and record drainage.	*Removes suction pressure, so canister can be emptied*

If Using Canister Suction

- Loosen seal and remove cap (disconnect tubing leading to NG tube if

Action	**Rationale**

    disposable lining is
    used).
- Empty contents into
   graduated container
   and rinse canister (or
   discard plastic liner
   and obtain fresh one).
- Reseal cap and recon-
   nect NG tubing.

If Using Vacuum Suction
- Open door to suction
   machine (Omnibus).
- Remove bag.
- Remove cap from bag
   port.
- Pour contents into grad-
   utated container.
- Replace cap and place
   bag into suction
   machine.
- Reseal door to suction
   machine.
- Reset and initiate
   appropriate suction
   pressure.

15. Every 24 hours (or per   *Reduces accumulation of micro-*
    agency policy) client/   *organisms*
    caregiver should replace
    drainage bag (if used)
    and clean canister.

16. Discard supplies and   *Reduces contamination*
    wash hands.

Procedure 5.17 Nasogastric Tube Discontinuation

1. Explain procedure to   *Decreases anxiety*
   client.
2. Place client in semi-   *Opens glottis for easy removal*
   Fowler's position.
3. Don gloves.   *Reduces contamination*
4. Remove tape securing   *Facilitates smooth removal of*
   tube to cheek or attaching   *tube*
   tube to gown and remove
   or loosen tape across
   bridge of nose.

Action	Rationale
5. Remove tube:	
- Place towel under nose and drape over tube.	*Shields appearance of tube from client during removal*
- Clamp tube by pinching off or folding over.	*Prevents aspiration while withdrawing the tube (accidental leaking of gastric contents from tube into lungs)*
- Slowly withdraw tube until completely removed.	
- Wrap tube in towel and place in trash bag.	
6. Clean nares and apply ointment.	*Promotes skin integrity*
7. Perform mouth care.	
8. Position client with head of bed elevated 45 degrees.	*Facilitates comfort and gastric drainage*
9. Encourage client to call if nausea or discomfort is experienced.	*Facilitates early detection of gastric distention or distress*
10. Instruct client/caregiver to monitor bowel sounds and note flatulence.	*Indicates adequate bowel activity*
11. Measure drainage (if a drainage bag present) and discard bag and tubing in trash. Wash measuring container.	

Evaluation

Were desired outcomes achieved?

DOCUMENTATION

The following should be noted on the visit note:

- Type of NG tube and therapy (suction or tube feeding)
- Status of tubing patency and security
- Type and amount of drainage (or of residual if tube feeding)
- Time of NG tube removal
- Client tolerance of continued therapy or tube removal

Sample Documentation

DATE	TIME	
2/5/98	1400	Nasogastric tube connected to bedside bag. Thick green drainage noted, with scant amounts this visit. Sump tube intact in right naris with surrounding skin intact. Bilateral nares cleaned with petroleum jelly.
2/5/98	1800	NG tube removed per orders. Mouth care performed with mouthwash. Active bowel sounds noted. Sips of water provided and tolerated without nausea.

*N*ursing *P*rocedure 5.18

Gastric Feeding Tube Maintenance

☒ EQUIPMENT

- ½ strength peroxide (optional)
- Soap and water
- Antibiotic ointment (if applicable)
- 4 × 4 Wicker gauze (precut)
- Tape (paper or silk)
- Zinc oxide/lubricating jelly (if ordered)
- Cotton-tipped applicator (optional)
- Irrigation tray with 30–60 mL syringe
- 4 × 4 gauze (multi-pack)
- Tap water (tepid)
- Clean gloves
- Karaya/Stomahesive
- Moisture-proof bag

Purpose

Prevent skin redness, irritation, and excoriation from seepage of gastric or jejunal fluids onto the skin.

Desired Outcomes (sample)

Tube insertion site is free from irritation and infection.

Family and/or caregiver demonstrate consistence in the performance of the procedure.

Family and/or caregiver demonstrate proper disposal of used supplies and utilize asepsis.

Assessment

Assessment should focus on the following:

Doctor's orders for use of gastrointestinal tube and tube maintenance

Skin integrity and patency of the tube

Client, family member, or caregiver's reliability to perform tube maintenance

Outcome Identification and Planning

Key Goals and Sample Goal Criteria

The client and/or caregiver will:

Demonstrate consistent ability to perform the procedure
Demonstrate knowledge of treatment plan and prevention of infection
Demonstrate proper disposal of used supplies

Special Considerations

Because a gastrostomy is often a small catheter inserted at the skin surface, the stoma forms a seal when the catheter is removed. If the anchoring balloon ruptures or is dislodged, a 14Fr. Foley catheter can be inserted as a replacement.

A percutaneous endoscopic gastrostomy (PEG), however, is placed via percutaneous endoscopy. A retention disk and bumper secure the tube. If PEG tube is accidentally dislodged it has to be surgically replaced.

Geriatric

When tube is long term, included in the plan of care is replacement of the tube by physician orders to avoid complications such as adhesions.

Economic

If finances are a factor, consult community resources and national organizations to assist the client with purchase of supplies.

HINT

If the gastrointestinal tube becomes clogged, two methods can be used to clear it: milking the tube in an upward or downward fashion; and instilling cola or cranberry juice via tube until the tube is cleared.

IMPLEMENTATION

Action	Rationale
1. Wash hands and gather equipment.	*Reduces transmission of micro-organisms*
2. Apply clean gloves.	*Prevents contact with bodily fluids*
3. Observe the tube site	*Determines presence of*

Action	Rationale
for redness, swelling, drainage, and abdominal distention.	*infection and complications*

Routine Tube Maintenance
(before and after use of tube)

Action	Rationale
4. Check the tube for kinks or evidence of drainage obstruction and failure of the tube to flush (if obstructed flush to clear).	*Changes in position of the distal tip could push drainage port against mucosa causing the tube not to flush*
5. Move client to one side of the bed and place a clean towel on the other side of the bed.	*Provides a clean field*
6. Peel open multipack 4 × 4 gauze and empty container onto the towel; leave gauze from plastic container on the towel.	*Provides a container for cleaning of tube*
7. Place tepid water and soap, or half strength peroxide, in the empty plastic gauze container.	
8. Open precut 4 × 4 Wicker gauze.	*Provides dressing that fits closely around the tube*
9. Tear tape and hang from nearby table.	*Facilitates easy access to tape*
10. Open antibiotic ointment and cotton-tipped applicator (if ordered).	
11. Open irrigation tray and fill container with tepid tap water.	
12. Tape moisture-proof bag within reach.	*Promotes proper disposal of soiled and used supplies*
13. Fold 4 × 4 gauze into a swab and moisten with soap and water (or half strength peroxide).	
14. Clean tube insertion site utilizing a circular motion; remember not to cross the same area twice.	*Prevents recontamination of skin surface*
15. Discard gauze in moisture-proof bag.	

Action	Rationale
16. Repeat process, with new 4 × 4 each repetition, until area is clean. NOTE: Clean around tube insertion site with moistened cotton-tipped applicator if tube fits snugly.	
17. Cleanse the exterior of the tube with soap and water starting at the base of the tube working upward with moistened 4 × 4s.	*Promotes cleanliness*
For gastrostomy/PEG insertion site care: Apply protective ointment or skin barrier (Karaya) as ordered to protect skin from gastric juices.	
For jejunostomy insertion site care: Apply zinc oxide or lubricating jelly as ordered to skin for protection against intestinal juices.	
18. Dry area and tube thoroughly with remaining 4 × 4 gauze.	
19. Cover insertion site with precut 4 × 4 gauze dressing and tape to secure in place.	*Maintains the stability and dryness of the tube*
20. Apply antibiotic ointment, if ordered, with cotton-tipped applicator, using circular motion.	
21. Clean irrigation set with soap and water, store in designated area.	
22. Store ointments, peroxide, 4 × 4s, and tape in designated area.	

Action	Rationale

23. Check and reorder supplies for client if supplies are low.

Evaluation

Were desired outcomes achieved?

DOCUMENTATION

The following should be noted on the visit note:

- Signs and symptoms of infection (redness, warmth, swelling, and drainage)
- Improper displacement of tube
- Leakage around tube insertion site
- Tube patency and actions taken for blockage, if present

Sample Documentation

DATE	TIME	
2/6/98	1000	Observed family and/or caregiver performing feeding tube maintenance with no assistance needed. Family member and or caregiver report tube insertion site free from infection. Family member and/or caregiver demonstrate eagerness to learn maintenance technique, maintaining infection-free environment. PLAN: Will continue to instruct on feeding maintenance when deficits appear. Transfer to the care of family member and/or caregiver when services no longer required.

Nursing **P**rocedure **5.19**

🖐 *Tube Feeding Management/Medication by Nasogastric or Gastrointestinal Tube*

❌ EQUIPMENT

- Ordered nutritional supplement
- Syringe
- Appropriate feeding bag and tubing for pump
- Glass or cup
- Nonsterile gloves

Purpose

Provides nutritional support using the gastrointestinal tract

Desired Outcomes (sample)
Tube feeding is infused at appropriate volume and rate.
Client has no complaints of nausea or signs of aspiration.
Client gains ½ to 1 kg per week.

Assessment

Assessment should focus on the following:

Nutritional status (skin turgor, urine output, weight, caloric intake)
Elimination pattern (diarrhea, constipation, date of last stool)
Response to previous nutritional support

Outcome Identification and Planning

Key Goals and Sample Goal Criteria
The client will:

Maintain current weight or gain ½ to 1 kg per week
Have decreased edema
Show albumin level within normal limits

Special Considerations

If the client has a tracheostomy tube and is receiving NG tube feedings, check tracheostomy cuff inflation. If cuff is deflated, inflate and maintain for 30 minutes after feeding to prevent aspiration.

Many tube feeding formulas cause diarrhea, thus volume and concentration are increased slowly. If diarrhea persists, report to doctor and administer antidiarrhea medication, if ordered.

Be careful with gastrostomy tube irrigations. Depending on the surgery, irrigation may be contraindicated. Verify this with the doctor.

IMPLEMENTATION

Action	Rationale
1. Wash hands and organize supplies.	*Reduces contamination* *Promotes efficiency*
2. Explain procedure to client and caregiver and insert feeding tube, if needed (see Procedure 5.15).	
3. Verify tube placement: - Apply gloves. - Aspirate and check for gastric contents (or old tube feeding if reinsertion), or - Pinch tube off at the end and connect syringe with 15 to 20 mL air to tube and push air in while listening with stethoscope over epigastric area for gurgling.	*Indicates tube is in stomach* *Prevents infusion of tube feeding into pharynx or pulmonary tree*
4. Prior to feeding or every 4 hours for client/caregiver: - Check for residual: slowly aspirate gastric contents, and note amount of residual—may be difficult with small feeding tubes. (If residual is greater than specified amount per doctor's orders	*Determines degree of absorption of feeding* *Prevents distension of abdomen and possible aspiration*

Action	Rationale

[commonly 100 mL], discard aspirated volume to stomach, cease feedings, and notify doctor).

- Monitor bowel sounds in all abdominal quadrants.

Determines presence of bowel activity (peristalsis)

- Perform mouth care.

Freshens mouth
Prevents accumulation of microorganisms

5. Assist client to position with head elevated 30 to 45 degrees and maintain throughout feedings.

Decreases aspiration of feeding into lungs

6. Determine amount of water, if any, to be infused and pour into glass or cup.

7. Attach syringe to NG tube and aspirate small amount of contents to fill tube and lower portion of syringe.

Prevents infusion of air into stomach

8. Infuse feeding or medication (see steps 12–15):

Assists flow of feeding by gravity

 - Hold syringe 6 inches above tube insertion site (nose or abdomen; Fig. 5.19.1)
 - Fill syringe with feeding and allow to flow slowly into NG tube; follow with water (30-mL flush if no water is ordered). DO NOT ALLOW SYRINGE TO EMPTY UNTIL FEEDING AND WATER INFUSION ARE COMPLETED.

Prevents entrance of air into tubing and stomach

9. Clamp NG or gastrostomy tube and place client in semi-Fowler's position.

Decreases reflux of feeding and possible aspiration into lungs

10. Teach client and caregiver

Detects loss of or decrease in GI

Action	Rationale

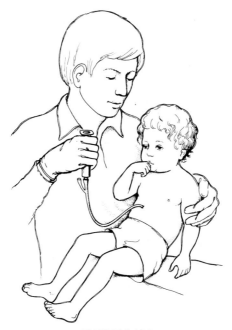

FIGURE 5.19.1

to monitor bowel sounds, stools, and residual.	*function*
11. Client/caregiver should check NG tube placement and residual prior to each tube feeding.	*Prevents aspiration of secretions into tracheobronchial tree*

Medication Administration Through NG Tube

12. Check tube placement.	*Prevents obstruction of tube with large medication particles or thick solution*
13. Crush pill (if crushable) and mix with fluid to make a thin solution with small sediment. (*Note:* Be sure guidelines for drug	

Action	Rationale
administration are being followed.)	
14. Mix viscous solutions with water or saline (30 to 60 mL).	*Prevents clogging of tube*
15. Follow medication infusion with 30 mL saline or water.	*Prevents obstruction of tubing*
16. Teach client/caregiver medication administration procedure and monitor progress.	

Evaluation

Were desired outcomes achieved?

DOCUMENTATION

The following should be noted on the visit note:

- Type of NG tube and tube feeding
- Status of tubing patency and security
- Type and amount of residual
- Client tolerance of tube feeding or tube removal

Sample Documentation

DATE	TIME	
7/8/98	1400	Tube feeding initiated at 0800 with Ensure, 150 mL infused per Dobhoff feeding tube. Active bowel sounds noted; no complaints of nausea. Residual of 30 mL noted 4 hours after prior feeding. Tubing flushed with 30 mL water. Caregiver performed procedure with assistance.

Chapter 6

Elimination

OVERVIEW

▶ Adequate elimination of body waste is an essential function to sustain life.

▶ Inadequate bladder and bowel elimination ultimately affects the body's delicate balance of fluid, electrolyte, and acid–base level.

▶ Various means are available clinically to help assess and maintain adequate elimination status.

▶ Factors that affect bowel and bladder elimination status include food and fluid intake; age; psychological barriers; medications; personal hygiene habits; educational level; cultural practices; pathology of the renal, urinary, or gastrointestinal system; surgery; hormonal variations; muscle tone of supporting organs and structures; and concurrent medical problems, such as decreased cardiac output or motor disturbances.

▶ Alterations in bowel and bladder elimination mandate careful assessment and monitoring of the upper and lower abdomen, as well as amounts and appearance of body excretions.

▶ Procedures related to adequate bladder elimination usually require the use of sterile technique to prevent contamination to the highly susceptible urinary tract.

▶ Because clients on hemodialysis are using final means of adequate renal excretion, it is crucial that the nurse perform these procedures with precision.

▶ Various concentrations of dialysate affect osmolality, rate of fluid removal, electrolyte balance, solute removal, and cardiovascular stability.

▶ Elimination is very personal to the client; therefore, privacy and professionalism should be maintained when assisting clients with elimination needs.

▶ Clients with colostomies frequently experience body-image and self-concept alterations. Psychological support and teaching are crucial in resolving these problems.

▶ All procedures involving elimination of body waste require use of gloves and occasionally other protective barriers.

▶ Before planning a procedure, the nurse should determine if same-sex or opposite-sex contact with genitalia is culturally offensive to the client.

*N*ursing *P*rocedure 6.1

🖐 *Midstream Urine Collection*

⊠ EQUIPMENT

- Basin of warm water
- Soap
- Washcloth
- Towel
- Antiseptic swabs or cotton balls
- Sterile specimen collection container
- Specimen container labels
- Bedpan, urinal, bedside commode, or toilet
- Nonsterile gloves
- Pen

Purpose

Obtains urine specimen by aseptic technique for microbiological analysis

Desired Outcomes (sample)

Client shows no signs or symptoms of urinary tract infection.
Client verbalizes relief of discomfort within 3 days.

Assessment

Assessment should focus on the following:

Characteristics of the urine
Symptoms associated with urinary tract infections (eg, pain or discomfort on voiding, urinary frequency)
Temperature increase
Ability of client to follow instructions for obtaining specimen
Time of day of specimen collection
Fluid intake and output

Outcome Identification and Planning

Key Goal and Sample Goal Criterion

The client will:

Demonstrate no signs of urinary tract infection (such as discomfort upon voiding, elevated temperature, abnormal urine constituents, and abnormal urine characteristics) within 3 days.

Special Considerations

Midstream urine collection is frequently performed by the client; however, instructions for the procedure must be clear to obtain reliable laboratory results. Perhaps the most frequent error the client commits is poor cleaning technique. Be certain women understand to cleanse from the front to the back of the perineum, and men from the tip of the penis downward.

If possible, a specimen should be obtained upon first voiding in the morning.

IMPLEMENTATION

Action	Rationale
1. Wash hands.	*Reduces microorganism transfer*
2. Explain procedure to client.	*Decreases anxiety*
3. Provide for privacy.	*Decreases embarrassment*
4. Don clean gloves.	*Reduces nurse's exposure to body secretions*
5. Wash perineal area with soap and water, rinse, and pat dry.	*Reduces microorganisms in perineal area*
6. Cleanse meatus with antiseptic solution in same manner as for catheterization in males (see Procedure 6.3, steps 15 to 17) and females (see Procedure 6.4, steps 23 and 24).	*Reduces microorganisms at urethral opening*
7. Ask client to begin voiding.	*Flushes organisms from urethral opening*
8. After stream of urine begins, place specimen container in place to obtain 30 mL of urine.	*Collects urine at point in which urine is least contaminated*
9. Remove container before client stops voiding.	*Prevents end stream organisms from dripping into container*

Action	Rationale
10. Allow client to complete voiding using urinal, bedpan, or toilet.	
11. Wash perineal area again if stain-producing antiseptic was used.	*Removes antiseptic solution* *Promotes general comfort*
12. Label specimen container with date and time as well as client identification information.	
13. Discard equipment and gloves.	*Reduces spread of infection*
14. Wash hands.	*Reduces contamination*

Evaluation

Were desired outcomes achieved?

DOCUMENTATION

The following should be noted on the visit note:

- Signs or symptoms of urinary infection
- Amount, color, odor, and consistency of urine obtained
- Specimen collection time
- Total amount voided
- Teaching performed regarding technique for cleaning genitalia

Sample Documentation		
DATE	**TIME**	
1/11/98	1100	Clean-catch urine specimen obtained and taken to laboratory—30 mL of cloudy, yellow urine with slight foul odor noted. Client reports slight perineal burning.

*N*ursing *P*rocedure   **6.2**

🖐 *Urine Specimen Collection From an Indwelling Catheter*

❌ EQUIPMENT

- Sterile 3-mL syringe with 23- or 25-gauge needle
- Nonsterile gloves
- Alcohol swab
- Sterile specimen container
- Container labels
- Pen
- Catheter clamp or rubber band
- Antiseptic (such as povidone)

Purpose

Obtain sterile urine specimens for microbiological analysis

Desired Outcomes (sample)

Client shows no signs of urinary tract infection.
Client verbalizes lack of perineal discomfort within 3 days.

Assessment

Assessment should focus on the following:

Characteristics of the urine
Symptoms associated with urinary tract infections (pain or discomfort)
Temperature increase
Fluid intake and output

Outcome Identification and Planning

Key Goals and Sample Goal Criteria
The client will:

Demonstrate no signs of urinary tract infection (ie, perineal discomfort, elevated temperature, abnormal urine constituents, and abnormal urine characteristics)

Verbalize lack of perineal discomfort within 3 days

Special Considerations

If a specimen is needed and a new catheter is to be inserted, obtain the specimen during catheter insertion procedure. See Procedure 6.3, Male Catheterization, or Procedure 6.4, Female Catheterization.

Geriatric

If a specimen is needed from a confused client who is unable to follow directions, obtain assistance to maintain sterility of the specimen and catheter.

IMPLEMENTATION

Action	Rationale
1. Wash hands.	*Reduces microorganism transfer*
2. Explain procedure to client.	*Decreases anxiety*
3. Provide for privacy.	*Decreases embarrassment*
4. Don clean gloves.	*Reduces nurse exposure to body secretions*

Proceed to step 12 for open-system method

Closed-System Method

5. Fold or clamp drainage tubing about 4 inches below junction of drainage tubing and catheter.	*Facilitates trapping of urine in tubing at specimen port*
6. Allow urine to pool in drainage tubing; if urine does not pool in tubing immediately, leave it clamped for urine to collect over period of time (usually 10 to 30 minutes).	*Allows urine to pool in tubing at specimen port*
7. Cleanse specimen collection port of drainage tubing with alcohol swab or antiseptic solution recommended by agency. (If no collection port is visible, catheter tubing is probably designed with a self-	*Reduces microorganisms at insertion port*

Action	Rationale

sealing material so that specimen may be obtained from catheter itself by cleansing and piercing catheter tubing close to junction. However, check package label and instructions. If catheter tubing is self-sealing, cleanse catheter tubing close to junction of drainage tubing.)

8. Carefully insert sterile needle of syringe into specimen-collection port or self-sealing catheter tubing at a 45-degree angle; insert needle slowly, taking care not to puncture other side of catheter tubing (Fig. 6.2).

Prevents accidental puncture of drainage tubing or catheter

9. Pull back on plunger of syringe and obtain 3 to 10 mL of urine.

Draws urine into syringe

10. Slowly squirt urine into collection container; do not touch inside of specimen container.

Places urine in container maintaining sterility of container and specimen

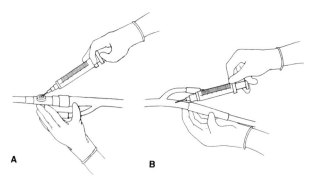

A

B

FIGURE 6.2

Action	Rationale

11. Complete steps 20 to 24.

Open-system Method

12. Place linen saver under tubing at junction of catheter and drainage tubing. — *Prevents soiling linen*

13. Remove cap from specimen bottle and place bottle on linen saver.

14. Cleanse junction with antiseptic solution such as Povidone (or antiseptic recommended by agency). — *Reduces microorganisms*

15. Carefully disconnect catheter from drainage tubing at junction. Hold drainage tubing and catheter 1.5 to 2 inches from junction, being careful not to contaminate either end. — *Disconnects catheter to allow for specimen collection* / *Avoids system contamination*

16. Place specimen container under catheter opening and allow urine to run into container; do not allow catheter tip to touch container. — *Allows urine to run into container* / *Avoids contamination*

17. Place specimen container on bedside table after urine is obtained. — *Prevents contamination of catheter line*

18. Wipe catheter and drainage tubing again with antiseptic solution. — *Reduces microorganism transfer*

19. Firmly reconnect drainage tubing and catheter at junction. — *Reconnects to close system*

20. Replace top of specimen container. — *Prevents urine waste*

21. Label container with date and time of collection as well as client identification information. — *Eliminates errors in client identification*

22. Fill out agency requisition form for specimen. — *Facilitates proper logging and charging in lab*

Action	Rationale
23. Discard gloves and wash hands.	*Prevents spread of micro-organisms*
24. Transport immediately after visit.	*Avoids sending old specimen in which urine constituents may have changed*

Evaluation

Were desired outcomes achieved?

DOCUMENTATION

The following should be noted on the visit note:

- Amount, color, odor, and consistency of urine obtained
- Specimen collection time
- Total amount of urine collected
- Signs or symptoms of urinary infection
- Disposition of specimen to lab

Sample Documentation

DATE	TIME	
1/3/98	1100	Sterile urine specimen obtained via indwelling catheter and taken to laboratory. Specimen is 30 mL of cloudy, yellow urine with slight foul odor noted. Client reports slight perineal burning.

Nursing Procedure **6.3**

Male Catheterization

X EQUIPMENT

- Urethral catheterization set (includes sterile gloves, specimen-collection container, catheter, two drapes, graduated measurement receptacle, antiseptic solution, cotton balls, forceps, lubricating jelly)
  or
- Indwelling catheterization set (all of the items in urethral catheterization kit, except the graduated measurement receptacle, plus a drainage-collection system [tubing and bag that connect to the catheter] and a prefilled saline syringe for inflation)
- Basin of warm soapy water
- Washcloth
- Large towel
- Nonsterile gloves
- Sheet for draping
- Linen saver or plastic bag
- Roll of tape
- Bedpan, urinal, and second collection container
- Specimen container, if specimen is needed

Purpose

Facilitates emptying of bladder
Facilitates obtaining sterile urine specimens
Facilitates determining amount of residual urine in bladder
Allows for continuous, accurate monitoring of urinary output
Provides avenue for bladder irrigations

Desired Outcomes (sample)

A urine output of at least 250 mL per 8 hours is attained and maintained.
Client verbalizes relief of lower abdominal pain within 1 hour of catheter insertion.

Assessment

Assessment should focus on the following:

Type of catheterization ordered (straight, Foley, residual)
Status of bladder (distension prior to catheter insertion)
Abnormalities of genitalia or prostate gland
History of conditions that may interfere with smooth insertion
(eg, prostate enlargement, urethral stricture)
Client allergy to iodine-based antiseptics (eg, povidone)

Outcome Identification and Planning

Key Goals and Sample Goal Criteria
The client will:

Attain and maintain a urine output of at least 250 mL every 8
hours
Verbalize relief of lower abdominal pain within 1 hour of
catheter insertion

Special Considerations
Never force a catheter if it does not pass through the urethral
canal smoothly. If the catheter still does not pass smoothly after using the suggested troubleshooting methods, discontinue
the procedure and notify the physician. Forcing the catheter
may result in damage to the urethra and surrounding structures.
Because indwelling catheterization is used on a long-term basis
for the homebound client, potential is high for infection. Be
alert for early signs and symptoms of infection and adhere to
a strict schedule for changing catheters.
Explore the possibility of an external catheter as an alternative
to the indwelling catheter.

Geriatric

A common pathologic feature in elderly men is enlargement of
the prostate gland. The enlargement frequently makes inserting a catheter difficult.

 Cost-cutting

If replacing a Foley catheter, note the size of the previous
catheter to avoid wastage from insertion of too small a
catheter. This occurs frequently with clients on long-term
catheterization.

IMPLEMENTATION

Action	Rationale
1. Wash hands.	*Reduces microorganism transfer*
2. Explain procedure to client.	*Decreases anxiety*
3. Determine if client is allergic to iodine-based antiseptics.	*Avoids allergic reactions*
4. Provide for privacy.	*Decreases embarrassment*
5. Don nonsterile gloves.	*Reduces nurse's exposure to body secretions*
6. If catheterization is for residual urine, ask client to void in urinal, and measure and record the amount voided; empty urinal.	*Determines amount of urine client is able to void without catheterization* *Determines exact amount*
7. Place linen saver under buttocks.	*Avoids wetting linens*
8. Wash genital area with warm water, rinse, and pat dry with towel.	*Decreases microorganisms around urethral opening*
9. Discard gloves, bath water, wash cloth, and towel; then wash hands.	*Decreases clutter* *Reduces microorganism transfer*
10. Drape client so that only penis is exposed.	*Provides privacy* *Reduces embarrassment*
11. Set up work field: - Open catheter set and remove from outer plastic package.	*Removes kit without opening inner folds*
- Tape outer package to bedside table with top edge turned inside.	*Provides waste bag*
- Place catheter kit beside client's knees and carefully open outer edges.	*Places items within easy reach*
- Ask client to open legs slightly.	*Relaxes pelvic muscles*
- Remove full drape from kit with fingertips and place across thighs, plastic side down, just below penis; keep other side sterile.	*Provides sterile field*

Action	Rationale
- If catheter and bag are separate, use sterile technique to open package containing bag and place bag on work field.	
12. Don sterile gloves.	*Avoids contaminating other items in kit*
13. Prepare items in kit for use during insertion as follows:	
- Pour iodine solution over cotton balls.	*Prepares cotton balls for cleaning*
- Separate cotton balls with forceps.	*Promotes easy manipulation*
- Lubricate 6 to 7 inches of catheter tip and place carefully on tray so that tip is secure in tray.	*Prevents local irritation of meatus on catheter insertion* *Promotes ease of insertion*
- If inserting indwelling catheter, attach prefilled syringe of sterile water to balloon port of catheter.	*Connects to balloon port the syringe needed to inflate balloon*
- Inject 2 to 3 mL of sterile water from prefilled syringe into balloon and observe balloon for leaks as it fills.	*Tests balloon for defects*
- Discard and obtain another kit if any leaks are noted.	*Prevents catheter dislodgment after insertion*
- Deflate balloon and leave syringe connected.	*Leaves syringe within reach*
- Attach catheter to drainage container tubing (or if drainage tubing is already attached to the catheter, place tubing and bag securely on sterile field, close to the other equipment.	*Facilitates organization while maintaining sterility*
- Check clamp on collection bag to be sure it is closed. Place catheter and collection tray close to perineum.	*Prevents loss of urine prior to measurement*

Action	Rationale
- Open specimen collection container and place on sterile field.	*Places container within easy reach for specimen*
14. Remove fenestrated drape from kit and place penis through hole in drape with nondominant hand. KEEP DOMINANT HAND STERILE.	*Expands sterile field*
15. Pull penis up at a 90-degree angle to client's supine body.	*Straightens urethra*
16. With nondominant hand, gently grasp glans (tip) of penis; retract foreskin, if necessary.	*Provides grasp of penis preventing contamination of sterile field later*
17. With forceps in dominant hand, cleanse meatus and glans with cotton balls, beginning at urethral opening and moving toward shaft of penis; make one complete circle around penis with each cotton ball, discarding cotton ball after each wipe (Fig. 6.3).	*Cleanses meatus without cross-contaminating or contaminating sterile hand*
18. After all cotton balls have been used, discard forceps.	*Prevents contamination of sterile field*
19. With thumb and first finger, pick catheter up about 1.5 to 2 inches from tip.	*Gives nurse good control of catheter tip (which easily bends)*

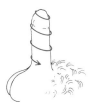

FIGURE 6.3

Action	Rationale
20. Carefully gather additional tubing in hand.	*Gives nurse good control of full catheter length*
21. Ask client to bear down as if voiding and take slow, deep breaths; encourage him to continue to breathe deeply until catheter is fully inserted.	*Opens sphincter. Relaxes sphincter muscles of bladder and urethra*
22. Insert tip of catheter slowly through urethral opening 7 to 9 inches (or until urine returns).	*Inserts catheter*
23. Lower penis to about a 45-degree angle after catheter is inserted about halfway and hold open end of catheter over collection container (if it is not connected to a drainage bag).	*Places penis in position for urine to be released into collection container so that accurate amount is measured*
24. If resistance is met: - Stop for a few seconds.	*Allows sphincters to relax and reduces anxiety*
- Encourage client to continue taking slow, deep breaths.	
- Do not force; remove catheter tip and notify doctor if above sequence is unsuccessful.	*Prevents injury to prostate, urethra, and surrounding structures*
25. After catheter has been advanced an appropriate distance, advance another 1 to 1.5 inches. If unable to obtain urine perform the Credé technique.	*Ensures catheter advances far enough not to dislodge* *Facilitates urine flow*
26. For straight catheterization: - Obtain urine specimen in specimen container, if ordered.	*Obtains sterile specimen*
- Allow urine to drain until it stops or UNTIL MAXIMUM NUMBER OF MILLILITERS SPECIFIED BY AGENCY (usually 1000 to 1500 mL) have drained into	*Empties bladder* *Obtains residual urine amount*

Action	Rationale
container; use second container, bedpan, or urinal, if necessary.	
27. For an indwelling catheter, inflate balloon with attached syringe and gently pull back on catheter until it stops (catches).	*Secures catheter placement*
28. Secure catheter loosely with tape to lower abdomen on side from which drainage bag will be hanging (preferably away from door); make certain that tubing is not tangled or obstructed.	*Stabilizes catheter* *Prevents accidental dislodgment*
29. Clear bed of all equipment.	*Removes waste from bed*
30. Reposition client for comfort and replace linens for warmth and privacy.	*Promotes general comfort*
31. Measure amount of urine in collection container or drainage bag and discard.	*Provides assessment data*
32. Gather all additional equipment and discard with gloves.	*Promotes clean environment*
33. Wash hands.	*Reduces microorganism transfer*

Evaluation

Were desired outcomes achieved?

DOCUMENTATION

The following should be noted on the visit note:

- Presence of distension prior to catheterization
- Assessment of genitalia, if abnormalities noted
- Type of catheterization
- Size of catheter
- Amount, color, and consistency of urine returned on catheterization

- Amount of urine returned prior to catheterization (if residual urine catheterization)
- Difficulties encountered, if any, in passing the catheter smoothly
- Reports of unusual discomfort during insertion
- Specimen obtained

Sample Documentation

DATE	TIME	
4/6/98	1100	Catheter (#16 French Foley) inserted without resistance or report of discomfort. Procedure yielded 700 mL straw-colored urine without sediment or foul odor.

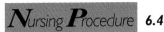

Female Catheterization

EQUIPMENT

- Urethral catheterization set (includes sterile gloves, specimen collection container, catheter, two drapes, graduated measurement receptacle, antiseptic solution, cotton balls, forceps, lubricating jelly)
  or
- Indwelling catheterization set (all of the items in urethral catheterization kit, except the graduated measurement receptacle, plus a drainage-collection system [tubing and bag that connect to the catheter] and a prefilled saline syringe for balloon inflation)
- Basin of warm soapy water
- Washcloth
- Large towel
- Nonsterile gloves
- One sheet for draping
- Linen saver or plastic bag
- Roll of tape
- Bedpan, urinal, or second collection container
- Specimen container, if specimen is needed
- Extra lighting

Purpose

Facilitates emptying of bladder
Facilitates obtaining sterile urine specimens
Facilitates determining amount of residual urine in bladder
Allows for continuous, accurate monitoring of urinary output
Provides avenue for bladder irrigations

Desired Outcomes (sample)

A urine output of at least 250 mL per 8 hours is attained and maintained.
Client verbalizes relief of lower abdominal pain within 1 hour of catheter insertion.

Assessment

Assessment should focus on the following:

Type of catheterization ordered (straight, Foley, residual)
Status of bladder (distension prior to catheter insertion)
Abnormalities of genitalia
Client allergy to iodine-based antiseptics (eg, Povidone)

Outcome Identification and Planning

Key Goals and Sample Goal Criteria
The client will:

Attain and maintain a urine output of at least 250 mL every 8
  hours
Verbalize relief of lower abdominal pain within 1 hour of
  catheter insertion

Special Considerations
When indwelling catheterization is used on a long-term basis,
  there is a high potential for infection: Be alert for early signs
  and symptoms of infection and adhere to a strict schedule for
  changing catheters.

 Cost-cutting Tips

- For female clients, time and money may be saved by using
  clean gloves to locate the meatus *before* opening the sterile kit.
  This minimizes the chance of sterile glove contamination.
- If replacing a Foley, note the size of the previous catheter to
  avoid waste from insertion of too small a catheter. This occurs
  frequently with clients on long-term catheterization.

IMPLEMENTATION

Action	Rationale
1. Wash hands.	*Reduces microorganism transfer*
2. Explain procedure to client, emphasizing need to maintain sterile field.	*Decreases anxiety*
3. Determine if client is allergic to iodine-based antiseptics.	*Avoids allergic reactions*
4. Provide for privacy.	*Decreases embarrassment*
5. Don nonsterile gloves.	*Reduces nurse's exposure to body secretions*
6. If catheterization is for residual urine, ask client to void in urinal, and	*Determines amount of urine client is able to void without catheterization*

Action	Rationale
measure and record the amount voided; empty urinal.	*Determines exact amount* *Promotes tidiness*
7. Place linen saver under buttocks.	*Avoids wetting linens*
8. Place light to enhance visualization.	*Promotes clear identification of anatomical parts*
9. Separate labia to expose urethral opening:	*Allows nurse to identify ure- thral opening clearly before area is cleansed*
- If using dorsal recumbent position (Fig. 6.4.1*A*), separate labia with thumb and forefinger by gently lifting upward and out- ward (Fig. 6.4.2 illustrates	*Subtle variations in location of structures of female geni- talia often cause a delay that increases chance of contami- nation of field*

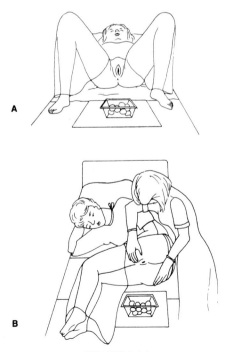

A

B

FIGURE 6.4.1

Action	Rationale

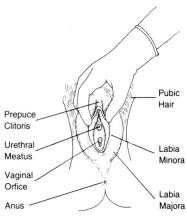

Prepuce Clitoris
Urethral Meatus
Vaginal Orfice
Anus

Pubic Hair
Labia Minora
Labia Majora

FIGURE 6.4.2

this technique and identifies parts of the female perineum).

- If using side-lying position, pull upward on upper labia minora as shown in Fig. 6.4.1B).

10. Wash genital area with warm water, rinse, and pat dry with towel.

11. Discard gloves, bath water, washcloth, and towel; then wash hands.

12. If inserting an indwelling catheter in which the drainage apparatus is separate from catheter (not preconnected):
- Check for closed clamp on collection bag.
- Secure drainage collection bag on bed.

Decreases microorganisms around urethral opening

Decreases clutter
Reduces microorganisms

Places drainage tubing within immediate and easy reach, decreasing chance of catheter contamination once inserted

Action	Rationale
- Check to be sure tubing will not get tangled with client movement.	
13. Position client in dorsal recumbent or side-lying position with knees flexed (Fig. 6.4.1*A* and *B*); in side-lying position, slide client's hips toward edge of bed.	*Exposes labia*
14. Drape client so that only perineum is exposed.	*Provides privacy* *Reduces embarrassment*
15. Remove gloves and wash hands.	*Reduces microorganism transfer* *Prevents client from falling* *Reduces embarrassment*
16. Carefully open catheter set and remove it from plastic outer package.	*Removes kit without opening inner folds*
17. Tape outer package to bedside table with top edge turned inside.	*Provides waste bag*
18. Places catheter kit between client's knees and carefully open outer edges (if using side-lying position, place kit about 1 foot from perineal area near thighs).	*Places items within easy reach*
19. Remove full drape from kit with fingertips and place, plastic side down, just under buttocks by having client raise hips; keep other side sterile.	*Provides work field*
20. Don sterile gloves.	*Avoids contaminating other items in kit*
21. Prepare items in kit for use during insertion as follows:	
- Pour iodine solution over cotton balls.	*Prepares cotton balls for cleaning*
- Separate cotton balls with forceps.	*Promotes easy manipulation*
- Lubricate 3 to 4 inches of catheter tip and place carefully on tray such	*Prevents local irritation of meatus on catheter insertion* *Promotes ease of insertion*

Action	Rationale
that tip is secure in tray.	
- If inserting indwelling catheter, attach prefilled syringe to balloon port of catheter by twisting syringe in clockwise direction.	*Connects syringe needed to inflate balloon to balloon port*
- Push plunger in and inject 2 to 3 mL of sterile water from prefilled syringe into balloon and observe balloon for leaks as it fills.	*Tests balloon for defects*
- Discard and obtain another kit if any leaks are noted.	*Prevents catheter dislodgment after insertion*
- Deflate balloon and leave syringe connected.	*Leaves syringe within reach*
- If inserting closed indwelling system with drainage tubing already attached to catheter, move tubing and bag close to other equipment on work field, making certain that drainage system is on the sterile field only. (Check clamp on collection bag to be sure it is closed)	*Facilitates organization while maintaining sterility*
	Prevents loss of urine prior to measurement
- Open specimen collection container and place on sterile field.	*Places container within easy reach for specimen*
22. Remove fenestrated drape from kit and place on perineum such that only labia is exposed (or discard the drape if you prefer).	*Expands sterile field*
23. Separate labia minora with nondominant hand in same manner as in step 9 and hold this position until catheter is inserted	*Exposes urethral opening*

Action	Rationale

(*Note:* Dominant hand is only hand sterile now; contaminated hand continues to separate labia).

24. Using forceps, cleanse meatus with cotton balls:
    - Making one downward stroke with each cotton ball, begin at labia on side farthest from you and move towards labia nearest you.
    - Afterwards, wipe once down center of meatus.
    - Wipe once with each cotton ball and discard (Fig. 6.4.3).

Cleanses meatus without cross-contaminating

25. After all cotton balls have been used, remove forceps from field.

Prevents contamination of sterile field

26. Move cleaning tray to end of sterile field and move collection container and catheter closer to client.

Facilitates organization
Prevents accidental contamination of system

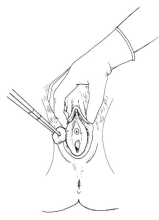

FIGURE 6.4.3

Action	Rationale
27. With thumb and first finger, pick catheter up about 1.5 to 2 inches from tip.	*Gives nurse good control of catheter (which easily bends)*
28. Carefully gather additional tubing in hand.	*Gives nurse good control of full catheter length*
29. Ask client to bear down as if voiding and take slow, deep breaths; encourage her to take deep breaths until catheter is fully inserted.	*Opens sphincter* *Relaxes sphincter muscles of bladder and urethra*
30. Insert tip of catheter slowly through urethral opening 3 to 4 inches (or until urine returns), releasing tubing from hand as insertion continues; direct open end of catheter into collection container.	*Inserts catheter*
31. After catheter has been advanced an appropriate distance (3 to 4 inches or until urine returns), advance another 1 to 1.5 inches.	*Ensures catheter advances far enough not to dislodge*
32. Grasp catheter with thumb and first finger of nondominant hand and hold steady.	*Keeps catheter from being forced out by sphincter muscles* *Avoids contamination*
33. If straight catheterization: - Obtain urine specimen in specimen container, if ordered, and replace open end of catheter in collection container.	*Obtains sterile specimen*
- Allow urine to drain until it stops or UNTIL MAXIMUM NUMBER OF MILLILITERS SPECIFIED BY AGENCY (usually 1000 to 1500 mL) have drained into container; use second container,	*Empties bladder* *Obtains residual urine amount* *Prevents temporary hypovolemic shock state*

Action	Rationale
bedpan, or urinal if necessary.	
- Remove catheter.	
34. If indwelling catheter is being used, inflate balloon with attached syringe, and gently pull back on catheter until it stops (catches).	*Secures catheter placement*
35. If the indwelling catheter is separate from bag and tubing, remove protective cap from end of tubing and attach drainage tubing to end of catheter.	*Converts system to closed system*
36. Secure catheter loosely with tape to thigh on side from which drainage bag will be hanging (preferably away from door); make certain that tubing is not caught.	*Stabilizes catheter Prevents accidental dislodgment*
37. Clear bed of all equipment, reposition client for comfort, and replace linens for warmth and privacy.	*Promotes clean environment, comfort, and safety*
38. Measure amount of urine in collection container or drainage bag and discard.	*Provides assessment data*
39. Gather up all additional equipment and discard with gloves.	*Promotes clean environment*
40. Wash hands.	*Reduces microorganism transfer*

Evaluation

Were desired outcomes achieved?

DOCUMENTATION

The following should be noted on the visit note:

- Assessment of lower abdomen prior to catheterization

- Assessment of genitalia, if abnormalities noted
- Types of catheterization
- Size of catheter
- Amount, color, and consistency of urine returned on catheterization
- Amount of urine returned prior to catheterization (if residual urine was collected)
- Difficulties encountered, if any, in passing catheter smoothly
- Reports of unusual discomfort during insertion
- Specimen obtained

Sample Documentation

DATE	TIME	
1/5/98	1000	Catheter (#16 French Foley) inserted without resistance or report of discomfort. Procedure yielded 700 mL of straw-colored urine without sediment or foul odor. Instructed patient on care of catheter.

◢N◣ursing ◢P◣rocedure *6.5*

Intermittent Self-catheterization

◢X◣ EQUIPMENT

- #14 to #16 French straight catheter
- Water-soluble lubricant
- Mirror (females only)
- Soap, water, clean washcloths
- Container for draining urine if toilet is not available
- Plastic bag for used catheter

Purpose

To empty the bladder at regular intervals without the risks of an indwelling urinary catheter

Desired Outcomes (sample)

Client has independence in urinary control.

Client develops no skin breakdown.

Intermittent catheterization is incorporated into client's lifestyle.

Client is free from urinary tract infection.

Assessment

Assessment should focus on the following:

Doctor's order for the procedure

Client's knowledge of the procedure

Status of the bladder before and after the procedure

Client's cognitive status, vision, and manual dexterity

Family member's or significant other's reliability to assist with procedure

Outcome Identification and Planning

Key Goals and Sample Goal Criteria

The client and/or caregiver will:

Demonstrate consistent ability to perform procedure

Adhere to schedule for intermittent catheterization

Demonstrate ability to safely clean, sterilize, and store catheters for reuse

Identify signs of UTI (fever, cloudy or foul-smelling urine) to report immediately

Special Considerations

Never force a catheter. Forcing a catheter may result in damage to the urethra and surrounding structures.

Have the client attempt to void before the procedure by applying moderate pressure on the lower abdomen, stroking the thighs, or running water to induce urination.

Female

There are various positions that may be used to facilitate perineal exposure considering the client's physical condition and preference. Alternate positions are semirecumbent with legs abducted, squatting, seated on the toilet, standing with one foot on the toilet, or using the posterior approach.

Geriatric

Elderly women often find lying on the left side, with the right knee and thigh drawn up, if possible, more comfortable than the dorsal recumbent position.

Economic

In the home, clean technique is easier and less expensive for the client than sterile technique.

IMPLEMENTATION

Action	Rationale
1. Explain procedure to client.	*Decreases anxiety*
2. Have client or caregiver wash hands.	*Avoid transfer of microorganisms*
3. Organize equipment within reach.	*Promotes efficiency*
4. Squeeze a generous amount of lubricant on clean paper towel.	
5. Position client sitting on edge of bed, chair, or toilet. Men may stand. Women should be positioned with	*To aid in emptying the bladder*

Action	Rationale

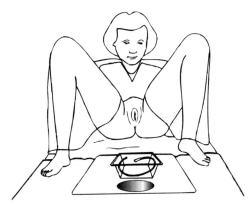

FIGURE 6.5

mirror between legs (Fig. 6.5).

6. Have the female client
   - Separate the folds of the vulva with the non-dominant hand and thoroughly wash perineal area with soap and warm water using front to back strokes; pat area dry with washcloth.

   Exposes urethral opening, decreases microorganisms around the urethral opening and avoid contamination with fecal material

   - Roll the first three inches of the catheter in the lubricant.

   Reduce friction and damage to the meatus and urethra.

   - Put one end of the catheter in the container or toilet. Spread the lips of vulva with the ring and index finger of the non-dominant hand.
   - With the dominant hand, insert the tip of the catheter into the urethral meatus until urine begins to flow.

   A mirror may be propped between the legs to identify the urethral meatus

Action	Rationale
- Apply slight pressure to abdominal muscles.	*Facilitates emptying the bladder*
- When the catheter stops draining, pinch it closed and remove it.	*Prevents leakage of urine into the urethra*
- Rinse the used catheter in cold water. Wash in warm soapy water, rinse, then boil for 20 minutes in a pan of water. Allow to air dry on clean paper towels, then store in a clean jar or freshly laundered towel.	*Proper cleansing of catheters prolongs their effective use*
- Discard hard or brittle catheters.	*Avoids damage to the urethra and surrounding structures*
7. Have the male client	
- Retract foreskin if necessary and wash the penis thoroughly with soap and warm water. Pat dry with washcloth.	*Decreases microorganisms around the urethral opening*
- Lubricate 6 to 7 inches of catheter tip.	*Prevents local irritation of meatus on catheter insertion*
- Hold penis at a right angle to the body.	*Straightens urethra*
- Bear down as if voiding and take slow deep breaths.	*Relaxes sphincter muscles of bladder and urethra*
- Insert tip of catheter into urethra 7 to 9 inches or until urine begins to flow.	
- Allow urine to drain in toilet or container. Have the client cough or deep breathe if it is necessary to overcome resistance at the sphincter.	
- When the catheter stops draining, pinch it closed and remove it.	*Prevents leakage of urine into the urethra*
8. Assist the client to dress, provide comfort measures, and dispose of the urine.	*Promotes general comfort*
9. Clean and replace equipment.	*Promotes clean environment*

Evaluation

Were desired outcomes achieved? Are additional services needed? (social worker for assistance with finances; occupational therapy to assist with increasing manual dexterity)

DOCUMENTATION

The following should be noted on the visit note:

- Teaching done
- Return demonstration of self-catheterization
- Functional limitations that interfere with performance of procedure
- Client tolerance of procedure
- Adherence to recommended frequency of catheterization
- Quality and quantity of urine
- Status of urinary control
- Intake and output
- Condition of skin
- Plans for future visits
- Discharge planning

Sample Documentation

DATE	TIME
9/26/98	1000

Catheter (#16 French Straight) inserted without resistance or report of discomfort. Procedure yielded 600 mL of amber-colored urine without sediment or foul odor. Verbal instruction and assistance needed with insertion of catheter. Demonstrates eagerness and ability to learn but has difficulty with identifying urethral meatus. Expresses concerns about buying disposable catheters. PLAN: Will contact MD re: need for social worker to assist with financial concerns impacting care. Continue to instruct in intermittent self-catheterization. Discharge from home health service when able to demonstrate self-care.

*N*ursing *P*rocedure 6.6

Care of the Indwelling Catheter

☒ EQUIPMENT

- 2 pair disposable gloves
- 2 clean washcloths
- Soap
- Basin of warm water
- Towel

Purpose

To prevent buildup of debris around insertion site
To prevent urinary tract infection
To provide adequate hygiene

Desired Outcomes (sample)

Client maintains clean catheter without buildup of debris.
Client/caregiver verbalizes/demonstrates appropriate technique for cleaning catheter.
Client verbalizes signs and symptoms of urinary tract infection (UTI).

Assessment

Assessment should focus on the following:

Client/caregiver manual dexterity
Client/caregiver knowledge of procedure and signs of urinary tract infection
Client/caregiver knowledge of UTI prevention
Appearance of meatus and overall perineal area
Appearance of urine

Outcome Identification and Planning

Key Goals and Sample Goal Criteria

The client will:

Demonstrate ability to clean indwelling catheter correctly.
Verbalize signs and symptoms of UTI.

Special Considerations

Geriatric
Many elderly clients are prone to the development of UTIs.

IMPLEMENTATION

Action	Rationale
1. Wash hands.	*Reduces microorganisms*
2. Explain procedure to client and caregiver.	*Reduces anxiety*
3. Assist the client into supine position.	*Positions client; allows optimal visualization of perineal area*
4. Assess color, amount, and consistency of urine.	*Notes if urine appearance is normal*
5. Don gloves.	*Prevents transfer of micro-organisms*
6. Expose and assess the perineum (female) or meatus (males). For the uncircumcised male, the foreskin should be retracted to clean the glans, then replace the foreskin. (Note: If unable to replace the foreskin after it has been retracted, notify physician immediately.)	*Determines if irritation or signs of infection present* *Avoids swelling from constriction of blood vessels. This could cause local tissue damage and necrosis.*
7. Perform perineal care. Females: Wash front to back. Males: Wash from tip of penis back. Rinse and pat dry.	*Cleanses perineum*
8. Change water and gloves.	*Prepares for cleaning of catheter*
9. Gently grasp tip of catheter at insertion site and wipe from tip of catheter down (toward drainage tubing), until reaching drainage tubing. Take care in holding catheter tip so that it is not dislodged.	*Prevents pulling organisms toward meatus* *Prevents dislodgment*

Action	Rationale
When handling catheter tubing, always hold in manner that urine does not flow back into bladder.	*Prevents cross-contamination*
- Repeat several times, rewetting washcloth with soap and water each time.	
- Rinse and pat dry in the same manner.	
10. Dry catheter from tip downward.	*Prevents undue moistness which sets up medium for infection*
11. Replace clothing.	
12. Discard, clean, and replace equipment properly.	
13. Wash hands.	
14. Teach client/caregiver the following in regard to maintaining the catheter between visits:	
- Correct cleansing technique for female/male perineal care	*Teaches appropriate care and maintenance of procedure, and prevention of cross-contamination with subsequent UTI*
- Perform catheter care at least once per day, and preferably more with morning and evening bath. Also perform care after bowel movements.	
- Do not hold catheter tubing so that urine flows back into bladder.	
- If insertion site redness or abnormal urine is noted, notify nurse.	

Evaluation

Were desired outcomes achieved?

DOCUMENTATION

The following should be noted on the visit note:

- Procedure performed and taught
- Color, amount, and consistency of urine
- Appearance of meatus and perineum
- Complaints of client discomfort
- Ability/inability of client/caregiver to perform procedure
- Disposition of specimen, if obtained

Sample Documentation

DATE	TIME	
2/20/99	1800	Catheter care performed on client. Urine cloudy yellow, foul odor, volume 600 mL. Slight redness noted at catheter insertion site. Perineal care given prior to catheter care. Will return for observation of daughter performing procedure tomorrow and teaching of signs of UTI.

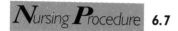

*N*ursing *P*rocedure **6.7**

Bladder Scanning

⊠ EQUIPMENT

- Bladder scanning device (Fig. 6.7)
  (BVI for home use)
- Ultrasound gel pad (or gel)
- Washcloth
- Soap

Purpose

Evaluates bladder volume noninvasively to determine need for
  catheterization to empty bladder
Assists in evaluating general bladder function

Desired Outcomes (sample)

Clients maintain urine output of at least 250 mL per 8 hours.
Client verbalizes no lower abdominal pain.
Client achieves residual volume of less than 100 mL.

Assessment

Assessment should focus on the following:

Medical diagnosis (urinary retention, urinary incontinence,
  stroke, spinal cord injury, or other pertinent diagnosis)
Physician order for use of bladder scanning
Bladder palpation for fullness
Patterns of urine amounts on previous voidings or catheteriza-
  tions
Previous residual urine volumes, if applicable
Time of last bladder emptying
Incontinent episodes

Outcome Identification and Planning

Key Goals and Sample Goal Criteria
The client will:

Maintain urine output of at least 250 mL per 8 hours

Verbalize relief of abdominal pain
Maintain a nonpalpable bladder
Residual volume of less than 100 mL.

Special Considerations

Bladder scanning has been associated with less urinary tract infections (UTIs) in some research studies.

Geriatric

Urinary incontinence is a significant problem for many elderly clients. Bladder scanning is used in many geriatric rehabilitation settings, as they are prone to the development of UTIs.

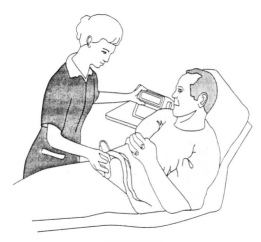

FIGURE 6.7

IMPLEMENTATION

Action	Rationale
1. Wash hands.	*Reduces microorganisms*
2. Explain procedure to client.	*Reduces anxiety*
3. Have client void, if applicable, then assist the client into supine position.	*Used as part of the procedure for determining post-void residual* *Positions client for obtaining accurate readings*

Action	Rationale
4. Expose the lower abdomen.	*Accesses location of bladder*
5. Palpate the symphysis pubis.	*Identifies starting point for scan*
6. Apply gel pad over bladder area.	
7. Press scan button (see Fig. 6.7).	*Obtains bladder volume*
8. Check aiming screen.	*Verifies correct position of scanhead*
9. Note the final calculated volume reading on the display screen in 10 seconds.	*Obtains calculated bladder volume*
10. Turn machine off.	
11. Wash gel off client.	*Removes gel*
12. Lower clothing top.	*Reclothes client*
13. Clean and store bladder scanning device according to manufacturer's instructions.	

Evaluation

Were desired outcomes achieved?

DOCUMENTATION

The following should be noted on the visit note:

- Status of bladder on palpation
- Volume amount indicated on bladder scan readings
- Complaints of client discomfort
- Disposition of catheterization as intervention for bladder emptying

---

Sample Documentation

DATE	TIME	
2/20/99	1800	Client has not voided since 1200. Bladder scanning reading volume amount of 450 mL. Straight catheterization done with 450 mL clear yellow urine return.

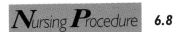

6.8

Care of Nephrostomy Tubes

◼ EQUIPMENT

- Clean drainage bag and connecting tube
- Disposable gloves
- Alcohol swabs
- Sterile gauze pads
- Adhesive tape
- Paper bag for disposal of soiled dressing

Purpose

Allows urine to drain from the kidney to a drainage bag in cases of ureters obstructed by tumors, calculi, strictures, or fistulae

Desired Outcomes (sample)

Maintenance of adequate urine output.
Maintenance of nephrostomy tube without infection or skin breakdown.
Resumption of a high level of independent functioning.

Assessment

Assessment should focus on the following:

Continuous flow of urine
Doctor's order for dressing change
Client's knowledge of the procedure
Rise in temperature, purulent discharge at insertion site, odorous urine, flank pain, integrity of skin around the insertion site
Appearance of urine
Client's cognitive status, vision, and manual dexterity
Family member's or significant other's reliability to care for the tube successfully

Outcome Identification and Planning

Key Goals and Sample Goal Criteria

The client will:

Demonstrate no signs of tube displacement, infection, or skin breakdown

Maintain an adequate urine output

The client and/or caregiver will:

Demonstrate consistent ability to change the dressing, tubing, and drainage bag

Demonstrate consistent ability to irrigate the tube when irrigation is indicated

Demonstrate consistent ability to properly clean used equipment

Verbalize when to call for assistance

Special Considerations

Instruct the patient to notify the health care provider immediately if the tube comes out. The tract closes quickly in 2 to 3 hours.

Keep the drainage bag lower than the nephrostomy tube to enhance gravitational flow.

NEVER IRRIGATE THE NEPHROSTOMY TUBE UNLESS ORDERED.

IMPLEMENTATION

Action	Rationale
1. Explain procedure to client.	*Decreases anxiety*
2. Wash hands.	*Avoids transfer of micro-organisms*
3. Organize equipment within reach.	*Promotes efficiency*
4. Put on disposable gloves.	*Minimizes exposure to body secretions*
5. Disconnect the nephrostomy tube from the used tubing and drainage bag. Clean end of the nephrostomy tube with an alcohol swab.	*Reduces microorganism transfer*
6. Attach the ends of the nephrostomy tube and the connecting tube securely. Don't touch the ends of the tubes.	*Maintains the sterility of system*
7. Check the tubing for kinks.	*Maintains patency of system*

Action	Rationale
8. Change the dressing (Teach client/caregiver to change dressing daily according to doctor's order). Dispose of soiled dressing appropriately.	*Removes medium for micro-organism growth*
9. Gently wash around the nephrostomy tube.	*Decreases microorganisms around the nephrostomy tube*
10. Inspect the skin around the tube. Note color and character of any drainage.	*Redness or white, yellow, or green drainage may indicate infection. Drainage that smells like urine may indicate tube displacement. Either condition should be reported to the doctor immediately.*
11. Fold several gauze pads in half and place them around the base of the nephrostomy tube. Secure the pads with tape. Cover the nephrostomy tube entry site with a dry sterile 4 × 4 and tape securely.	*Protects the skin and is more comfortable for the client*
12. Bring all the tubing forward and tape securely to the body.	*Allows the client to turn without obstructing urine flow or dislodging the tube from the kidney*
13. Keep separate output records for each kidney, if both have tubes.	*Promotes more accurate assessment of kidney function*
14. Irrigate the tube gently with 5 mL of sterile warm saline solution if ordered.	*To determine patency. Alert doctor immediately if tube is not patent.*
15. Wash the used bag and connecting tubing with a weak detergent (Instruct client/caregiver to wash daily). Rinse with plain water and hang on clothes hanger to air dry.	*A biodegradable or chlorine product may erode the bag*
16. Twice weekly client/caregiver should wash the bag and tubing with a solution of 1 part white vinegar to 3 parts water.	*Avoids crystalline buildup*

Evaluation

Were desired outcomes achieved? Are additional services needed?

DOCUMENTATION

The following should be noted on the visit note:

- Teaching done
- Functional limitations that interfere with performance of procedure
- Client tolerance of procedure
- Condition of the insertion site
- Quality and quantity of urinary output
- Plans for future visits
- Discharge planning

Sample Documentation
DATE
9/26/98

Left flank nephrostomy tube site care given and sterile dressing applied. Observed continuous clear amber urine flow. Denies flank pain. Temperature 98.8°F. No redness or drainage noted at insertion site.

*N*ursing *P*rocedure **6.9**

🖐 *Bladder/Catheter Irrigation*

❎ EQUIPMENT

- Two-way indwelling catheter set
  or
- Three-way indwelling catheter set
- Solution ordered for irrigation
- Catheter irrigation kit
  - Large catheter-tip syringe with protective cap
  - Sterile linen saver
  - Graduated irrigation container
- Medication additives, as ordered
- Medication labels
- Two pairs of clean gloves
- Basin of warm water
- Soap
- Washcloth
- Towel
- Linen saver or plastic bag with towel
- Betadine (or recommended antiseptic solution for cleansing irrigation port)
- Catheter clamp or rubber band

Purpose

Maintains bladder and catheter patency by removing or minimizing obstructions such as clots and mucous plugs in bladder
Prevents or treats local bladder inflammation or infection
Instills medications for local bladder treatments

Desired Outcomes (sample)

Client verbalizes decrease in lower abdominal discomfort within 24 hours.
Client maintains urine output of at least 250 mL per 8 hours.

Assessment

Assessment should focus on the following:

Type of irrigation order
Characteristics of urine prior to irrigation, such as hematuria
Amount of urine output
Distension, pain, or tenderness of the lower abdomen
Signs of inflammation or infection of bladder and perineal
   structures
Status of catheter (if already inserted) prior to irrigations

Outcome Identification and Planning

Key Goals and Sample Goal Criteria
The client will:

Verbalize a decrease in lower abdominal discomfort within 2
   days
Demonstrate an absence of bladder obstruction by passing a
   minimum of 250 mL of urine every 8 hours

Special Considerations
When calculating urine output for a client receiving bladder irrigations, subtract the amount of irrigation solution infused
   within a designated period of time from the total amount of
   fluid accumulated within the bag.

IMPLEMENTATION

Action	Rationale
Bladder Irrigation:	
1. Wash hands.	*Reduces microorganism transfer*
2. Explain procedure to client.	*Decreases anxiety*
3. Determine if client is allergic to iodine-based antiseptics or additives to be injected into irrigation fluid.	*Avoids allergic reactions*
4. Provide for privacy.	*Decreases embarrassment*
5. If three-way catheter is ordered and has not already been inserted, don clean gloves, place linen saver under buttocks, and wash and dry perineal area.	*Reduces microorganisms in local perineal area before catheter insertion*

Action	Rationale
6. Discard gloves, bath water, washcloth, and towel; then wash hands.	*Decreases bedside clutter* *Reduces microorganism transfer*
7. Insert catheter using Procedure 6.3 for men or Procedure 6.4 for women.	*Inserts catheter for irrigation*
8. Don clean gloves.	*Reduces nurse's exposure to body secretions*
9. Cleanse irrigation port of catheter with antiseptic solution recommended by agency.	*Removes microorganisms from port* *Decreases contamination*

Catheter Irrigation:
For catheter irrigation using a two-way catheter

1. Open catheter irrigation kit.	
2. Remove catheter-tip syringe from sterile container. Remove sterile cap and place syringe back into sterile container. Hold cap between fingers, being careful not to contaminate the open end.	*Ensures continued sterility of syringe tip while allowing use of sterile cap to protect drainage tubing tip*
3. Fill container with saline or ordered irrigant and fill syringe.	*Prepares syringe for irrigation process*
4. Disinfect the drainage tubing–catheter connection using an antimicrobial agent recommended by the agency.	*Decreases microorganisms at the connection site*
5. Open sterile linen saver and spread onto bed near catheter.	*Provides sterile field*
6. Disconnect catheter and drainage tubing. If 3-way catheter is present, use the irrigation port. Place cap over drainage tube tip, being careful to keep catheter end sterile. Lie capped tubing onto linen saver.	*Maintains sterility of drainage tubing for reconnection*

Action	Rationale
7. Remove syringe from container and insert tip securely into catheter using sterile technique or port.	*Re-establishes closed sterile system for irrigation*
8. Slowly infuse irrigant into catheter until full amount of ordered fluid has been infused or patient complains of inability to tolerate additional fluid infusion.	*Minimizes discomfort caused by rapid or excessive fluid infusion*
9. Clamp catheter by bending end above syringe tip and remove the syringe. Disinfect the catheter end with antimicrobial agent. Remove cap from the drainage tubing and insert it into catheter end.	*Prevents leakage of irrigant from catheter* *Minimizes microorganisms at connection site*
10. Repeat irrigation at frequency ordered.	*Re-establishes closed bladder drainage system*
11. Remove linen saver.	
12. Discard gloves and wash hands.	
13. Record urinary output on intake and output flow sheet.	

Evaluation

Were desired outcomes achieved?

DOCUMENTATION

The following should be noted on the visit note:

- Amount, color, and consistency of fluid obtained
- Type and amount of irrigation solution and medication additives administered
- Infusion rate
- Abdominal assessment
- Urine output (total fluid volume measured minus irrigation solution instilled)
- Discomfort verbalized by client

Sample Documentation

DATE	TIME	
7/6/98	1330	Three-way irrigation catheter inserted. Bladder irrigated with 200 mL sterile normal saline irrigant in 60 mL increments. Client reports "cramping sensation in lower abdomen as if having spasms." Urine and irrigant clear without sediment or evidence of blood clots.

*N*ursing *P*rocedure 6.10

🖐 *Hemodialysis Shunt, Graft, and Fistula Care*

ⓧ EQUIPMENT

- Nonsterile gloves
- Two pairs of sterile gloves
- Antiseptic cleansing agent or antiseptic swabs
- Topical antiseptic, if ordered
- Sterile 4 × 4-inch gauze pads
- Kling wrap
- Cannula clamps

Purpose

Maintains patency of access for dialysis
Detects complications of a hemodialysis access site related to infection, occlusion, or cannula separation

Desired Outcomes (sample)

A bruit is present on auscultation, a thrill is palpable. There is no edema, redness, pain, drainage, or bleeding at the hemodialysis access site.

Assessment

Assessment should focus on the following:

Status of fistula, graft, or cannula site and dressing
Location of shunt, fistula, or graft
Vital signs
Pulses distal to shunt, fistula, or graft
Color and temperature of extremity in which access is located
Presence of pain or numbness in extremity in which access is located
Time of last dressing change

Outcome Identification and Planning

Key Goals and Sample Goal Criterion

The client will:

Maintain a functional access site as evidenced by the presence of a bruit on auscultation and a thrill on palpation and by the absence of edema, redness, pain, drainage, or bleeding

Special Considerations

A potential complication related to the presence of the shunt is cannula separation. Hemorrhage can occur if the shunt is not clamped off until a new cannula is inserted; therefore, a pair of cannula clamps should be kept with the client at all times.

HINT

To enable client to change dressings between nursing visits, secure the dressing with a stockinette dressing that the client can roll down over Kerlix and remove old dressing and roll up to secure new dressing.

IMPLEMENTATION

Action	Rationale
1. Wash hands.	*Reduces microorganism transfer*
2. Explain procedure to client.	*Decreases anxiety*
3. Open several 4 × 4 packages and soak several gauze pads with antiseptic solution *or* open antiseptic swabs and position for easy access. Keep one package of gauze 4 × 4s dry.	*Facilitates cleaning process; provides gauze to cover shunt*
4. Don clean gloves.	*Reduces nurse's exposure to body secretions*
5. Remove old dressing, if present, and check access site.	*Exposes access site*
6. Discard dressing and gloves.	*Removes contaminated items*
7. Wash hands and don sterile gloves.	*Avoids site contamination*

Action	Rationale
8. Cleanse access area with antiseptic agent recommended by agency: for shunt care, begin at exit areas and work outward, discarding antiseptic swab or folded gauze pad after each wipe.	*Reduces contamination*
9. Lightly place two or three fingertips over access site and assess for presence of thrill (a palpable vibration should be present); assess site for extreme warmth or coolness.	*Tests for adequate blood flow through shunt*
10. Apply topical ointment, if ordered.	*Prevents infection*
11. Place dry sterile gauze pads over access site.	*Reduces site contamination*
12. For shunt, apply Kerlix or Kling wrap over gauze pads and around extremity (wrap firmly enough that dressing is secure but not so tight as to occlude blood flow) and tape securely; leave small piece of shunt tubing visible.	*Prevents accidental dislodgment of cannula* *Allows for visualization of continuous blood flow*
13. Discard equipment and gloves; then wash hands.	*Reduces spread of infection*
14. Instruct client/caregiver to assess status of dressing, access site, and pulses in affected extremity every 2 hours.	*Monitors frequently for complications*
15. During early postoperative period, inform client, family, and staff of the following care instructions: - If shunt is in arm or leg, keep extremity elevated on pillow until instructed otherwise.	*Prevents unnecessary loss of access site due to occlusion, infection, or cannula separation*

Action	Rationale
- Keep extremity as still as possible.	
- Do not apply pressure to or lift heavy objects with extremity. (If shunt is in leg, crutches will be used for a short while when client becomes ambulatory)	*Prevents rupture and pain*
- Do not allow access area to get wet during showering, bathing, or swimming.	
16. Inform client and caregiver of the following care instructions:	*Facilitates cooperation with care of site, reduces fear, and prevents undue injury*
- Do not allow the performance of the following procedures on the affected extremity:	
(1) Blood pressure assessment or any procedure that might occlude blood flow	*Prevents occlusion of blood flow*
(2) Venipuncture or any procedure involving a needlestick.	*Prevents injury, clotting, and infection*
- Avoid restricting blood flow of affected extremity with tight-fitting clothes, watches, name bands, knee-high stockings, antiembolytic hose, restraints, and so forth.	*Prevents restriction of blood flow and injury to graft/ shunt/fistula area*
- Notify nurse or doctor immediately if bleeding or cannula disconnection is noted.	*Prevents excessive bleeding*

Evaluation

Were desired outcomes achieved?

DOCUMENTATION

The following should be noted on the visit note:

- Location of access site
- Status of site and dressing
- Vital signs
- Status of pulses distal to access area
- Color and temperature of extremity in which access is located
- Presence of pain or numbness in extremity in which access is located

Sample Documentation		
DATE	**TIME**	
2/6/98	1115	Left forearm Goretex-graft site care given. Radial pulse normal (3+) in left arm. Left fingers pink with 2-second capillary refill. Client denies pain or numbness of left arm. Thrill palpable at graft site. Site cleaned with Beta-dine solution and sterile dressing applied.

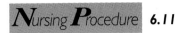

*N*ursing *P*rocedure **6.11**

Fecal Impaction Removal

EQUIPMENT

- Three pairs of nonsterile gloves
- Packet of water-soluble lubricant
- Bedpan
- Linen saver or plastic bag with towel
- Basin of warm water
- Soap
- Washcloth
- Towel
- Air freshener

Purpose

Manually removes hardened stool blocking normal evacuation
    passage in lower part of colon
Relieves pain and discomfort
Facilitates normal peristalsis
Prevents rectal and anal injury

Desired Outcomes (sample)

Client has normal bowel movement within 24 hours.
Client verbalizes pain relief within 1 hour.

Assessment

Assessment should focus on the following:

Agency policy and physician's order regarding performance of
    procedure
Status of anus and skin surrounding buttocks (ie, presence of
    ulcerations, tears, hemorrhoids, and excoriation)
Indicators of impaction (ie, lower abdominal and rectal pain,
    seepage of liquid stools, inability to pass stool, general malaise,
    urge to defecate without being able to do so, nausea and vomit-
    ing, shortness of breath)
Abdominal status
Vital signs before, during, and after removal
Time of last bowel movement and usual bowel evacuation pat-
    tern

History of factors that may contraindicate or present complications during impaction removal (such as cardiac instability or spinal cord injury)

Client history regarding dietary habits (ie, intake of bulk and liquids), changes in activity pattern, frequency of use of laxatives or enemas

Client knowledge regarding promotion of normal bowel elimination

Medications that decrease peristalsis, such as narcotics

Outcome Identification and Planning

Key Goals and Sample Goal Criteria
The client will:

Have bowel movement within 24 hours of impaction removal
Verbalize relief of pain within 1 hour of impaction removal

Special Considerations
Digital removal of impacted stool stretches the anal sphincter causing vagal stimulation. As a result, electrical impulses may be inhibited at the sinoatrial node of the heart causing a decrease in pulse rate as well as dysrhythmias. This procedure is, therefore, contraindicated in cardiac clients.

Certain tube feeding formulas (hypertonic) promote constipation and fecal impaction. Check medication record and nutritional supplement list if impaction occurs.

Geriatric

Many elderly clients are especially prone to dysrhythmias and palpitations related to vagal stimulation because of chronic cardiac problems. Observe such clients closely during procedure.

Many elderly clients are especially prone to fecal impaction because of decreased metabolic rate, decreased activity levels, inadequate dietary intake, and tendency to overuse laxatives and enemas as a routine means of promoting bowel evacuation. A thorough history related to these factors should be obtained.

IMPLEMENTATION

Action	Rationale
1. Wash hands.	*Reduces microorganism transfer*
2. Explain procedure to	*Reduces anxiety*

Action	Rationale
client, admitting that the procedure will cause some discomfort.	
3. Assess blood pressure and rate and rhythm of pulse.	*Provides baseline data in case of complications*
4. Provide privacy; drape client so that only buttocks are exposed.	*Reduces embarrassment*
5. Don gloves, placing one on nondominant hand and two gloves on dominant hand.	*Decreases nurse's exposure to body secretions in case hardened fecal mass tears glove*
6. Position client in side-lying position with knees flexed.	*Allows good exposure of anal opening*
7. Place linen saver under buttocks.	*Prevents soiling of linens*
8. Place bedpan on bed within easy reach.	*Facilitates disposal of fecal mass*
9. Generously lubricate first two gloved fingers of dominant hand.	*Prevents injury to anus and rectum*
10. Gently spread buttocks with nondominant hand.	*Exposes anal opening*
11. Instruct client to take slow, deep breaths through mouth.	*Relaxes sphincter muscles facilitating entry*
12. Insert index finger into rectum (directed toward umbilicus) until fecal mass is palpable (Fig. 6.11).	*Prevents rectal trauma*
13. Gently break up hardened stool and remove one piece at a time until all of stool is removed; place stool in bedpan as it is removed.	*Manually removes impacted stool*
14. Observe client for untoward reactions or unusual discomfort during stool removal.	*Prevents complications from vagal stimulation*
15. Obtain pulse and blood pressure if unusual reaction is suspected.	

Action	Rationale

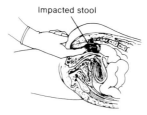

Impacted stool

FIGURE 6.11

Action	Rationale
16. Remove finger, wipe excess lubricant from perineal area, and release buttocks.	*Promotes comfort*
17. Empty bedpan and discard gloves.	*Promotes clean environment*
18. Wash hands.	*Reduces microorganism transfer*
19. Don new pair of gloves.	
20. Wash, rinse, and dry buttocks.	
21. Reposition client.	*Promotes comfort and safety*
22. Leave bedpan within easy reach.	*Impaction removal may have stimulated defecation reflex*
23. Discard bathwater and gloves.	*Promotes clean environment*
24. Spray air freshener at bedside.	*Eliminates odor*
25. Wash hands.	*Reduces microorganism transfer*

Evaluation

Were desired outcomes achieved?

DOCUMENTATION

The following should be noted on the visit note:

- Color, consistency, and amount of stool removed
- Condition of anus and surrounding area
- Status of vital signs before and after removal
- Description of adverse reactions during removal
- Abdominal assessment before and after removal

- Presence of discomfort after removal
- Client teaching regarding prevention of fecal impaction

Sample Documentation

DATE	TIME	
6/6/98	1100	Large, dark brown, impacted stool removed manually with no signs of adverse effects. Pulse, 75 and regular before removal and 68 and regular afterwards. Bowel sounds auscultated in four quadrants after removal. Abdomen soft and nondistended. Discussed with client factors preventing constipation and impaction. Factors verbalized by client.

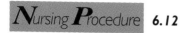

Nursing Procedure 6.12

Enema Administration

☒ EQUIPMENT

- Two pairs of nonsterile gloves
- Enema set-up (administration bag or bucket with rectal tubing, castile soap, protective plastic linen saver, packet water soluble lubricant)
- Solution for enema (for adults, 750 to 1000 mL)
- Bath thermometer (or use wrist)
- Bedpan
- Linen saver or plastic bag with towel
- Basin of warm water
- Soap
- Washcloth
- Towel
- Air freshener

Purpose

Relieves abdominal distension and discomfort
Stimulates peristalsis
Resumes normal bowel evacuation
Cleanses and evacuates colon

Desired Outcomes (sample)

Client evacuates moderate to large stool.
Client verbalizes pain relief within 1 hour.

Assessment

Assessment should focus on the following:

Physician's order for type of enema
Agency policy and physician's order regarding performance of procedure
Status of anus and skin surrounding buttocks (ie, presence of ulcerations, tears, hemorrhoids, and excoriation)
Indicators of constipation (ie, lower abdominal pain or hard, small stools)
Abdominal status

Vital signs before, during, and after enema

Time of last bowel movement and usual bowel evacuation pattern

History of factors that may contraindicate enema or present complications during enema administration (such as cardiac instability)

Client history regarding dietary habits (eg, intake of bulk and liquids), changes in activity pattern, frequency of use of laxatives or enemas

Client knowledge regarding promotion of normal bowel evacuation

Client medications that decrease peristalsis, such as narcotics

Outcome Identification and Planning

Key Goals and Sample Goal Criteria

The client will:

Evacuate moderate to large amount of stool after enema

Verbalize relief of pain within 1 hour after enema

Special Considerations

Geriatric

Many elderly clients are especially prone to dysrhythmias and palpitations related to vagal stimulation because of chronic cardiac problems. Observe such clients closely during procedure.

Many elderly clients are especially prone to constipation and impaction because of decreased metabolic rate, decreased activity levels, inadequate dietary intake, and tendency to overuse laxatives and enemas as a routine means of promoting bowel evacuation. A thorough history related to these factors should be obtained.

If anal sphincter control is weak, may want to cut tip of a baby bottle nipple, then insert enema tubing through nipple. This will facilitate solution retention.

 Cost-cutting Tip

If bath thermometer is not available to test solution temperature, use the inner aspect of your forearm to test the temperature.

IMPLEMENTATION

Action	Rationale
1. Wash hands.	*Reduces microorganism transfer*
2. Explain procedure to client, admitting that the procedure may cause some mild discomfort.	*Reduces anxiety*
3. Prepare solution, making certain that temperature of solution is lukewarm (about 105°F to 110°F). May use wrist to test temperature.	*Reduces abdominal cramping during procedure*
4. Prime tubing with fluid and close tubing clamp.	*Prevents distension of colon and abdominal discomfort from air*
5. Hold container of solution (or hang on door hook) so that enema solution hangs no more than 18 to 24 inches above buttocks (Fig. 6.12).	*Slows rate of fluid infusion and prevents cramping*
6. Provide privacy by draping client so that only buttocks are exposed.	*Reduces embarrassment*
7. Don gloves.	*Decreases nurse's exposure to body secretions*
8. Place linen saver under buttocks.	*Prevents soiling of linens*
9. Position client in side-lying position with knees flexed, if not contraindicated. Left side is preferable.	*Allows good exposure of anal opening*
10. Lubricate 4 to 5 inches of catheter tip.	*Reduces anorectal trauma*
11. Place bedpan on bed within easy reach.	*Facilitates disposal of enema solution*
12. Obtain pillows to place on edge of bed as shield from falling.	*Prevents injury due to fall*
13. Gently spread buttocks with nondominant hand.	*Exposes anal opening*
14. Instruct client to take slow, deep breaths through mouth.	*Relaxes sphincter muscles, facilitating entry*
15. With dominant hand, in-	*Prevents rectal trauma*

Action	Rationale

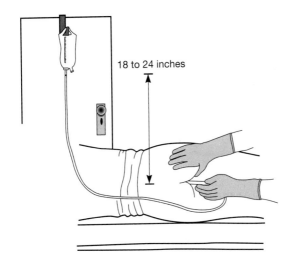

18 to 24 inches

FIGURE 6.12

sert rectal tube into rectum (directed towards umbilicus) about 3 to 4 inches and hold in place with dominant hand.

Places tube in far enough to effect cleansing of colon

16. Release tubing clamp.

Allows solution to flow

17. Allow solution to flow into colon slowly, observing client closely.

Avoids cramping

18. If cramping, extreme anxiety, or complaint of inability to retain solution occurs:
    - Lower solution container.
    - Clamp or pinch tubing off for a few minutes.
    - Resume instillation of solution.

Decreases or stops solution flow to allow client to readjust and gain composure

Action	Rationale
19. Administer all of solution or as much as client can tolerate; be sure to clamp tubing just before all of solution clears tubing.	*Delivers enough solution for proper effect* *Prevents infusion of air*
20. Slowly remove rectal tubing while gently holding buttocks together.	*Prevents accidental evacuation of solution*
21. Remind client to hold solution for amount of time appropriate for type of enema.	*Ensures optimal effect*
22. Reposition client.	*Facilitates comfort*
23. Place bedpan or bedside commode within easy reach.	*Provides means of contacting nurse* *Provides receptacle for enema solution*
24. Discard or restore equipment appropriately.	*Promotes clean environment*
25. Wash hands.	*Reduces microorganism transfer*
26. Check client every 5 to 10 minutes.	*Reassesses client condition and results of enema*
27. Assist client on bedpan or toilet after retention time has expired.	*Facilitates evacuation of solution*
28. Spray air freshener after evacuation.	*Eliminates odor*
29. Wash hands.	*Reduces microorganism transfer*

Evaluation

Were desired outcomes achieved?

DOCUMENTATION

The following should be noted on the visit note:

- Type and amount of solution used
- Color, consistency, and amount of stool return
- Condition of anus and surrounding area
- Status of vital signs before and after enema
- Description of adverse reactions during enema
- Abdominal assessment before and after enema
- Presence of discomfort after enema
- Client teaching regarding prevention of constipation

Sample Documentation

DATE	TIME	
2/6/98	2200	Soap suds enema (750 mL) given. Large, dark brown stool returned from enema. No signs of adverse effects. Bowel sounds auscultated in four quadrants. Abdomen soft and nondistended. Discussed factors for promoting normal bowel evacuation with client. Factors verbalized by client.

*N*ursing *P*rocedure **6.13**

✍ *Colostomy Stoma Care*

⊠ EQUIPMENT

- Two pairs of peristomal gloves (add pair for client, if desired)
- Graduated container
- Two linen savers or plastic bags with towel
- Basin of warm water
- Mild soap (without oils, perfumes, or creams)
- Washcloth
- Towel
- Air freshener
- New pouch appliance
- Scissors
- Pen or pencil
- Mirror
- Peristomal skin paste or powder
- Ostomy pouch deodorizer
- Toilet paper

Purpose

Maintains integrity of stoma and *peristomal* skin (skin surrounding stoma)
Prevents lesions, ulcerations, excoriation, and other skin breakdown caused by fecal contaminants
Prevents infection
Promotes general comfort
Promotes positive self-concept

Desired Outcomes (sample)

No redness, edema, swelling, tears, breaks, ulceration, or fistulas appear at stoma area.
Client performs procedure with 100% accuracy.

Assessment

Assessment should focus on the following:

Appearance of stoma and peristomal skin (should be pink and shiny)
Characteristics of fecal waste

Abdominal status
Teaching needs, ability, and preference of client for self-care

Outcome Identification and Planning

Key Goals and Sample Goal Criteria

The client will:

Maintain intact skin integrity of stoma and peristomal skin, as evidenced by absence of tears, excoriation, ulcerations, redness, edema, and pain

Demonstrate with 100% accuracy self-care of stoma within 2 weeks

Special Considerations

Once client (or family member) shows readiness to begin learning how to perform ostomy care, supervise client performance of procedure until it is accomplished accurately and comfortably.

Ostomy care alters an individual's self-concept significantly; perform care unhurriedly, and discuss care in a positive manner with the client.

The United Ostomy Association is a good resource for ostomy clients and families.

HINT

Clients may dry the skin after cleaning the stoma by using a hair dryer on a low setting.

IMPLEMENTATION

Action	Rationale
1. Wash hands.	*Reduces microorganism transfer*
2. Explain general procedure to client.	*Reduces anxiety*
3. Explain each step as it is performed, allowing client and caregiver to ask questions or perform any part of the procedure.	*Reinforces detailed instructions client will need to perform self-care*
4. Provide privacy.	*Reduces embarrassment*
5. Position mirror	*Permits client to observe and learn procedure*

Action	Rationale
6. Don gloves.	*Avoids nurse's exposure to body secretions*
7. Place linen saver on abdomen around and below stoma opening.	*Prevents seepage of feces onto skin*
8. Carefully remove pouch appliance (bag and skin barrier) and place in plastic waste bag; remove pouch and skin barrier by gently lifting corner with fingers of dominant hand while pressing skin downward with fingers of nondominant hand; remove small sections at a time until entire barrier wafer is removed.	*Avoids tearing skin*
9. Empty pouch; measure, discard, and record amount of fecal contents (see Procedure 6.15).	*Maintains records*
10. Wash hands and reglove.	*Reduces contamination*
11. Gently clean entire stoma and peristomal skin with gauze or washcloth soaked in warm soapy water (if some of fecal matter is difficult to remove, leave wet gauze or cloth on area for a few minutes before gently removing fecal matter); rinse and pat dry.	*Removes fecal matter from skin and stoma opening*
12. Dry skin thoroughly and apply new pouch device (see Procedure 6.14).	*Provides skin protection from fecal contaminants*
13. Remove gloves and restore or discard all equipment appropriately.	*Promotes clean environment*
14. Spray room deodorizer, if needed.	*Eliminates unpleasant odor*
15. Wash hands.	*Reduces microorganism transfer*

Evaluation

Were desired outcomes achieved?

DOCUMENTATION

The following should be noted on the visit note:

- Color, consistency, and amount of feces in pouch
- Condition of stoma and peristomal skin
- Abdominal assessment
- Emotional status of client
- Verbal and nonverbal indicators of altered self-concept during procedure
- Verbal and nonverbal indicators of readiness to perform self-care
- Teaching and client participation in performance of procedure
- Additional teaching needs of client

Sample Documentation		
DATE	**TIME**	
2/3/98	1600	Stoma care performed by client with 50% accuracy. Discarded large amount of semiformed brown stool. Stoma pink without excoriation or abnormal discharge. New pouch applied. Additional instruction needed.

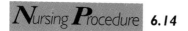

Nursing Procedure 6.14

Colostomy Pouch Application

EQUIPMENT

- Three pairs of peristomal gloves
- Graduated container
- Two linen savers
- Basin of warm water
- Mild soap (without oils, perfumes, or creams)
- Washcloth
- Towel
- Air freshener
- New pouch appliance
- Scissors
- Pen or pencil
- Mirror
- Peristomal skin paste or powder
- Ostomy pouch deodorizer

Purpose

Provides clean ostomy pouch for fecal evacuation
Reduces odor from overuse of old pouch
Promotes positive self-image

Desired Outcomes (sample)

No seepage of fecal material from pouch occurs.
Pouch is secured without dislodgment.
Client demonstrates application of new pouch appliance with
   100% accuracy.

Assessment

Assessment should focus on the following:

Appearance of stoma and peristomal skin
Characteristics of fecal waste
Type of appliance needed for type of colostomy, nature of
   drainage, and client preference
Teaching needs, ability, and preference of client for self-care

Outcome Identification and Planning

Key Goals and Sample Goal Criteria

The client will:

Show no signs of seepage of fecal contents onto skin
Maintain an intact pouch without accidental disconnection
Demonstrate with 100% accuracy self-application of ostomy
pouch

Special Considerations

A wide variety of ostomy appliances is available to meet clients'
personal preferences and needs. Minor variations in techniques of application may be needed to ensure adequate skin
protection and pouch security. Some ostomy appliances are
permanent and should be discarded only every few months.
Consult appliance manuals for complete information regarding application and recommended usage time for the pouch.

The United Ostomy Association is a good resource for ostomy
clients and families.

Once client (or family member) shows readiness to learn how to
perform ostomy care, supervise client performance of the procedure until it is accomplished accurately and comfortably.

Ostomy care alters an individual's self-concept significantly.
Perform care unhurriedly and discuss care in a positive manner with the client.

DO NOT USE ASPIRIN in pouch—this could cause stomal irritation and bleeding.

IMPLEMENTATION

Action	Rationale
1. Wash hands.	*Reduces microorganism transfer*
2. Explain general procedure to client.	*Reduces anxiety*
3. Explain each step as it is performed, allowing client to ask questions or perform any part of the procedure.	*Reinforces detailed instructions client will need in order to perform self-care*
4. Provide privacy.	*Reduces embarrassment*
5. Don gloves and offer client gloves.	*Avoids nurse's exposure to body secretions*
6. Place towel or linen saver around stoma pouch close to stoma, remove old	*Removes old pouch for new pouch application* *Maintains clean environment*

Action	Rationale
pouch, and discard contents; discard gloves.	
7. Wash hands and don fresh gloves.	*Reduces microorganism transfer*
8. Assess stoma and peristomal skin.	*Provides assessment data*
9. Perform stoma care (see Procedure 6.13)	
10. Wash hands.	*Reduces microorganism ransfer*
11. Position mirror.	*Allows client to observe and learn procedure*
12. Reglove.	
13. Place linen saver in client's lap or on bed under client's side where colostomy tubing is located.	*Protects skin and linens during pouch change*
14. Measure stoma with measuring guide.	*Provides for accurate fit of pouch appliances*
15. Leaving intact adhesive covering of skin-barrier wafer (a flat platelike piece, without pouch attached, that fits on skin around stoma), draw a circle on adhesive liner the same size as stoma; cut out circle.	*Cuts barrier to size appropriate for stoma*
16. Cut circular adhesive back of ostomy pouch so that it measures about ⅛ inch larger than actual stoma size.	*Allows pouch to be placed over and around stoma without adhering to stoma membrane*
17. Open bottom of pouch and apply a small amount of pouch deodorizer, if client prefers; reclose pouch securely.	*Reduces odor and embarrassment* *Avoids leakage of feces*
18. Remove adhesive covering of skin-barrier wafer and place wafer on skin with hole centered over stoma; HOLD IN PLACE FOR ABOUT 30 SECONDS.	*Adheres barrier wafer to skin* *Warmth of skin and fingers enhances adhesiveness once wafer makes contact with skin*

Action	Rationale
19. Apply stomal paste or powder to any exposed skin between skin-barrier wafer and stoma.	*Prevents skin irritation of uncovered peristomal skin*
20. Remove adhesive covering of back of pouch and center pouch over stoma, and place on skin-barrier wafer. (If pouch has a flange, snap pouch onto circular flange on barrier wafer as in Fig. 6.14).	*Secures pouch for collection of feces*
21. Remove gloves; restore or discard all equipment appropriately.	*Promotes clean environment*
22. Spray room freshener, if needed.	*Eliminates unpleasant odor*
23. Wash hands.	*Reduces microorganism transfer*

Evaluation

Were desired outcomes achieved?

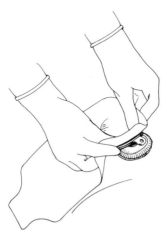

FIGURE 6.14

DOCUMENTATION

The following should be noted on the visit note:

- Color, consistency, and amount of feces in pouch
- Condition of stoma and peristomal skin
- Abdominal assessment
- Emotional status of client
- Verbal and nonverbal indicators of altered self-concept during procedure
- Verbal and nonverbal indicators of readiness to perform self-care
- Teaching and client participation in performance of procedure
- Additional teaching needs of client
- Type of appliance client prefers

Sample Documentation

DATE	TIME	
2/3/98	1100	New colostomy pouch applied by client with 100% accuracy. Discarded large amount of semi-formed brown stool. Stoma pink without excoriation or abnormal discharge. Client verbalized anxiety about how wife will accept assisting with his care and stated preference for pouch appliance with flange rings.

Nursing **P**rocedure *6.15*

🖐 *Colostomy Pouch Evacuation and Cleaning*

☒ EQUIPMENT

- Three pairs of peristomal gloves
- Bedpan and/or graduate container
- Two linen savers or plastic bags with towel
- Air freshener
- Two washcloths
- Mirror
- Ostomy pouch deodorizer
- Toilet paper
- Paper towels

Purpose

Removes fecal material from ostomy pouch
Cleans pouch for reuse
Maintains integrity of stoma and peristomal skin
Promotes general comfort
Promotes positive self-concept

Desired Outcomes (sample)

No redness, edema, swelling, tears, breaks, ulceration, or fistulas are present in stoma area.
Client performs procedure with 100% accuracy within 2 weeks.
Client verbalizes feelings about fecal diversion.

Assessment

Assessment should focus on the following:

Appearance of stoma and peristomal skin (should be pink and shiny)
Characteristics of fecal waste
Abdominal status
Type of ostomy appliance (permanent or temporary) and condition of appliance
Teaching needs, ability, and preference of client for self-care

Outcome Identification and Planning

Key Goals and Sample Goal Criteria

The client will:

Maintain skin integrity of stoma and peristomal area, as evidenced by absence of tears, excoriation, ulcerations, redness, edema, and pain

Demonstrate self-care of stoma within 2 weeks with 100% accuracy

Verbalize feelings about the colostomy

Special Considerations

Instruct females to carry waist-size piece of elastic in purse to position clothing out of way when not at home.

Once client (or family member) shows readiness to learn how to perform ostomy care, supervise client performance of the procedure until it is accomplished accurately and comfortably.

Ostomy care alters an individual's self-concept significantly. Perform care unhurriedly and discuss care in a positive manner with the client.

The United Ostomy Association is a good resource for ostomy clients and families.

IMPLEMENTATION

Action	Rationale
1. Wash hands.	*Reduces microorganism transfer*
2. Explain general procedure to client.	*Reduces anxiety*
3. Explain each step as it is performed, allowing client to ask questions or perform any part of the procedure.	*Reinforces detailed instructions client will need to perform self-care*
4. Provide privacy.	*Reduces embarrassment*
5. Position mirror.	*Allows client to observe and learn procedure*
6. Don gloves.	*Avoids nurse's exposure to body secretions*
7. Place linen saver on abdomen around and below pouch.	*Prevents seepage of feces onto skin*
8. If using toilet, seat client on toilet or in a chair fac-	*Positions client so that feces drain into receptacle*

Action	Rationale
ing toilet, with pouch over toilet; if using bedpan, place pouch over bedpan.	
9. Remove clamp on bottom of pouch and place within easy reach.	*Promotes efficiency*
10. Slowly unfold end of pouch and allow feces to drain into bedpan or toilet (Fig. 6.15.1).	*Removes feces from pouch*

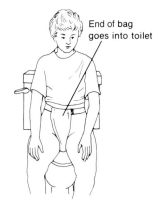

End of bag
goes into toilet

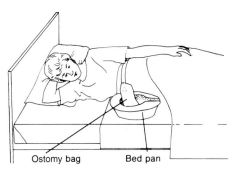

Ostomy bag   Bed pan

FIGURE 6.15.1

Action	Rationale
11. Press sides of lower end of pouch together (Fig. 6.15.2).	*Expels additional feces from pouch*
12. Open lower end of pouch and wipe out with toilet paper.	*Removes excess feces from lower end of pouch*
13. Determine if pouch is suitable for reuse; if not, discard and apply new pouch to skin-barrier wafer.	*Prevents embarrassment due to pouch odor or leakage*
14. Flush toilet or, if using bedpan, take time to resecure end of pouch with rubber band and then empty bedpan. If client has not established good bowel control, go to step 18.	*Reduces client embarrassment and room odor*
15. If client has established good bowel control: - Carefully remove pouch from skin-barrier wafer and wash entire	*Cleanses pouch collector*

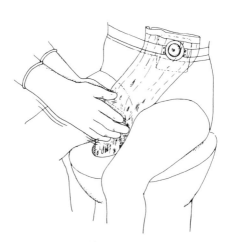

FIGURE 6.15.2

Action	Rationale
pouch out with soap and water	
- Rinse and dry with paper towels	
- Complete steps 16, 17, and 19 through 24.	
16. Wash hands and reglove.	*Reduces microorganism transfer*
17. Wash clamp while in bathroom and dry with paper towel. Proceed to step 19.	*Cleans exterior clamp*
18. Reopen end of pouch and wipe out inside of lower end of pouch with wet washcloth or paper towels.	*Cleans bottom of pouch*
19. Apply pouch deodorizer to lower end of pouch.	*Reduces unpleasant odor*
20. Reclamp pouch with cleaned clamp.	*Prevents leakage of feces*
21. Wipe outside of pouch with clean, wet wash-cloth; be sure to wipe around clamp at bottom of pouch.	*Completes cleaning of pouch*
22. Remove gloves and re-store or discard all equip-ment appropriately.	*Promotes clean environment*
23. Spray room freshener, if needed.	*Eliminates unpleasant odor*
24. Wash hands.	*Reduces microorganism transfer*

Evaluation

Were desired outcomes achieved?

DOCUMENTATION

The following should be noted on the visit note:

- Color, consistency, and amount of feces in pouch
- Condition of stoma and peristomal skin
- Abdominal assessment
- Emotional status of client

- Verbal and nonverbal indicators of altered self-concept during procedure
- Verbal and nonverbal indicators of readiness to perform self-care
- Teaching and client participation in performance of procedure
- Additional teaching needs of client

Sample Documentation

DATE	TIME	
8/31/98	1430	Ostomy pouch cleaning and evacuation performed by client with 100% accuracy. Discarded large amount of semiformed brown stool. Stoma pink without excoriation or abnormal discharge.

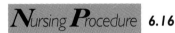 **6.16**

 Colostomy Irrigation

EQUIPMENT

- IV pole or wall hook
- Irrigation bag and tubing
- Irrigation cone
- Water-soluble lubricant
- Commode or commode chair
- Warm saline or tap water
- Antiseptic (optional)
- Bath thermometer
- Two towels
- Two washcloths
- Linen savers
- Bath basin or sink
- Fresh pouch
- Nonsterile gloves

Purpose

Facilitates emptying of colon

Desired Outcomes (sample)

Stool passes freely through stomal opening.
Client demonstrates correct procedure.
Client experiences no excessive cramping or pain during irrigation.

Assessment

Assessment should focus on the following:

Doctor's order for frequency of irrigation and type and amount of solution
Type of colostomy and nature of drainage
Client's ability and preference to perform colostomy care
Client teaching needs

Outcome Identification and Planning

Key Goals and Sample Goal Criteria

The client will:

Show unobstructed passage of stool
Demonstrate correct technique for irrigation
Show no adverse physical reactions to irrigation

Special Considerations

If no stool returns and irrigant is retained, reposition client, apply drainable pouch, if needed. You may have client ambulate, if permissible. Notify doctor if there is no return or if abdominal distension is noted.

If client plans to irrigate colostomy while sitting on commode, teach client the proper procedure and have him or her demonstrate it to you. Correct client's technique, if necessary.

IMPLEMENTATION

Action	Rationale
1. Explain procedure to client and family.	*Reduces anxiety*
2. Wash hands and organize equipment.	*Reduces microorganism transfer and promotes efficiency*
3. Obtain extra lighting, if needed.	
4. Provide for warmth and privacy.	*Promotes comfort and reduces embarrassment*
5. Prepare irrigating solution as follows:	*Ensures proper preparation of solution and tubing*
- Obtain irrigation bag and solution (usually tepid water); use 250 to 500 mL for initial irrigation, 500 to 1000 mL for subsequent irrigations (minimal amounts are recommended).	*Allows bowel to adjust to fluid pressure*
- Check temperature of solution (should feel warm to touch but not hot).	*Prevents injury from hot solution or cramping from cold solution*
- Close tubing clamp.	*Allows better fluid control*
- Fill bag with tap water or ordered solution at	

Action	Rationale
appropriate tempera-ture.	
- Open clamp and expel air from tubing.	*Prevents air infusion into bowel*
- Close off clamp.	
- Hang bag and tubing on pole or hook.	*Permits drainage by gravity*
- Lubricate 3 to 4 inches of tubing tip with water-soluble gel and cover end of tubing.	*Prevents irritation of stomal tissue*
6. Don gloves.	*Prevents nurse's contact with body secretions*
7. Place client comfortably in any of the following positions (place linen saver under client if per-forming procedure in bed):	
- On commode	
- Sitting on chair facing toilet	*Provides for effective irrigation*
- In side-lying position, turned towards side of stomal opening, with head of bed elevated 30 to 45 degrees	
- In supine position	
8. Gently remove existing pouch from stomal area.	*Avoids skin irritation or injury*
9. Assess site for redness, swelling, tenderness, and excoriation.	*Determines need for other skin care measures*
10. Gently wash stomal area with warm soapy water.	*Removes secretions*
11. Rinse with clear water and dry thoroughly.	
12. Apply irrigation sleeve and belt:	*Holds irrigation bag in place to prevent spillage*
- Round opening of irri-gation sleeve fits over stoma	
- Belt fits around waist	
13. Position irrigation bag (with tubing attached) at a height of 18 inches	*Avoids undue pressure on mucosal tissues from rushing of fluid*

Action	Rationale
above stoma (approximately shoulder level).	
14. Place lower end of *drainage* sleeve into toilet or large bedpan and unclamp.	*Provides receptacle for and begins flow of irrigant*
15. Expose stoma through upper opening of sleeve.	
16. Lubricate tip of cone and gently ease into stomal opening (Fig. 6.16.1).	*Prevents escape of bowel content onto skin*
17. Gently insert 3 to 4 inches of irrigation tubing through cone opening into stoma; if tubing does not ease into opening, do not force (Fig. 6.16.2).	*Prevents injury to stomal or bowel tissue*
18. Release irrigation tubing clamp and allow solution to infuse over 10 to 15 minutes.	*Slow infusion prevents cramping from over-distension*
19. Encourage client to take slow, deep breaths as solution is infusing.	*Relaxes client and decreases cramping of bowel*
20. If client complains of cramping, stop infusion for several minutes; then resume infusion slowly.	*Allows bowel time to adjust to fluid*

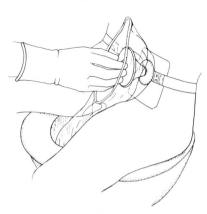

FIGURE 6.16.1

Action	Rationale

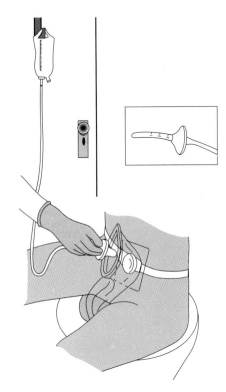

FIGURE 6.16.2

21. Observe for return of fecal material and solution and assess drainage.

Indicates effectiveness of irrigation

22. Remove bottom of sleeve from drainage receptacle and flush toilet or empty bedpan.

Restores room cleanliness

23. Dry bottom of sleeve and clamp.

Prevents soiling and collects further drainage

24. Encourage client to move about for the next 30 to 45

Allows irrigant to loosen remaining bowel contents

Action	Rationale
minutes (or assist, as needed, for safety during mobility).	
25. Repeat steps 14, 21, and 22.	
26. Clean bedpan.	*Restores room cleanliness and order*
27. Remove irrigation sleeve and belt.	*Concludes irrigation procedure*
28. Discard or restore equipment.	*Promotes clean, organized environment*
29. Discard old gloves and don new pair.	*Reduces contamination*
30. Wash, rinse, and dry stoma area.	*Cleanses peristomial area*
31. Apply antiseptic, if ordered.	*Prevents infection*
32. Apply new dressing or ostomy pouch, if needed.	
33. Wash hands.	*Reduces microorganism transfer*

Evaluation

Were desired outcomes achieved?

DOCUMENTATION

The following should be noted on the visit note:

- Condition of stoma site
- Amount of irrigant infused
- Amount and nature of drainage
- Client tolerance for procedure
- Client teaching accomplished and/or neeeded

Sample Documentation

DATE	TIME	
3/23/98	1250	Colostomy irrigation done with 600 mL tap water infused. Approximately 800 mL soft and liquid brown drainage noted. Client tolerated procedure without cramping or pain. Client demonstrated correct technique.

> **N**ursing **P**rocedure **6.17**

Stool Testing for Occult Blood With Hemoccult Slide

⊠ EQUIPMENT

- Stool specimen
- Hemoccult specimen collection card
- Chemical reagent (developer)
- Tongue blade
- Nonsterile gloves
- Stop watch or watch with second hand
- Specimen container labels
- Pen

Purpose

Obtains stool specimen to detect occult blood related to gastrointestinal (GI) bleeding and anemia

Serves as a preliminary screening test for colorectal cancer

Desired Outcome (sample)

Signs and symptoms of GI bleeding (bloody or dark black stools, fatigue, decreased bowel sounds, abdominal discomfort) are detected early.

Assessment

Assessment should focus on the following:

Specific orders regarding specimen collection
Characteristics of stool
Manifestations associated with GI bleeding or anemia
History of GI bleeding or anemia
Dietary intake of food or drugs that could alter test reliability
Intake of medications that cause occult bleeding

Outcome Identification and Planning

Key Goal and Sample Goal Criterion

The client will:

Have no undetected signs and symptoms of GI bleeding

Special Considerations

Some vitamins and minerals (such as vitamin C and iron) can cause erratic test results. Consult a pharmacy reference for a complete listing of such preparations and the amounts necessary to alter results.

Many clients are placed on special diagnostic diets 2 to 3 days before Hemoccult testing. Emphasize to client the importance of adhering to diet restrictions.

IMPLEMENTATION

Action	Rationale
1. Wash hands.	*Reduces microorganism transfer*
2. Explain procedure to client.	*Decreases anxiety*
3. Provide for privacy.	*Decreases embarrassment*
4. Don clean gloves.	*Reduces nurse's exposure to body secretions*
5. Obtain stool specimen with tongue blade and smear thin specimen onto guaiac test paper: - Smear specimen onto slot A on front of card. - Smear a second specimen from another part of stool onto slot B. - Close card.	*Prepares specimen for test*
6. Turn card over and open back window; apply two drops of reagent to slot over each specimen and wait 60 seconds.	*Activates chemical components necessary for results (alpha guaiacoconic and hydrogen peroxide)*
7. Read results (consult product instructions for visual comparison): - If either slot has bluish discoloration, test is positive.	*Determines if results are positive or negative*

Action	Rationale
- If there is no bluish discoloration, test is negative.	
8. Restore or discard equipment appropriately (test card may be discarded).	*Promotes clean environment*
9. Wash hands.	*Reduces microorganism transfer*

Evaluation

Were desired outcomes achieved?

DOCUMENTATION

The following should be noted on the visit note:

- Amount, color, odor, and consistency of stool obtained
- Specimen collection time
- Signs and symptoms consistent with GI bleeding

Sample Documentation		
DATE	**TIME**	
3/2/98	1100	Second stool tested for occult blood with Hemoccult slide. Results negative. Stool is dark brown, large, and formed. Client reports no discomfort during defecation.

Activity and Mobility

OVERVIEW

▶ The ability to remain physically active and mobile is essential in maintaining health and well-being.
▶ Immobility may pose psychological as well as physiological hazards.
▶ Nurses should be alert for such physical complications of immobility as the following:
- Hypostatic pneumonia
- Pulmonary embolism
- Thrombophlebitis
- Orthostatic hypotension
- Decubitus ulcers or pressure areas
- Decreased peristalsis with constipation and fecal impaction
- Urinary stasis with renal calculi formation
- Contractures and muscle atrophy
- Altered fluid and electrolyte status

▶ Proper positioning and correct support surfaces are important factors in managing tissue loads for clients in bed.

▶ Psychological hazards of immobility may range from mild anxiety to psychosis.

▶ Improper use of body mechanics when moving a client could result in injury to client and nurse. Knowledge of principles of body mechanics and proper body alignment is essential to injury prevention.

▶ Nurses are the occupational group documented as most frequently absent from work with back injury for more than 3 days.

▶ Proper body mechanics, with prevention of injury, serves to conserve time and energy expenditure, as well as, prevent financial expense resulting from injury.

▶ Substitution for needed equipment may be made using household items (see Appendix).

*N*ursing *P*rocedure 7.1

✋ *Using Principles of Body Mechanics*

❌ EQUIPMENT

- Equipment needed to move client or lift object (eg, Hoyer lift, trapeze bar)
- Turn sheets
- Chair, stretcher such as one used with a Hoyer lift, or bed for client
- Adequate lighting
- Positioning equipment (eg, trochanter rolls, pillows, footboards)
- Nonsterile gloves
- Visual and hearing aids needed by client
- Appropriate assistance from others (assistive personnel or family)

Purpose

Prevents physical injury of caregiver and client

Promotes correct body alignment

Facilitates coordinated, efficient muscle use when moving clients

Conserves energy of caregiver for accomplishment of other tasks

Desired Outcomes (sample)

Client displays no evidence of physical injury, such as new bruises, tears, or skeletal trauma after moving.

Client demonstrates proper use of body mechanics to be used in performing major lifting and moving tasks at home.

Assessment

Assessment should focus on the following:

Presence of deformities or abnormalities of vertebrae

Physical characteristics of client and caregiver that will influence techniques used (weight, size, height, age, physical limitations and abilities, condition of target muscles to be used in moving client, problems related to equilibrium)

Characteristics of object to be moved during client care (eg, weight, height, shape)

Immediate environment (amount of space available to work in; distance to be traveled; presence of obstructions in pathway; condition of floor; placement of chairs, stretchers, and other equipment being used; lighting)

Adequacy of function and stability of all equipment to be used

Extent of knowledge of assisting personnel, client, and family regarding proper use of body mechanics and body alignment

Status of equipment attached to client that must be moved (eg, IV machines, tubes, drains)

Outcome Identification and Planning

Key Goals and Sample Goal Criteria

The client/caregiver will:

Experience no physical injury related to improper use of body mechanics during moving, lifting, turning, or repositioning and will reveal no new bruises, tears, or skeletal trauma following these procedures

Demonstrate proper use of body mechanics to be used in performing major lifting and moving tasks at home by the time of discharge from home health care services

Special Considerations

Secure as much additional assistance as is needed for safe moves. NEVER BECOME SO IMPATIENT THAT UNSAFE RISK IS TAKEN WITH ANY TYPE OF MOVE. As a general rule of thumb, if mechanical equipment is available that will make lifting, turning, pulling, or positioning easier, use it.

Check all equipment to be used, including chairs, for adequate function and stability.

If physical injury of personnel is sustained because of performance of any work-related activity, follow agency policies regarding follow-up medical attention and completion of incident report forms. This provides for proper care and ensures financial assistance as needed.

The client's home environment should be assessed adequately to determine the need to rearrange furniture and other items and to secure mechanical equipment to ensure the safety of client and family as they perform care.

Geriatric

If client is restless, agitated, confused, or has a condition that causes loss of muscle control, secure assistance to prevent injury during the moving process.

IMPLEMENTATION

Action	Rationale
1. Wash hands.	*Reduces microorganism transfer*
2. Determine factors indicating need for additional personnel such as: - Equipment attached to client - Does move require persons of approximately the same height?	*Promotes efficiency*
3. Restore client's glasses and hearing aids if client is able to assist at all.	*Enables client to assist in making a safe move*
4. Explain required movement techniques to assisting personnel, family, and client; instruct and allow client to do as much as possible.	*Facilitates coordinated movement and prevents physical injury* *Promotes independence*
5. Don gloves as needed if contact with body fluids is likely.	*Prevents exposure to body secretions*
6. Organize equipment so that it is within easy reach, stabilized, and in proper position: - If moving client to chair, place chair so that back of chair is in same direction as head of bed. - If placing client on stretcher, align stretcher with side of bed.	*Avoids risks once movement begins* *Keeps number of actions needed for the move to a minimum*
7. If medical bed, raise or lower bed and other equipment to comfortable and suitable height.	*Prevents use of back muscles in performing tasks*
8. Maintain proper body alignment by using the following principles when handling equipment and when moving, lifting, turning, and positioning clients: - Stand with back, neck, shoulders, pelvis, and	*Maintains proper body alignment*

Action	Rationale
feet in as straight a line as possible; knees should be slightly flexed and toes pointed forward (Fig. 7.1.1).	
- Keep feet apart to establish broad support base; keep feet flat on floor (Fig. 7.1.2).	*Provides greater stability*
- Flex knees and hips in order to lower center of gravity (heaviest area of body) close to object to be moved (Fig. 7.1.3).	*Establishes more stable position* *Prevents pulling on spine*
- Move close to object to be moved or adjusted; do not lean or bend at waist.	*Promotes use of muscles of extremities rather than of spine* *Prevents improper alignment and inefficient muscle use*
- Use smooth, rhythmic motions when using bedcranks or any equipment requiring a pumping motion.	

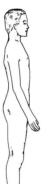

Head up

Eyes straight ahead

Neck straight

Chest out

Back straight

Arms relaxed at sides

Abdomen in

Knees slightly flexed

FIGURE 7.1.1

Action | Rationale

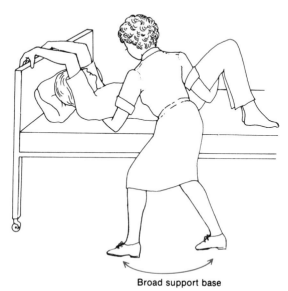

Broad support base

FIGURE 7.1.2

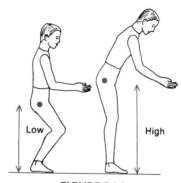

Low | High

FIGURE 7.1.3

Action	Rationale
- Use arm muscles for cranking or pumping, and arm and leg muscles for lifting.	*Avoids use of spine and back muscles*
9. Secure all tubes, drains, traction equipment, and so forth by whatever means are needed for proper functioning during moving, lifting, turning, and positioning.	*Prevents dislodgment of tubes and reflux of contaminants into body*
10. Move client close to edge of bed in one unit, or move client to side of bed at any time during procedure, moving one unit of the body at a time from top to bottom or vice versa (ie, head and shoulders first, trunk and hips second, and legs last). Coordinate move so that everyone exerts greatest effort on count of "three"; the individual carrying the heaviest load should direct the count.	*Maintains correct alignment* *Facilitates comfort* *Prevents physical injury*
11. Use the following principles to move a heavy object or client:	
a. Review each move again before move is made.	*Reinforces original plan*
b. Face client or object to be moved.	*Allows full use of arm and leg muscles*
c. Place hands or arms fully under client or object; lock hands with assistant on opposite side, if necessary.	*Provides extra leverage*
d. Prepare for move by taking in a deep breath, tightening abdominal and gluteal muscles, and tucking chin to-	*Facilitates use of large muscle groups*

Action	Rationale
wards chest. (If client is unable to provide assistance, instruct client to cross arms on chest.)	
e. Allow adequate rest periods, if needed.	*Prevents fatigue and subsequent physical injury*
f. When performing move, keep heaviest part of body within base of support.	*Promotes stability*
g. Perform pulling motions by leaning backward and pushing motions by leaning forward, maintaining wide base of support with feet, keeping knees flexed and one foot behind the other; pushing and pulling (use instead of lifting, whenever possible) should be done with muscles of the arms and legs, not back.	*Prevents injury to vertebrae and back muscles*
h. Always lower head as much as permissible.	*Avoids pulling against gravity*
i. When moving from a bending to standing position, stop momentarily once in standing position before completing next move. When getting clients into a chair, stop to allow client and self to stand to establish stability before pivoting into chair.	*Allows time to straighten spine and re-establish stability*
j. Move in as straight and direct a path as possible, avoiding twisting and turning of spine.	*Avoids vertebral and back injury related to rotating and twisting spine*

Action	Rationale

    k. When turning is un-
avoidable, use a pivot-
ing turn; when
positioning client in
chair or carrying client
to a stretcher, pivot to-
ward chair or stretcher
together.

12. Position props and body
parts for appropriate
body alignment of client
after move is completed:
- When client is sitting,
hips, shoulders, and
neck should be in line
with trunk; knees, hips,
and ankles should be
flexed at a 90-degree
angle and toes should
be pointed forward.
- When client is in bed,
neck, shoulders, pelvis,
and ankles should be in
line with trunk, and
knees and elbows
should be slightly
flexed.

13. After move is completed,
provide for comfort and
safety of client with the
following actions, if ap-
plicable:
- Raise protective rails,   *Prevents falls*
if applicable.
- Apply safety belts on   *Promotes safety*
wheelchairs.
- Lower height of bed, if   *Promotes safety*
possible.
- Elevate head properly.   *Supports airway clearance*
- Restore all tubes,   *Re-establishes proper func-*
drains, and equipment   *tioning of equipment*
being used by client to
proper functioning and
placement.
- Place pillows and   *Promotes proper body align-*

Action	Rationale
position equipment properly.	ment and supports airway
- Replace covers.	Provides warmth and privacy
- Place items of frequent use within client reach.	Enhances comfort and general satisfaction
- Instruct client/family on how to move client with return demonstration.	Prevents injury
14. Discard gloves and wash hands.	Reduces microorganism transfer

Evaluation

Were desired outcomes achieved?

DOCUMENTATION

The following should be noted on the visit note:

- Amount of assistance given by client
- Position client was placed in (eg, in chair, returned to bed)
- Reports of discomfort, dizziness, or faintness during or after move
- Re-establishment of proper functioning of equipment
- Safety belts applied
- Status of side rails, if applicable
- Auxiliary equipment used
- Status of equipment being used to maintain alignment

Sample Documentation

DATE	TIME	
10/19/98	1030	Assisted client into chair. Client able to provide partial assistance; reported slight dizziness when standing. IV remains intact and infusing correctly. Posey vest reapplied. Family instructed on appropriate use of body mechanics when assisting in transfer from bed to chair.

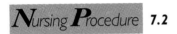

*N*ursing *P*rocedure **7.2**

🖐 *Body Positioning*

❎ EQUIPMENT

- Support devices required by client (eg, trochanter roll, foot-board, heel protectors, sandbags, hand rolls, restraints)
- Pillow for head and extra pillows needed for support

Purpose

Positions client for comfort and body alignment
Positions client for a variety of clinical procedures

Desired Outcome (sample)

Client's skin is warm, dry, intact, and without discoloration over pressure points.

Assessment

Assessment should focus on the following:

Client's age and medical diagnosis
Physical ability of client to maintain position
Integumentary assessment
Length of time client has maintained present body positioning
Doctor's orders for specific restrictions in positioning client or for special position required by impending procedure
Client/family knowledge regarding positioning techniques

Outcome Identification and Planning

Key Goal and Sample Goal Criterion

The client will:

Maintain skin integrity without pressure areas or decubitus ulcers during confinement

Special Considerations

To avoid injury when positioning clients, it is important that body alignment of the client and nurse or assistant be supported and that appropriate body mechanics be used. (Procedure 7.1 presents the principles of body mechanics.) Secure additional assistance as needed for the safe repositioning of the client and for protection of your back. NEVER BECOME SO IMPATIENT THAT RISKS ARE TAKEN.

In the home, pillows, sofa cushions, or rolled linen may be used for positioning. A recliner may be used to maintain a Fowler's or semi-Fowler's position.

Foot drop, pressure ulcers, shoulder subluxation, and internal and external rotation of large joint areas are preventable complications if the client is positioned and supported correctly. Be sure that pillows, trochanter rolls, footboards, and other supportive equipment are positioned to maintain body alignment; that joint and ligament pulling is prevented; that head, feet, and hands do not droop; that large joint areas do not rotate internally or externally; and that excess pressure on any body area is avoided.

Immobile clients with existing pressure ulcers who are at risk for new pressure ulcers should not be positioned directly on their trochanters.

Geriatric

Bedridden elderly clients are particularly susceptible to impaired skin integrity when they are not repositioned frequently; this is due to a decreased amount of subcutaneous fat and to skin that is less elastic, thinner, drier, and thus more fragile than that of a younger person.

IMPLEMENTATION

Action	Rationale
1. Wash hands.	*Reduces microorganism transfer*
2. Explain procedure to client, emphasizing importance of maintaining proper position.	*Decreases anxiety* *Increases compliance*
3. Provide for privacy.	*Decreases embarrassment*
4. If medical bed, adjust to comfortable working height.	*Prevents back and muscle strain in nurse*
5. Place or assist client into appropriate position (various positions are illus-	

Action	Rationale
trated in Fig. 7.2 and described in Table 7.2).	
6. Use the following guidelines in repositioning client:	
- Place all equipment, lines, and drains attached to client so that dislodgment will not occur.	*Prevents accidental dislodgment and client injury*
- Close off drains, if necessary, and remember to reopen them after positioning client.	*Prevents reflux of drainage*
- Be sure that an assistant is designated to handle extremities bound by heavy stabilizers (such as casts and traction) and heavy equipment that must be moved with client (such as traction apparatus).	*Maintains stability of body part to prevent injury and pain*
- Maintain head elevation for clients prone to dyspnea when flat; allow brief rest periods, as needed, during procedure.	*Facilitates breathing and reduces anxiety* *Prevents exertion*
- When moving client to side of bed, move major portions of the body sequentially, from top to bottom or vice versa (eg, head and shoulders first, trunk and hips second, legs last).	*Maintains body alignment* *Facilitates comfort*
- Use pillows, trochanter rolls, and special positioning supports as needed to maintain body alignment and normal position of extremities.	*Prevents injury and promotes comfort*
- Be certain that client's face is not pressed into bed or pillows while turning and that body	*Maintains adequate respirations*

Action   Rationale

A. High Fowler's

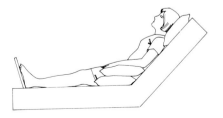

B. Supine

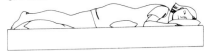

C. Prone

D. Side-lying

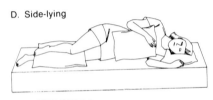

FIGURE 7.2

Action	Rationale

E. Sims'

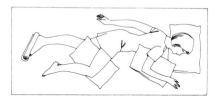

F. Lithotomy

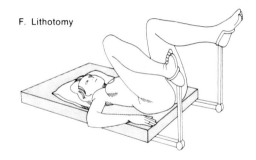

G. Dorsal Recumbent

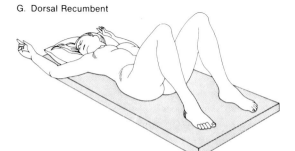

FIGURE 7.2 (cont.)

TABLE 7.2 Body Positioning

Position	Purpose	Description
Fowler's (low to high)	Improves breathing capacity Prevents aspiration Promotes comfort	Head of bed up 30 to 90 degrees Client in a semisitting position Knees slightly flexed
Supine	Prevents bending at crucial areas, such as groin or spine, after diagnostic procedures	Client flat on back in bed Body straight and in alignment Feet protected with footboard to support 90-degree flexion
Prone	Serves as positioning alternative in turning procedure for immobilized clients	Client flat on abdomen with knees slightly flexed Head turned to side Arms flexed at sides, hands near head Feet over end of mattress or protected with footboard to support normal flexion
Side-lying (lateral)	Serves as position for some procedures and alternative position for turning procedure	Client lying on side with upper leg flexed at hip and knee Top arm flexed Lower arm flexed and shoulder positioned to avoid pulling and excessive weight of body or shoulder
Sims'	Serves as position for some procedures and alternative position for turning procedure	Client halfway between side-lying and prone positions with bottom knee slightly flexed Knee and hip of top leg flexed (about 90 degrees) Lower arm behind back Upper arm flexed, hand near head
Lithotomy	Places client in position for vaginal or anorectal exams	Client on back with legs flexed 90 degrees at hips and knees Feet up in stirrups
Dorsal recumbent	Places client in position for vaginal exams and insertion of catheters	Client on back with legs flexed at hips and knees Feet flat on mattress
Modified Trendelenburg's	Places client in "shock" position to increase	Client flat on back with legs straight and elevated at hips

Action	Rationale
position does not prevent full expansion of diaphragm.	
- Use appropriate body mechanics (see Procedure 7.1).	*Prevents injury*
7. Assess status of client comfort and character of respirations; recheck client periodically.	*Prevents injury*
8. Lift side rails and place bed in low position, if applicable. If traction apparatus is being used, be certain weights are not dragging on floor or touching bed.	*Prevents falls*
9. Move bed table close to bed and place items of frequent use close to client.	*Places items used frequently within easy reach*
10. Wash hands.	*Decreases microorganism transfer*

Evaluation

Were desired outcomes achieved?

DOCUMENTATION

The following should be noted on the visit note?

- Client's position
- Client reports of pain, dyspnea, discomfort
- Exertion or dyspnea observed during repositioning
- Abnormal findings on integumentary assessment
- Status of equipment needed for stabilization of body parts (eg, traction, casts)
- Teaching regarding importance of maintaining position and positioning techniques

Sample Documentation

DATE	TIME	
10/5/98	1430	Client repositioned into right side-lying position. Slight shortness of breath reported during repositioning. Client given a brief rest period and no further shortness of breath reported. No redness, breaks, or discoloration noted over bony prominences. Family (daughter) instructed on techniques for positioning client.

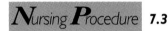 **7.3**

Hoyer Lift Usage

X EQUIPMENT

- Hoyer lift (should include base, canvas mat, two pairs of canvas straps)
- Large chair with arm support for client to sit in

Purpose

Helps move and transfer heavy clients who are unable to assist mover

Prevents undue strain on mover's body

Desired Outcome (sample)

Client is moved from and returned to bed by Hoyer lift without injury.

Assessment

Assessment should focus on the following:

Medical diagnosis

Doctor's activity orders (positions contraindicated and number and amount of time client may be up)

Client ability to keep head erect

Chart to determine previous tolerance of client to sitting position (eg, orthostatic hypotension, amount of time client tolerated sitting up)

Client's need for restraints while sitting up

Room environment (ie, adequate lighting, presence of clutter and furniture in pathway between chair and bed)

Condition of Hoyer device, hooks, and canvas mats

Family knowledge of operation of Hoyer

Outcome Identification and Planning

Key Goal and Sample Goal Criterion

The client will:

Experience no injury during transfer

Special Considerations

It is important for the nurse to be familiar with the Hoyer lift in
order to operate it correctly (parts of the lift are labeled in Fig.
7.3). Practice using the lift without a client on the mat if you
are unfamiliar with this device.

Organization is crucial when performing numerous moving
procedures on heavy clients to avoid client exertion and physical injury to the movers. Plan activities such as changing bed
linens while client is out of bed; encourage client to use bedside toilet once out of bed.

Help family obtain the equipment, if needed. Educate the family
on the use of the equipment and on proper body mechanics.

Geriatric

Chronic conditions in elderly clients require extra caution when
moving them using the Hoyer lift. Clients with chronic cardiopulmonary conditions should be observed closely while
sitting up and during transfer for exertion, respiratory difficulty, chest pain, and general discomfort.

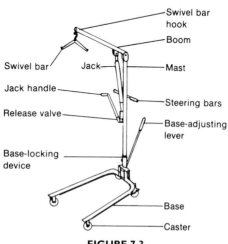

Swivel bar hook
Boom
Swivel bar
Jack
Mast
Jack handle
Steering bars
Release valve
Base-adjusting lever
Base-locking device
Base
Caster

FIGURE 7.3

IMPLEMENTATION

Action	Rationale
1. Wash hands.	*Reduces microorganism transfer*
2. Explain procedure and assure client that precaution will be taken to prevent falls.	*Decreases anxiety*
3. Provide for and maintain privacy throughout procedure.	*Decreases embarrassment*
4. Place chair on side of bed client will be sitting on (lock wheels, if wheelchair).	*Places chair at close distance*
5. Adjust bed to comfortable working height, if using medical bed.	*Prevents back and muscle strain in nurse*
6. Lock bed if applicable.	*Prevents bed movement*
7. Place client on mat as follows:	*Centers heaviest parts of body on mat*
- Roll client to one side and place half of mat under client from shoulders to midthigh.	*Positions client on mat with minimal movement*
- Roll client to other side and finish pulling mat under client.	
- Be sure one or both side rails are up as you move from one side of bed to other if medical bed.	*Prevents accidental falls*
8. Roll base of Hoyer lift under side of bed nearest to chair with boom in center of client's trunk; lock wheels of lift.	*Moves mechanical part of lift to bedside* *Prevents lift from rolling*
9. Using base-adjustment lever, widen stance of base.	*Provides greater stability to lift*
10. Raise and then push jack handle in towards mast, lowering boom (this is accomplished with appropriate button or control device in the electric Hoyer).	*Lowers boom close enough to attach hooks*
11. Place the strap or chain	*Secures hook placement into mat*

Action	Rationale
hooks through the holes of mat (hooks of short straps go into holes behind back and hooks of long straps into holes at other end), making certain that hooks are not indenting client's skin.	holes *Attaches rest of device to mat*
12. Place all equipment, lines, and drains attached to client so that dislodgment will not occur and close off drains, if necessary (remember to reopen them after moving client).	*Prevents accidental dislodgment and client injury* *Prevents reflux of drainage*
13. Instruct client to fold arms across chest.	*Prevents accidental injury*
14. Using jack handle, pump jack enough for mat to clear bed about 6 inches and tighten release valve.	*Safely assesses client stability and centering on mat*
15. Determine if client is fully supported and can maintain head support. Provide head support as needed throughout the procedure.	*Assesses stability in relation to weight and placement*
16. Unlock wheels and pull Hoyer lift straight back and away from bed; instruct assistant to provide support for equipment and client's legs throughout procedure.	*Promotes stability*
17. Move toward chair with open end of lift's base straddling chair; continue until client's back is almost flush with back of chair.	*Moves and guides client into chair*
18. Lock wheels of lift.	*Provides Hoyer stability*
19. Slowly lift up jack handle and lower client into chair until hooks are slightly loosened from	*Lowers client fully into chair*

Action	Rationale
mat; guide client into chair with your hands as mat lowers. Avoid lowering client onto chair handles.	
20. Remove mat (unless difficult to replace or client's first time out of bed).	*Facilitates comfort*
21. Place tubes, drains, and support equipment for proper functioning, comfort, and safety:	*Prevents accidental dislodgment of tubes and drains and maintains necessary functions*
- Pillow behind head	*Ensures client stability in chair*
- Sheet over knees and thighs	
- Restraints, if needed (eg, Posey vest, sheet, arm restraints)	*Facilitates adequate support of other body parts*
- Phone and items of frequent use within close range	*Places items desired or needed by client within reach*
- Catheter hooked to lower portion of chair	*Facilitates communication*
- IV pole close enough to avoid pulling	
22. Assess client tolerance to sitting up.	*Reduces risk of falling*
23. Leave door to client's room open when leaving room, unless someone else will be with client.	*Allows visual observation of unattended client*
24. Instruct family on how to monitor client at intervals.	*Reduces risk of falling*
25. Return client to bed using above steps.	*Prevents injury and discomfort during transfer*
26. Wash hands and restore equipment.	*Reduces microorganism transfer* *Promotes clean environment*

Evaluation

Were desired outcomes achieved?

DOCUMENTATION

The following should be noted on the visit note:

- Status update with indication for continued use of mobility-assist device
- Time of client transfer and type of lift used
- Client tolerance of procedure
- Duration of time in chair
- Teaching on use of equipment

Sample Documentation

DATE	TIME	
7/15/98	1400	Client lifted out of bed using Hoyer lift. Placed in bedside chair. Client tolerated procedure well with respirations regular and nonlabored and is watching television. Door left partially open. Son instructed on use of Hoyer lift. Reinstruction needed.

*N*ursing *P*rocedure 7.4

Use of Assistive Devices for Ambulation

⊠ EQUIPMENT

- Appropriate-size crutches or walker
- Safety belt (gait belt)
- Well fitted shoes
- Eyeglasses or contacts, if worn

Purpose

Facilitates mobility and activity for client

Increases self-esteem by decreasing dependence

Decreases physical stress on weight-bearing joints and un-
healed skeletal injuries

Desired Outcomes (sample)

Client does not fall while using device.

Client demonstrates correct techniques for device maneuvers.

Assessment

Assessment should focus on the following:

Medical diagnosis

Doctor's orders for activity restrictions

Type of crutch–gait movement indicated

Neuromuscular status (muscle tone, strength, and range of motion of arms, legs, and trunk; gait pattern; body alignment
when walking; ability to maintain balance)

Focal point of injury and reason for device

Measurement parameters of device

Ability of client to comprehend instructions regarding use of
device

Additional learning needs of client

Nature of walking area (ie, presence of clutter, scatter rugs, adequacy of floor for good traction, proximity of adequate rest
area)

Outcome Identification and Planning

Key Goals and Sample Goal Criteria

The client will:

Experience no falls during use of device
Demonstrate correct use of device

Special Considerations

Walking on slippery, cluttered surfaces and on stairs can be hazardous. Clients should use railing of staircase (or walk close to walls) while using assistive device.

Clients with visual deficits should wear visual aids when using assistive device.

The client's home environment should be assessed carefully for hazards and adequate space. Assist client with arrangement of furniture and decorative items to eliminate hazards in the home while using crutches or walker.

Geriatric

Geriatric clients are especially prone to injuries from falls because of brittle or underdeveloped bones. Safety belts should always be used when assisting these clients with crutch walking and walker usage.

In elderly clients, extra time should be allotted because of decreased muscle strength, decreased coordination, and functional changes in vision.

Referral to physical therapy may be indicated if progress is not noted.

IMPLEMENTATION

Action	Rationale
1. Wash hands.	*Reduces microorganism transfer*
2. Explain procedure to client, emphasizing that it will take time to learn techniques; stress safety and the importance of moving slowly initially; when providing explanations, include demonstrations.	*Decreases anxiety and frustration* *Increases compliance* *Prevents injury*
3. Assist client into shoes that are comfortable, non-	*Prevents falls*

Action	Rationale

skid, hard soled, and low
heeled.

4. Assist client into house-
   coat or loose, comfortable
   clothes.

   Maintains privacy
   Facilitates comfort

5. Observe client for correct
   device fit:
   - Have client stand with
     elbows slightly flexed;
     note if client can stand
     upright while holding
     the device.

   Promotes correct body alignment
   *Avoids damage from crutches to
   brachial plexus, which can result in paralysis of extremity*

6. If using medical bed,
   lower height of bed, then
   lock wheels.

   Prevents falls

7. Slowly help client into sitting position; assess for
   dizziness, faintness, or
   decrease in orientation.

   *Prevents injury from sudden
   change in blood pressure when
   sitting up*

8. Apply safety belt.

   Prevents client injury

9. Assist client with maneuvers appropriate for type
   of gait and with other
   general device usage
   techniques. Initially, always have someone with
   client but allow greater
   independence as tech-
   niques are performed
   more proficiently and
   client demonstrates ability to crutch walk in all
   areas safely (encourage
   client to use rails and
   walk close to walls when
   climbing stairs).

   *Provides assistance and ensures
   client safety*

10. In general, demonstrate
    correct technique for type
    of gait to be used before
    client gets out of bed;
    have client demonstrate
    these techniques to you;
    reinforce instructions and
    make corrections as

    *Permits concentration on ma-
    neuvers before client attempts
    them*

Action	Rationale

client demonstrates walking with the device.

Crutch walking:
11. Begin demonstrating gait technique from tripod position with devices 6 inches to side and 6 inches to front of seat (Fig. 7.4.1).

Promotes stability and balance

a. Four-point gait: Advance right crutches, then left foot, then left crutch, then right foot (Fig. 7.4.2).

Places weight on legs while crutches provide stability

b. Three-point gait: Advance both crutches and affected extremity at same time; advance unaffected extremity (Fig. 7.4.3).

Places weight on unaffected leg and crutches, with light weight on affected leg

c. Two-point gait: Advance right crutch and left foot together, then left crutch and right foot together (Fig. 7.4.4).

Places partial weight on both legs

d. Swing-to or swing-through gait: Advance both crutches at same time and swing body

Provides additional stability for clients with bilateral leg disability

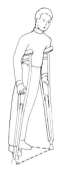

FIGURE 7.4.1

Action	Rationale

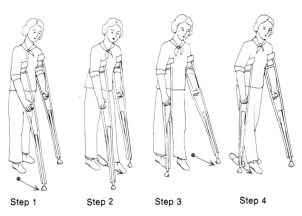

Step 1   Step 2   Step 3   Step 4

FIGURE 7.4.2

forward to crutches or
past them (Fig. 7.4.5).
12. Demonstrate correct
techniques for sitting,
standing, and stair walk-
ing with crutches (Display

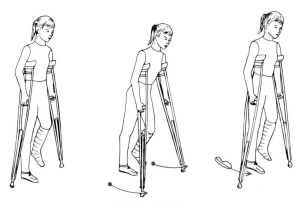

FIGURE 7.4.3

Action	Rationale

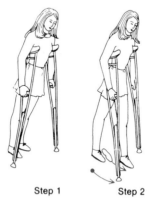

Step 1   Step 2

FIGURE 7.4.4

7.4), Figures 7.4.6 and
7.4.7 illustrate stair walking with crutches).

Walker Usage

13. Instruct client to stand
    straight, but not place all
    of weight on walker.

Prevents accidental slipping

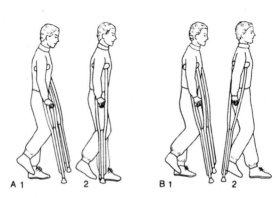

A 1   2   B 1   2

FIGURE 7.4.5

Action	Rationale

DISPLAY 7.4   Techniques for General Crutch-walking Maneuvers

Moving From Sitting to Standing	*Moving From Standing to Sitting*
• Place both crutches in hand on affected side (holding crutches together and even). • Push down on stable support base (locked bed, arm or seat of chair) with free hand, put weight on stronger leg, and lift body. • Stand with a straight back, bearing weight on stronger leg and crutches. • Place both crutches on same level as feet. • Advance unaffected leg to next step while bearing down on crutch handles. • Pull affected leg and crutches up to step while bearing weight on stronger leg.	• Inch back until backs of lower legs touch bed or center of chair. • Hold crutches together in hand on unaffected side. • Begin easing down onto chair or bed with back straight, using crutches and stronger leg as support. • When close enough, gently hold onto arm of chair and complete the move.
Walking Up Stairs (see Fig. 7.4.6)	*Walking Down Stairs (see Fig. 7.4.7)*
• Place both crutches on same level as feet. • Advance unaffected leg to next step while bearing down on crutch handles. • Pull affected leg and crutches up to step while bearing weight on stronger leg.	• Place both crutches on same level as feet. • Shift weight to stronger leg. • Lower affected leg and crutches to next step while bearing down on crutch handles. • Advance unaffected leg last.

Action	Rationale

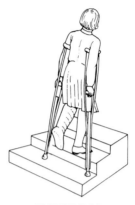

FIGURE 7.4.6

14. Instruct to advance the walker first at arms' length, then right followed by left leg and

Maintains balance and steady gait

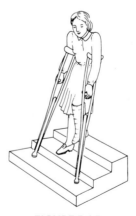

FIGURE 7.4.7

Action	Rationale

foot, advancing into the walker. Client should maintain straight back throughout (Fig. 7.4.8).

15. Observe return demonstrations and help client practice until proficiency in walker use is attained (provide intermittent praise and encouragement); encourage rest between activity periods, assisting client, as needed, to a comfortable position.

Ensures procedure has been learned

Provides avenue for feedback

16. Wash hands and properly store equipment.

Reduces microorganism transfer
Maintains order

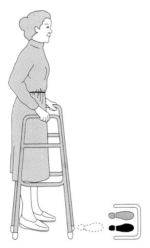

FIGURE 7.4.8

Evaluation

Were desired outcomes achieved?

DOCUMENTATION

The following should be noted on the visit note:

- Gait pattern used
- Steadiness of gait and amount of assistance needed
- Distance walked by client
- Client tolerance to procedure
- Teaching done and additional learning needs of client

Sample Documentation

DATE	TIME	
4/28/98	1200	Client completed first week of walking with crutches. Efficient with use of four-point gait pattern. Steady with good body alignment while on crutches. Walking entire house length 3 times per day without fatigue or reports of discomfort. Has not begun stair walking.

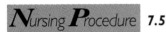

Nursing **P**rocedure **7.5**

Range-of-Motion Exercises

EQUIPMENT

- No equipment needed except gloves, if contact with body fluids is likely

Purpose

Maintains present level of functioning and mobility of extremity involved

Prevents contractures and shortening of musculoskeletal structures

Prevents vascular complications of immobility

Facilitates comfort

Desired Outcomes (sample)

Client's present range of motion is being maintained.

Range of motion of left elbow increased from 30- to 40-degree flexion.

No signs or symptoms of complications of immobility are present.

Assessment

Assessment should focus on the following:

Medical diagnosis

Doctor's orders for indications of specific restrictions

Present range of motion of each extremity

Physical and mental ability of client to perform the activity, including normal age-related changes

History of factors that contraindicate or limit the type or amount of exercise

Client and family knowledge of techniques

Outcome Identification and Planning

Key Goals and Sample Goal Criteria

The client will:

Maintain present level of functioning of joints that are not im-
mobilized by cast
Avoid complications of immobility, such as:
- Pressure ulcers or pressure areas
- Contractures
- Decreased peristalsis
- Constipation and fecal impaction
- Orthostatic hypotension
- Pulmonary embolism (evidenced by chest pain, dyspnea,
wheezing, increased heart rate)
- Thrombophlebitis (evidenced by redness, heat, swelling, or
pain in a local area)

Special Considerations

Decreased muscle mass, degenerative changes of joints, and degenerative connective tissue changes result in limited range of
motion.
A client able to perform all or part of a range-of-motion exercise
program should be allowed to do so and should be properly
instructed. Observe the client performing activities of daily
living to determine the limitations of movement and the need,
if any, for passive range-of-motion exercise to various joints.
When performing a range-of-motion exercise, a joint should be
moved *only to the point of resistance, pain, or spasm, whichever
comes first.*
Consult doctor's orders before performing a range-of-motion
exercise on a client with acute cardiac, vascular, or pulmonary
problems or a client with musculoskeletal trauma and acute
flare-ups of arthritis.
Instruct family members in performance of range-of-motion
techniques to be used during periods between nurse visits.

Geriatric

The presence of various chronic conditions in elderly clients requires the use of extra caution when performing range-of-motion exercises. Clients with chronic cardiopulmonary conditions should be observed closely during range-of-motion
activity for respiratory difficulty, chest pain, and general discomfort.

IMPLEMENTATION

Action	Rationale
1. Wash hands.	*Reduces microorganism transfer*
2. Explain procedure to client and family.	*Decreases anxiety*
3. Provide for privacy.	*Decreases embarrassment*

Action	Rationale
4. Adjust bed to comfortable working height if applicable.	*Prevents back and muscle strain in nurse*
5. Move client to side of bed closest to you.	*Facilitates use of proper body mechanics*
6. Beginning at top and moving downward on one side of body at a time, perform passive (or instruct client through active) range-of-motion exercises of joints in each of the following areas, as applicable for client (Fig. 7.5.1). - head and neck (A–B) - spine (C) - shoulder (D–F) - elbow (G) - forearm (H) - wrist (I) - fingers (J–K) - hips (L–N) - knees (O–P) - toes (Q–R) - ankles (S)	*Exercises all joint areas*
7. As maneuvers are performed, support body areas being exercised by holding the following in the rounded palms of your hands (Fig. 7.5.2). - Arms at elbow and wrist - Legs at knee and ankle - Head at occipital area and chin	*Prevents pulling and careless handling of extremity, which could result in pain or injury*
8. Slowly move each extremity through full range of positions 3 to 10 times or as tolerated by client (see Table 7.5 for definition of each motion).	*Provides adequate exercise of extremity*
9. Observe client for signs of exertion or discomfort while performing range-of-motion exercises.	*Alerts nurse for cues to terminate activity*

Action	Rationale

HEAD–NECK

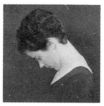

A   Flexion   Extension

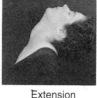

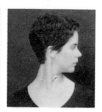

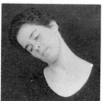
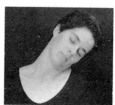

B   Lateral Flexion

FIGURE 7.5.1

Action	Rationale
10. Replace covers and position client for comfort and in proper body alignment.	*Promotes comfort*
11. Assess vital signs.	*Provides follow-up data regarding effects of activity on client*
12. Wash hands.	*Reduces microorganism transfer*

Action	Rationale

VERTICAL COLUMN

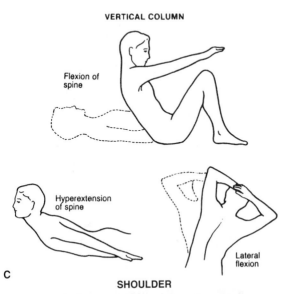

Flexion of spine

Hyperextension of spine

Lateral flexion

C

SHOULDER

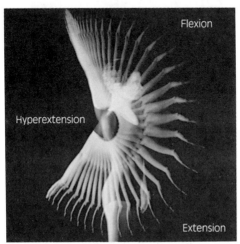

Flexion

Hyperextension

Extension

D

FIGURE 7.5.1 (cont.)

Action	Rationale

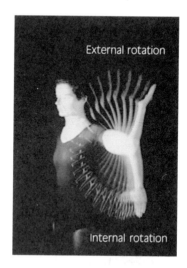

E

SHOULDER *(continued)*

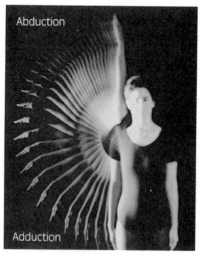

F

FIGURE 7.5.1 (cont.)

Action	Rationale

ELBOW

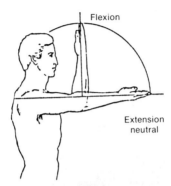

G

FOREARM

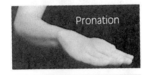

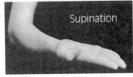

H

WRIST

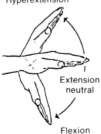

I

FIGURE 7.5.1 (cont.)

Action	Rationale

FINGERS

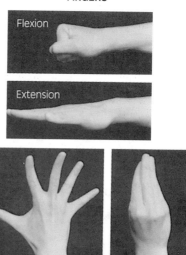

J

K

Abduction Adduction

HIPS

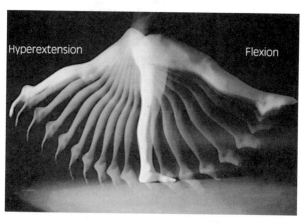

L

FIGURE 7.5.1 (cont.)

Action	Rationale

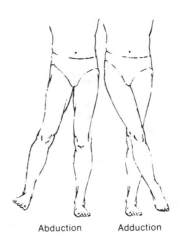

M   Abduction   Adduction

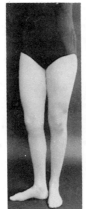 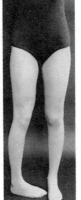

N   External   Internal
rotation   rotation

FIGURE 7.5.1 (cont.)

Action	Rationale

KNEE

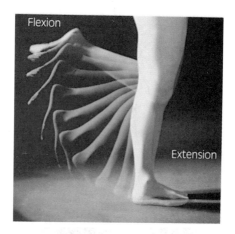

O

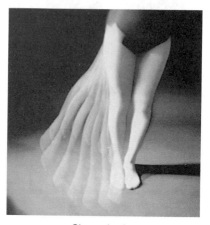

P   Circumduction

FIGURE 7.5.1 (cont.)

Action	Rationale

TOES

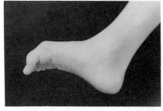

Flexion

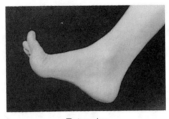

Q

Extension

FIGURE 7.5.1 (cont.)

Action	Rationale

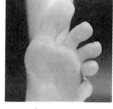 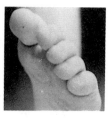

R

Abduction   Adduction

ANKLES

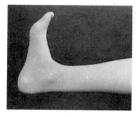 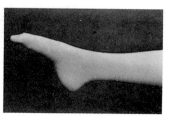

S

Dorsiflexion   Plantar flexion

FIGURE 7.5.1 (cont.)

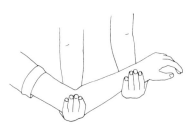

FIGURE 7.5.2

TABLE 7.5 Descriptions of Range-of-Motion Maneuvers

Maneuver	Description	Applicable Areas
Flexion	Bending joint at point of normal anatomic fold	All areas
Extension	Straightening joint into as straight a line as possible	All areas
Hyperextension	Straightening joint into extension, then moving past that point	Neck, fingers, wrists, toes, spine
Abduction	Moving extremity away from midline of body	Arms, legs, fingers, toes
Adduction	Moving extremity toward midline of body	Arms, legs, fingers, toes
Internal rotation	Rotating extremity toward midline of body	Hips, ankles, shoulders
External rotation	Rotating extremity away from midline	Hips, ankles, shoulders
Supination	Turning palm upward	Hands
Pronation	Turning palm downward	Hands
Circumduction	Rotating extremity in a complete circle	Shoulders, hips

Evaluation

Were desired outcomes achieved?

DOCUMENTATION

The following should be noted on the visit note:

- Areas on which range-of-motion exercises are performed
- Areas of limited range of motion and the degree of limitation
- Areas of passive versus active range of motion
- Reports of pain or discomfort
- Observations of physiologic intolerance to activity

Sample Documentation

DATE	TIME	
11/12/98	1400	Passive range-of-motion exercises performed on all extremities. Client has minimal range of motion of all joints and reports no pain or discomfort during exercise. No signs of intolerance of activity.

*N*ursing *P*rocedure **7.6**

General Muscle-Strengthening Exercises

☒ EQUIPMENT

- Unopened cans of food, of different sizes
- Well-fitted rubber-soled shoes, socks

Purpose

Promotes general increase in strength and activity

Desired Outcomes (sample)
The client will gradually recover general strength and endurance.

Assessment

Assessment should focus on the following:

Determination of functional limitations
Medical conditions that contraindicate general strengthening
Degree of client debilitation

Outcome Identification and Planning

Key Goals and Sample Goal Criteria
The client will:

Recognize debilitating effects of a recent decrease in activity, hospitalization, or change in condition
Verbalize understanding of the need to gradually increase strength and endurance
Participate in a safe and scheduled program of muscle strengthening

Special Considerations

HINT

ECONOMIC: For basic strengthening, purchased equipment is not necessary. Items found in the home may be used as weights. Such items include cans of soup or vegetables, or bags of flour or sugar.

HINT

Many clients seen in home health have recently been hospitalized or have experienced a decrease in activity, and have lost general strength and endurance. While their diagnosis may not justify physical therapy, they can benefit from basic exercise.

IMPLEMENTATION

Action	Rationale
1. Evaluate client ambulation ability, upper extremity strength, ability to transfer from sitting to standing.	*Allows the nurse to determine client needs, ability to perform exercises*
2. Discuss benefits of increased upper extremity strength to assist in transfer.	*Indicates to client that exercise has benefits*
3. Discuss importance of ambulation in terms of increased strength, general well-being, increased independence.	*Generates interest on the part of the client in participating in an exercise program*
4. Instruct and demonstrate upper extremity strengthening using small unopened cans of food (Fig. 7.6). Instruct to lift slowly to shoulder level, bending elbows. Have client demonstrate.	*Allows nurse to see client ability and understanding*
5. If appropriate to client, have client lift cans over	

Action	Rationale

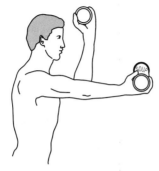

FIGURE 7.6

head to strengthen upper arms.

6. Specify number of repetitions and number of times per day to do exercises.

Promotes client participation by establishing a definite schedule

7. Gradually increase size and weight of cans, and number of repetitions. Note weight of can on label.

Allows client to see progress

8. For ambulation, determine client usual habits, ie, does client spend a lot of time watching TV or reading? Instruct client to ambulate a specified route, such as to the kitchen and back, during each commercial or after each chapter.

Connects exercise times with an already established habit, and improves client compliance

9. Gradually lengthen distance ambulated.

Indicates progress to client

10. Discuss available outpatient exercise programs, if applicable after discharge from services, other benefits of regular exercise.

Promotes ongoing healthy lifestyle

Evaluation

Were desired outcomes achieved?

DOCUMENTATION

The following should be noted on the visit note:

- Client limitations
- Exercise program established
- Client progress

Sample Documentation

DATE	TIME	
9/6/99	1100	Difficulty rising to a standing position, ambulates only 4 feet. General debilitation noted due to previous hospital bedrest exceeding 3 days. Instructed in basic strengthening, use of soup cans for upper extremities 4 times daily, 5 reps each arm. Instructed to stand and ambulate around living room at each TV commercial. Return demonstration of instructions by client. Will evaluate next visit and increase weight, reps, and ambulation distance if indicated.

*N*ursing *P*rocedure 7.7

📋 *Cast Care*

❎ EQUIPMENT

- Washcloth
- Towel
- Soap
- Basin of warm water
- Linen savers for bed (or plastic bags)
- Pen
- Roll of 1- or 2-inch tape
- Pillows wrapped in linen saver or plastic bag
- Bed linens with pull/turn sheet
- Sterile gloves

Purpose

Prevents neurovascular impairment of areas encircled by cast
Maintains cast for immobilization of treatment area
Prevents infection

Desired Outcomes (sample)

Signs of neurovascular deficits are detected early.
Client verbalizes actions necessary for cast maintenance by discharge.

Assessment

Assessment should focus on the following:

Medical diagnosis
Doctor's orders for special care of treatment area
Client's report of pain or discomfort
Integumentary status
Neurovascular indicators of health of extremities, particularly of areas distal to cast: color, temperature, capillary refill, sensation, pulse quality, ability to move toes or fingers
Indicators of infection (foul odor from cast, pain, fever, edema, extreme warmth over a particular area of cast)

Indicators of complications of immobility: decubitus ulcers or pressure areas; reduced joint movement; decreased peristalsis, constipation, and fecal impaction; signs of pulmonary embolism (chest pain, dyspnea, wheezing, increased heart rate); signs of thrombophlebitis (redness, heat, swelling, or pain in local area)

Outcome Identification and Planning

Key Goals and Sample Goal Criteria

The client will:

Have no undetected signs of developing neurovascular complications

Verbalize actions necessary for cast maintenance by discharge

Special Considerations

If client experienced traumatic injury to the extremity in the cast, watch for a sudden decrease in capillary refill and loss of pulse during first 24 to 48 hours due to development of compartment syndrome.

Inform the client that a wet cast may be dried with a hair dryer on the LOW setting.

Geriatric

Watch client closely during initial gait retraining: additional weight of cast could cause lack of balance and result in stress and fracture of fragile bones.

IMPLEMENTATION

Action	Rationale
1. Wash hands.	*Reduces microorganism transfer*
2. Place pull/turn sheet and linen savers on bed before client returns from casting area (place these items on bed with each linen change).	*Promotes ease of positioning client* *Prevents unnecessary pain when moving client*
3. Explain procedure to client, emphasizing importance of maintaining elevation of extremity, of not handling wet cast, and of frequent assessment;	*Decrease anxiety* *Increases compliance*

Action	Rationale
instruct client not to insert anything between cast and extremity.	*Prevents injury and infection*
4. Don gloves.	*Avoids contact with body fluids*
5. Provide for privacy.	*Decreases embarrassment*
6. Handle casted extremity or body area with *palms* of hands for first 24 to 36 hours, until cast is fully dry.	*Avoids dents that could ultimately result in edema and pressure areas*
7. If cast is slow to dry, place small fan directly facing cast (about 24 inches away). DO NOT PLACE LINEN OVER CAST UNTIL CAST IS DRY.	*Enhances speed of drying* *Allows air to circulate and assist in drying cast*
8. If cast is on extremity, elevate on pillows (cover pillow with linen savers or plastic bags) so that normal curvatures created with casting are maintained.	*Prevents edema* *Enhances venous return* *Prevents soiling of pillows* *Prevents flattened areas on cast as it dries and prevents pressure areas*
9. Wash excess antimicrobial agents (such as povidone) from skin. Rinse, and pat dry.	*Allows for clear skin and vascular assessment*
10. Perform and instruct family on procedure for observation of skin and neurovascular assessment at frequent intervals. If cast is on extremity, compare to opposite extremity	*Detects signs of abnormal neurovascular function, such as vascular or nerve compression* *Suggests possible nature of neurovascular deficit*
11. If breakthrough bleeding is noted on cast, circle area, then write date and time on cast; if moderate to large amount of bleeding, notify doctor (otherwise, follow orders as written for bleeding).	*Provides baseline data for amount of bleeding* *Facilitates early intervention and prevention of complications*
12. Assess for signs of infec-	*Detects infectious process at*

Action	Rationale
tion under cast; obtain temperature.	*early stage*
13. Instruct client and family on how to reposition client every 2 hours; if client has body or spica cast, secure assistants to help turn client.	*Prevents client discomfort* *Makes turning quick, efficient, and safe*
14. Provide back and skin care frequently.	*Prevents skin breakdown*
15. If flaking of cast around edges is noted, remove flakes, pull stockinette over cast edges, and tape down.	*Prevents accumulation of particles inside cast, which cause infection*
16. Place client with leg or body cast on fracture pan for elimination: for clients with good bowel and bladder control, temporarily line edge of cast close to perineal area with plastic; if client has little or no elimination control (eg, some elderly clients), maintain plastic lining on cast edges and change once every 8 hours.	*Provides for elimination needs* *Prevents soiling of cast*
17. Instruct client and family on how to perform range-of-motion exercises of all joint areas every 4 hours (except where contra-indicated).	
18. Instruct client to cough and deep breathe and reposition client (within guidelines for orders) every 2 hours.	*Prevents pneumonia, decubitus ulcers, and other complications of immobility*
19. Restore or discard equipment properly.	*Removes waste and clutter*
20. Wash hands.	*Removes microorganisms*

Evaluation

Were desired outcomes achieved?

Documentation

The following should be noted on the visit note:

- Data from neurovascular assessment
- Abnormal data indicating inflammation or infection
- Indicators of complications of immobility
- Frequency of body alignment and repositioning and positions into which client is placed
- Frequency and nature of skin care given
- Frequency of coughing and deep breathing exercises performed
- Frequency and nature of range-of-motion exercises performed
- Teaching completed and additional teaching needs of client

Sample Documentation

DATE	TIME	
12/19/98	1030	Fourth hour since cast applied. Left leg full-length cast remains cold and wet. Toes of both left and right feet are pink, warm, and dry. Client able to wiggle toes and identify which toe is being touched. Cough and deep breathing done. Repositioned every 2 hours. Active range-of-motion exercise performed to all extremities except left leg. Able to verbalize signs of infection and poor circulation in left leg.

Nursing Procedure 7.8

Traction Maintenance

EQUIPMENT

- Alcohol wipes
- Antimicrobial agent for cleaning pins (skeletal tractions)
- One sterile gauze pad (2 × 2 or 4 × 3) for each traction pin
- Sterile gloves
- Sterile dressings, if needed
- Equipment for supporting body positioning, eg, trochanter roll, pillows, sandbag, footboard)
- Traction setup

Purpose

Maintains traction apparatus with appropriate counterbalance
Prevents infection at site of insertion of traction pins

Desired Outcomes (sample)

No redness, swelling, pain, discharge, or odor occurs at pin site.
There is no evidence of complications of immobility.

Assessment

Assessment should focus on the following:

Medical diagnosis
Doctor's orders for traction weight and pin care
Type of skin traction or skeletal traction
Status of weights, ropes, and pulleys
Reports of pain or discomfort
Integumentary status
Neurovascular indicators distal to pin sites (skin color and temperature, capillary refill, sensation, presence of pulse, ability to move toes or fingers)
Indicators of complications of immobility: decubitus ulcers or pressure areas; contractures; decreased peristalsis, constipation, and fecal impaction; signs of pulmonary embolism (chest pain, dyspnea, wheezing, increased heart rate); signs of thrombophlebitis (redness, heat, swelling, or pain in local area)

Outcome Identification and Planning

Key Goals and Sample Goal Criteria

The client will:

Not develop infection from pin site, as evidenced by absence of redness, swelling, pain, discharge, and odor at site

Not develop complications of immobility, as evidenced by absence of signs and symptoms of complications such as decubitus ulcers, thrombophlebitis, and so forth

Special Considerations

If weights do not swing freely, traction can be counterproductive.

Assess status of weights frequently, particularly after moving client.

When the client is mobile, with intermittent traction on an extremity, install traction setup over a door with a measured source of weight (eg, flour bag with sand, rocks, bricks).

Geriatric

Elderly clients are particularly prone to the development of broken skin integrity when they are bedridden and not repositioned frequently; this tendency is due to a decreased amount of subcutaneous fat and to skin that is less elastic, thinner, drier, and more fragile than that of a younger person.

IMPLEMENTATION

Action	Rationale
1. Wash hands.	*Reduces microorganism transfer*
2. Explain procedure to client, emphasizing importance of maintaining counterbalance and position.	*Decreases anxiety*
3. Provide for privacy.	*Decreases embarrassment*
4. Assess traction setup (Fig. 7.8): - Weights hanging freely and not touching bed or floor - Ordered amount of weight applied - Ropes moving freely through pulleys	*Ensures accurate counterbalance and function of traction*

Action	Rationale

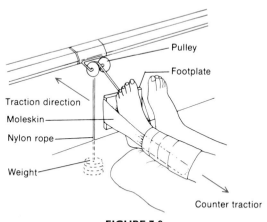

FIGURE 7.8

- All knots tight in ropes and away from pulleys
- Pulleys free of linens

5. Check client position (client's head should be near head of bed and properly aligned). *Maintains proper counter-balance*

6. Assess skin for signs of pressure areas or friction under skin traction belts. *Detects early signs of skin breakdown*

7. Assess neurovascular status of extremity distal to traction. *Detects neurovascular complications*

8. Assess site at and around pin for redness, edema, discharge, or odor. *Determines presence of infection*

9. Wash hands. *Reduces microorganism transfer*

10. Don gloves. *Prevents exposure to body fluids*

11. Wash, rinse, and dry skin thoroughly; if permissible, remove skin traction periodically to wash *Promotes circulation to skin*

Action	Rationale
under skin (check doctor's order and agency policy).	
12. Discard gloves, wash hands, and don sterile gloves.	*Prevents contamination*
13. Cleanse pin site and complete site care using sterile technique.	*Prevents infection*
14. Discard gloves and wash hands.	*Removes microorganisms*
15. Teach client to perform range-of-motion exercises on all joint areas, except those contraindicated, every 4 hours.	*Prevents pneumonia, decubitus ulcers, and complications of immobility*
16. Instruct client to cough and deep breathe and reposition client (within guidelines for orders) every 2 hours; use trochanter rolls and foot board to prevent internal and external hip rotation and footdrop.	*Prevents complications related to improper positioning*
17. Lift side rails, if using medical bed.	*Prevents falls*
18. Wash hands.	*Reduces microorganism transfer*

Evaluation

Were desired outcomes achieved?

DOCUMENTATION

The following should be noted on the visit note:

- Type of traction and amount of weight used
- Status of ropes, pulleys, and weights
- Body alignment of client
- Repositioning (frequency and last position)
- Pin care given
- Skin care given
- Coughing and deep breathing exercises performed

- Range-of-motion exercises performed
- Client teaching completed and additional teaching needs of client

Sample Documentation

DATE	TIME	
10/19/98	1030	Maintains intermittent pelvic traction with 20 pounds of weight. Traction removed about 4 times per day for client to go to restroom. Skin in pelvic area clean, warm, pink, and dry. Range-of-motion exercises of upper and lower extremities performed by client every 4 hours. Doing own coughing and deep breathing every 2 hours; breath sounds clear bilaterally. Client and family instructed on use of traction and safe operation.

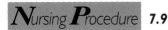 *Nursing Procedure* **7.9**

Antiembolism Hose/Pneumatic Compression Device Application

☒ EQUIPMENT

- Pneumatic compression equipment with comfort stockings or hose

or

- Antiembolic hose
- Washcloth
- Towel
- Soap
- Basin of warm water
- Tape measure (if not included in package)

Purpose

Promotes venous blood return to heart by maintaining pressure on capillaries and veins

Prevents development of venous thrombosis secondary to stagnant circulation

Desired Outcomes (sample)

Client states two ways to reduce risk of developing venous thrombosis.

Client remains free of signs of venous thrombosis.

Assessment

Assessment should focus on the following:

Medical diagnosis

Doctor's orders for hose length and frequency of application

Reports of pain or discomfort of lower extremities

Skin status of legs and feet

Neurovascular indicators of lower extremities (skin color and temperature, capillary refill, sensation, pulse presence and quality)

Indicators of venous disorders of lower extremities (redness, heat, swelling, or pain in local area)

Outcome Identification and Planning

Key Goals and Sample Goal Criteria
The client will:

Demonstrate no signs of venous thrombosis, as evidenced by absence of pain, redness, edema, and heat of lower extremities, prior to discharge

Demonstrate correct procedure for application and maintenance of hose

State two ways to reduce chances of developing venous thrombosis

Special Considerations
Clients with known or suspected peripheral vascular disorders should not wear hose because thrombus dislodgment may occur.

Poor maintenance of hose could result in circulatory restriction; hose must remain free of wrinkles, rolls, or kinks.

Geriatric

Elderly clients are particularly prone to development of venous disorders of lower extremities because of age-related physiological changes that occur in the tissue of veins. In addition, chronic cardiac and peripheral vascular dysfunctions also reduce venous return.

IMPLEMENTATION

Action	Rationale
1. Wash hands.	*Reduces microorganism transfer*
2. Explain procedure to client and family, emphasizing importance of maintaining hose on extremity for specified amount of time, wearing hose properly, and maintaining adequate circulation.	*Decreases anxiety* *Increases compliance*
3. Provide for privacy.	*Decreases embarrassment*
4. Measure for appropriate-size hose according to package directions (large,	*Promotes proper functioning of hose* *Prevents reduced circulation to*

Action	Rationale
medium, or small)	*legs*
or	
obtain vinyl sleeves and comfort stockings/hose.	
5. Wash, rinse, and dry legs; apply light talcum powder, if desired.	*Promotes comfort* *Promotes clean, dry skin*
6. Turn antiembolism hose (except foot portion) inside out.	*Promotes proper application of hose*
7. Place foot of hose over client's toes and foot; using both hands, slide hose up leg until completely on (smooth and straighten hose as it is pulled up); do not turn top of hose down.	*Applies hose, making certain that kinks and wrinkles are smoothed out* *Prevents tourniquet effect*
8. Apply second hose in same manner.	

Pneumatic Compression Device

9. Slide vinyl surgical sleeve over each calf (Fig. 7.9) *or* apply Velcro-secured vinyl compression hose by placing open hose under thigh and leg with knee-opening site under the popliteal area.	*Places source of intermittent compression over the veins of the extremities*

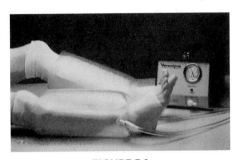

FIGURE 7.9

Action	Rationale
10. Establish the vinyl hose by overlapping the edges and securing the Velcro connectors.	*Establishes air pump source prepares unit for function*
11. Turn the power on to the unit.	
12. Monitor several inflation/deflation compression cycles.	*Permits early detection of excessive compression*
13. Replace covers.	*Provides privacy and warmth*
14. Instruct family to observe extremities 3–4 times/day to assess circulation and hose placement.	*Prevents complications*
15. Instruct client to remove hose twice a day for 20 minutes (ideally during morning and evening care).	*Allows for skin aeration and reassessment*
16. Wash hands and restore equipment.	*Reduces microorganism transfer Maintains organized environment*

Evaluation

Were desired outcomes achieved?

DOCUMENTATION

The following should be noted on the visit note:

- Size and length of hose applied
- Lower extremity skin color, temperature, sensation, capillary refill
- Status of pulses in lower extremities
- Presence of pain or discomfort in lower extremities
- Removal of hose twice daily
- Client teaching completed and additional teaching needs of client

Sample Documentation

DATE	TIME	
4/29/98	0830	Full-length embolic hose applied to lower legs—size, large/long. Skin of both lower extremities warm. No tears or abrasions noted. Toes pink with 2-second capillary refill. Bilateral pedal pulses 2+. Client stated purpose of hose and correctly related care measures. Able to verbalize signs of impaired/compromised circulation.

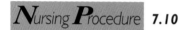

*N*ursing *P*rocedure **7.10**

Continuous Passive Motion (CPM) Device

▣ EQUIPMENT

- Continuous passive motion (CPM) device
- Softgoods kit (single patient use)
- Tape measure
- Goniometer

Purpose

Increases range of motion
Decreases effects of immobility
Stimulates healing of the articular cartilage
Reduces adhesions and swelling

Desired Outcomes (sample)

Client tolerates progressive increase in flexion and extension with CPM device.
Client demonstrates increasing mobility of affected extremity.

Assessment

Assessment should focus on the following:

Doctor's orders for degrees of flexion and extension
Neurovascular status of extremity prior to start of CPM
Presence of pulses and capillary refill in affected extremity
Skin color and temperature, sensation, and movement of extremity
Reports of pain or discomfort

Outcome Identification and Planning

Key Goals and Sample Goal Criteria
The client will:

Remain free of contractures
Maintain maximum mobility of extremities

Demonstrate increased tolerance to CPM device until prescribed goal is attained

Special Considerations

Geriatric

Elderly clients are particularly prone to the development of broken skin when they are immobilized.

HINT

ECONOMIC: Reimbursement for CPM equipment use in the home varies among payor sources.

Implementation

Action	Rationale
1. Wash hands. Organize equipment. Apply softgoods to CPM device (Fig. 7.10.1).	*Reduces microorganism transfer* *Promotes efficiency* *Prevents friction to extremity during motion*
2. Check doctor's order for degrees of flexion and extension. Speed will be determined by patient comfort. Begin with a midpoint setting.	*May change on a daily basis as the patient progresses*
3. Explain procedure to client.	*Decreases anxiety and facilitates cooperation*

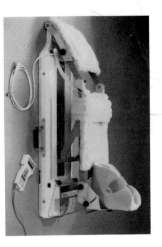

FIGURE 7.10.1

Action	Rationale
4. Using the tape measure, determine the distance between the gluteal crease and the popliteal space.	*Determines the distance to adjust the Thigh Length Adjustment knobs on the CPM device*
5. Measure the length of client's leg from the knee to ¼ inch beyond the bottom of the foot.	*Determines the distance to adjust the position of the foot-plate*
6. Position the client in the middle of the bed with the extremity in a slightly abducted position.	*Promotes proper body alignment Prevents CPM device from exerting pressure on opposite extremity*
7. Elevate client's leg and place in padded CPM device (Fig. 7.10.2).	*Prepares client for therapy*
8. Note proper anatomical placement of device: Client's knee should be at the hinged joint of the machine.	*Improper positioning of the device may cause injury*
9. Adjust the footplate to maintain the client's foot in a neutral position. Make certain that the leg is neither internally nor externally rotated.	*Improper positioning of the device may cause injury*
10. Apply the soft restraining straps under CPM device and around extremity	*The soft restraints maintain the extremity in position. Allowing several fingers to fit under*

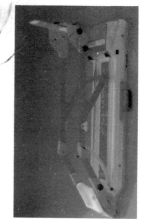

FIGURE 7.10.2

Action	Rationale

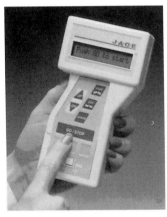

FIGURE 7.10.3

loosely enough to fit several fingers under it.

11. Turn unit on at main power switch. Set controls to levels prescribed by physician.

12. Instruct the client in the use of the GO/STOP button.

13. Set CPM device in the ON stage and press GO button (Fig. 7.10.3).

14. Determine angle of flexion when device has reached its greatest height using the goniometer. *Note:* If unit is not anatomical, there might be a slight difference between reading on the device and the actual angle of the patient's knee.

the restraint prevents pressure from restraint strap on affected extremity

Cannot adjust controls and setting unless power is on; prepares client for onset of therapeutic intervention

Client participates in care, thus decreasing anxiety

Initiates therapeutic intervention

Evaluation

Were desired outcomes achieved?

DOCUMENTATION

The following should be noted on the visit note:

- Onset of therapy
- Tolerance of procedure
- Degree of extension and flexion and speed of machine
- Amount of time client used device
- Neurovascular status of extremity
- Successive therapeutic aids, immobilizer, etc.

Sample Documentation

DATE	TIME	
8/4/98	1100	CPM device applied to left leg at 0 degrees of extension and 35 degrees of flexion started at slow speed. Verified by goniometer. Patient instructed in use of GO/STOP button. Denies need for pain medication at this time. Padding to all soft tissue near CPM device. Phone within reach.

Chapter 8

Rest and Comfort

OVERVIEW

► Each individual's perception of pain is unique.

► Cultural background may have a great impact on a client's pain threshold and pain tolerance, as well as on the client's expression of pain. The nurse must consider cultural impacts on the pain experience when planning care.

► Heat and cold may have special cultural significance for some clients (Asians or Hispanics, for example), who classify conditions accordingly and expect corresponding treatments (see Table 8.1).

► Nurses must be sensitive to alternative pain relief measures used by clients and the cultural significance of those measures. Efforts should be made to reconcile religious rituals, herbal remedies, or other alternate treatments with the established medical plan to facilitate culturally competent care.

► The assessment of pain should include its location, duration, intensity and its precipitating, alleviating, and associated factors.

► Appropriate duration of treatment is essential for the therapeutic use of heat and cold.

► The procedures in this chapter should be taught to client and caregiver(s).

413

TABLE 8.1 Hot–Cold Conditions*	
Hot Conditions	**Cold Conditions**
Fever	Arthritis
Infections	Colds
Diarrhea	Indigestion
Constipation	Joint pain
Rashes	Menstrual period
Tenesmus	Ear ache
Ulcers	Cancer
Kidney problems	Tuberculosis
Skin ailments	Headache
Sore throat	Paralysis
Liver problems	Teething
	Rheumatism
	Pneumonia
	Malaria

*The usual treatment for hot–cold conditions is thought to be use of a food or substance of the opposite temperature.

▶ Cold therapy causes vasoconstriction; reduces local metabolism, edema, and inflammation; and induces local anesthetic effects.
▶ Heat therapy causes vasodilatation, relieves muscle tension, stimulates circulation, and promotes healing.
▶ **DANGER—ADDITIONAL TISSUE DAMAGE CAN RESULT IF:**
  - Excessive temperature is used (hot or cold)
  - Overexposure of site to treatment occurs
  - Electrical equipment is not checked for safety

Nursing Procedure 8.1

🖐 *Aquathermia Pad*

❎ EQUIPMENT

- Aquathermia module (K-module) with pad (K-pad)
- Bedside table
- Disposable gloves
- Pillowcase
- Distilled water
- Tape

Purpose

Stimulates circulation, thus providing nutrients to tissues
Reduces muscle tension

Desired Outcomes (sample)

Client verbalizes increased comfort after treatment.
Client demonstrates increased mobility of affected extremity after treatment.

Assessment

Assessment should focus on the following:

Treatment order
Client's tolerance to last treatment
Status of treatment area (redness, tenderness, cleanliness, and dryness)
Temperature and pulse rate and rhythm
Degree of pain and position of comfort, if any
Mental status of client
Adequate functioning of heating device for proper functioning

Outcome Identification and Planning

Key Goal and Sample Goal Criterion

The client will:

State increased comfort after treatment

Special Considerations

Make sure lamp functions accurately and safely. DO NOT USE IF CORD IS FRAYED OR CRACKS ARE NOTED.

Schedule procedure when client can be assessed frequently.

IF A CLIENT IS CONFUSED OR UNABLE TO REMAIN ALONE WITH A HEATING DEVICE ON, REMAIN WITH THE CLIENT OR FIND SOMEONE TO DO SO.

Clients with decreased peripheral sensory perception, such as diabetics, must be monitored closely for heat overexposure.

Because a client will be using a K-module when a nurse is not present, teach the client or family how to use the module safely.

Geriatric

Elderly clients may be extremely sensitive to heat therapy. Assess more frequently because their skin is fragile.

 Transcultural

Determine cultural perspective regarding use of heat to treat the condition.

Discuss objections and incorporate hot/cold perception of illness and treatment.

Omit treatment if client objects, and consult physician.

IMPLEMENTATION

Action	Rationale
1. Wash hands and organize equipment.	*Reduces microorganism transfer* *Promotes efficiency*
2. Explain procedure to client.	*Decreases anxiety and promotes cooperation*
3. Place heating module on bedside table at a level above the client's body level (Fig. 8.1).	*Facilitates flow of fluid*
4. Fill module two thirds full with distilled water.	*Enables unit to function properly*
5. Turn module on low setting and allow water to begin circulating throughout the pad and tubing.	*Detects leakage of fluid or improper functioning before initiating therapy*
6. After water is fully circulating through the pad and tubing, check the pad with your hands to ascertain that it is warming.	*Checks for proper functioning and heating of unit*

Action	Rationale

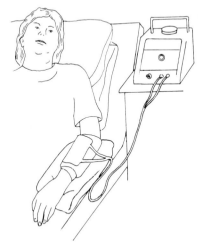

FIGURE 8.1

Action	Rationale
7. Don disposable gloves, if indicated.	*Decreases exposure to secretions*
8. Place pillowcase over the heating pad and position pad on or (if an extremity) around treatment area.	*Prevents direct skin contact with pad, minimizing danger of burn injury*
9. If placement of pad needs to be secured, use tape. DO NOT USE PINS.	*Prevents water leakage from possible puncture to pad*
10. After 60 seconds, assess for heat intolerance by: - Observing client's facial gestures - Asking if heat is too warm - Noting any dizziness, faintness, or palpitations - Removing pad and assessing for redness or tenderness; readjust temperature if necessary	*Prevents burn injury and complications of heat therapy*
11. Replace pad and secure	*Resumes treatment*

Action	Rationale
with tape, if needed.	
12. Instruct client NOT to alter placement of pad or heating module and to call if heat becomes too warm.	*Promotes client cooperation and continued optimum function of unit* *Prevents burn injury*
13. Recheck client every 5 minutes.	*Prevents burn injury*
14. After 20 minutes, turn module off and place pad on table with module.	*Terminates treatment*
15. Assist client to a comfortable position.	*Facilitates comfort*
16. Return equipment to proper area.	*Maintains organized environment*
17. Remove gloves and wash hands.	*Reduces microorganism transfer*

Evaluation

Were desired outcomes achieved?

DOCUMENTATION

The following should be noted on the visit note:

- Appearance of treatment area
- General response of client (weakness, faintness, palpitations, diaphoresis, extreme tenderness, if any)
- Duration of treatment
- Status of pain

Sample Documentation

DATE	TIME	
12/3/98	1400	K-module applied to right calf for 20 minutes. No redness, warmth, or tenderness to touch at treatment area. Vital signs stable during and after treatment. Family member assisted with and correctly verbalized steps to use of module.

*N*ursing *P*rocedure 8.2

Heat Therapy: Commercial Hot Pack/Moist Compresses

⊠ EQUIPMENT

- Prepackaged heat pack
- Tape
- Small towel or washcloth

or

- Warm compress
  - warmed solution, 43°C (110°F)
  - petroleum jelly
  - heating pad or aquathermia pad (optional)
  - distilled water (for aquathermia pad)
- Towel
- Plastic-lined underpad
- Clean basin
- Bath thermometer
- Pack of 4 × 4-inch gauze pads
- Bath blanket
- Two forceps (optional)
- Two pairs of nonsterile gloves

Purpose

Promotes comfort

Hot compress stimulates circulation and promotes localization of purulent matter in tissues

Desired Outcome (sample)

Client verbalizes pain is decreased within 1 hour after treatment.

Assessment

Assessment should focus on the following:

Treatment order, type of solution to be used, and response of client to previous treatments

Appearance of treatment area (edema, local bleeding)
Status of pain
Sensitivity of skin to heat treatment

Outcome Identification and Planning

Key Goals and Sample Goal Criteria

The client will:

Verbalize increased comfort within 1 hour after treatment
Show decreased redness at site within 3 days

Special Considerations

Schedule application of heat therapy when the client can be assessed at frequent intervals.

Determine with client the best body position for comfort and alignment.

If applying warm compresses, check heating device for safety and proper functioning.

If using aquathermia pad for warm compress, set up heating device according to the guidelines in Procedure 8.1.

Warn client that a clothing iron should NEVER be used as a heat source for a warm compress.

Schedule the treatment when the client can be checked every 5 to 10 minutes.

Do not use on clients with peripheral sensory deficits.

Geriatric

Elderly clients may require more frequent checks because skin may be more fragile.

   Transcultural

Determine cultural perspective regarding hot/cold perception of illness and appropriateness of treatment.

Incorporate client preference when possible.

Omit treatment if client objects and consult physician.

IMPLEMENTATION

Action	Rationale
1. Explain procedure to client.	*Decreases anxiety and promotes cooperation*
2. Wash hands and organize equipment.	*Decreases microorganism transfer*
	Promotes efficiency

Action	Rationale

For Commercial Hot Pack

3. Remove heat pack from outer package, if present.

Provides access to pack

4. Break the inner seal; hold pack tightly in the center in upright position and squeeze. DO NOT USE PACK IF LEAKING IS NOTED (CHEMICAL BURN MAY OCCUR).

Activates chemical ingredients to form "heat" pack

5. Lightly shake pack until the inner contents are lying in the lower portion of the pack.

Localizes activated chemicals

6. Proceed to Application Steps.

For Warm Moist Compress

1. Place gauze into basin half-filled with heated ordered solution.

Saturates gauze with solution

2. Assist client into position.

Facilitates compress placement

3. Place plastic pad under treatment area.

Prevents soiling of linens

4. Drape client.

Provides privacy

5. Wring one layer of wet gauze until it is dripless.

Removes excess solution

6. Proceed to Application Steps.

Application Steps

1. Don gloves.

Reduces microorganism transfer

2. Remove and discard old dressings, if present.

Provides access to treatment site

3. Remove and discard old gloves and don new gloves.

Reduces microorganism transfer

4. If necessary, clean and dry treatment area.

Facilitates effectiveness of treatment

For Hot Pack:

5. Place the hot pack lightly against treatment area.

Allows for gradual initiation of vasodilating effect

6. Remove pack and assess client for redness of skin or complaint of burning after 30 seconds.

Prevents burn injury

Action	Rationale
7. Replace pack snugly against the area if no problems are noted, and secure placement with tape (go to step 9).	*Resumes treatment* *Stabilizes cold-heat pack*
For Moist Compress	
5. Place compress on the wound for several seconds.	*Initiates vasoconstrictive or vasodilatation therapy*
6. Pick up edge of compress to observe initial skin response to therapy.	*Allows assessment of skin for adverse responses to therapy* *Promotes safety*
7. Replace compress gauze every 5 minutes, or as needed, to maintain warmth, assessing treatment area each time.	*Provides for reassessment of treatment area*
8. Place towel over compress (a heating device, if available, may be placed over) (proceed to step 9)	*Maintains heat of warm compress*
9. Reassess treatment area every 5 minutes by lifting the corners of the pack.	*Monitors effects of treatment over time*
10. After 20 minutes, terminate treatment and dry skin.	*Prevents local injury due to overexposure to treatment*
11. Apply new dressing over wound, if necessary.	*Promotes wound healing*
12. Assist client to a comfortable position.	*Facilitates comfort*
13. Remove all equipment from bedside.	*Maintains clean environment and facilitates asepsis*
14. Remove gloves and wash hands.	

Evaluation

Were desired outcomes achieved?

DOCUMENTATION

The following should be noted on the visit note:

- Size, location, and appearance of treatment area
- Status of pain
- Duration of treatment
- Client tolerance to treatment

Sample Documentation

DATE	TIME	
12/3/98	1300	Warm compress applied to right wrist for 20 minutes. Redness decreased from 2 to 1 cm. Site slightly warm to touch after treatment, capillary refill 3 secs. Client reports relief of pain.

Nursing **P**rocedure **8.3**

✋ *Cold Therapy: Ice Bag, Collar, Glove/Commercial Cold Pack/Moist Compresses*

❎ EQUIPMENT

- Ice bag/collar/glove or prepackaged cold pack

or

For cold compress:
- Plastic-lined linen saver
- Clean basin
- Bath thermometer
- Pack of 4 × 4 gauze pads
- Solution cooled with ice, 15°C (59°F)
- Cotton swab stick
- Tape
- Disposable gloves (2 pair)
- Small towel or washcloth
- Ice chips

Purpose

Reduces local edema, bleeding, and hematoma formation
Decreases local pain sensation

Desired Outcomes (sample)

Client states that pain is reduced or relieved after treatment.
No bleeding or hematoma is noted at treatment site.

Assessment

Assessment should focus on the following:

Treatment order and client's response to previous treatment, if used
Condition and appearance of treatment area (edema, local bleeding)
Status of pain

Outcome Identification and Planning

Key Goals and Sample Goal Criteria

The client will:

Verbalize decreased discomfort after treatment
Show decreased or no bleeding/hematoma at site
Show decreased edema from 2+ to 1+ cm within 36 hours

Special Considerations

Schedule the procedure when the client can be checked frequently.

A self-sealing plastic bag may be used as an ice bag, if necessary.

Geriatric

Elderly clients may require more frequent checks because skin may be fragile.

 Transcultural

Consider cultural perspectives and preference for cold therapy.
Consult physician if client objects to planned therapy.

IMPLEMENTATION

Action	Rationale
1. Explain procedure to client.	*Decreases anxiety*
2. Wash hands and organize equipment.	*Reduces microorganism transfer* *Promotes efficiency*

Ice Pack with Bag/Collar/Glove

1. Fill bag/collar/glove about three-fourths full with ice chips.	*Provides cold surface area*
2. Remove excess air from bag/collar/glove: - Place bag/collar/glove on flat surface. - Gently press until ice reaches the opening.	*Improves functioning of pack*
3. Contain ice securely by fastening end of the bag or collar; for plastic glove, tie end of glove itself.	*Prevents water seepage*
4. Cover body part with towel	*Promotes comfort*

Action	Rationale
or washcloth (if bag is made of a soft cloth exterior, this is not necessary).	
5. Proceed to Application Steps.	

Commercial Cold Pack

Action	Rationale
1. Remove ice pack from outer package, if present.	*Provides access to pack*
2. Break the inner seal; hold pack tightly in the center in upright position and squeeze. DO NOT USE PACK IF LEAKING IS NOTED (CHEMICAL BURN MAY OCCUR).	*Activates chemical ingredients to form "cold" pack*
3. Lightly shake pack until the inner contents are lying in the lower portion of the pack.	*Localizes activated chemicals*
4. Proceed to Application Steps.	

Moist Cold Compress

Action	Rationale
1. Place gauze into basin half-filled with chilled ordered solution.	*Saturates gauze with solution*
2. Assist client into position.	*Facilitates compress placement*
3. Place plastic pad under treatment area.	*Prevents soiling of linens*
4. Drape client.	*Provides privacy*
5. Wring one layer of wet gauze until it is dripless.	*Removes excess solution*
6. Proceed to Application Steps.	

Application Steps

Action	Rationale
1. Don gloves.	*Reduces microorganism transfer*
2. Remove and discard old dressings, if present.	*Provides access to treatment site*
3. Remove and discard old gloves and don new gloves.	*Reduces microorganism transfer*
4. If necessary, clean and	*Facilitates effectiveness of*

Action	Rationale
dry treatment area.	*treatment*

For Commercial Cold Pack

Action	Rationale
5. Place the pack lightly against treatment area.	*Allows for gradual initiation of vasoconstrictive effect*
6. Remove pack and assess client for redness of skin or complaint of burning after 30 seconds.	*Prevents burn injury*
7. Replace pack snugly against the area if no problems are noted, and secure placement with tape. Proceed to step 8.	*Resumes treatment* *Stabilizes cold pack*

For Moist Compress

Action	Rationale
5. Place compress on the wound for several seconds.	*Initiates vasoconstrictive therapy*
6. Pick up edge of compress to observe initial skin response to therapy.	*Allows assessment of skin for adverse responses to therapy* *Promotes safety*
7. Replace compress gauze every 5 minutes, or as needed, to maintain coolness, assessing treatment area each time. Proceed to step 8.	*Provides for reassessment of treatment area*
8. Reassess treatment area every 5 minutes by lifting the corners of the pack.	*Monitors effects of treatment over time*
9. After 20 minutes, terminate treatment and dry skin.	*Prevents local injury due to overexposure to treatment*
10. Apply new dressing over wound, if necessary.	*Promotes wound healing*
11. Assist client to position of comfort.	*Facilitates comfort and safety*
12. Remove all equipment from bedside.	*Maintains clean environment and facilitates asepsis*
13. Remove gloves and wash hands.	

Evaluation

Were desired outcomes achieved?

DOCUMENTATION

The following should be noted on the visit note:

- Size, location, and appearance of treatment area
- Status of pain
- Duration of treatment
- Client tolerance to treatment

Sample Documentation

DATE	TIME	
12/3/98	1300	Ice bag applied to right wrist for 20 minutes. Edema decreased from 2 to 1 cm. Site slightly cool to touch after treatment, capillary refill 3 secs. Client reports relief of pain.

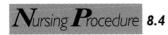

*N*ursing *P*rocedure 8.4

Sitz Bath

EQUIPMENT

- Clean bathtub filled with enough warm water to cover buttocks (or portable sitz tub, if available)
- Bath towel
- Bath thermometer, if available
- Rubber tub ring
- Bathroom mat
- Gown
- Small footstool
- Nonsterile gloves

Purpose

Promotes perineal and anorectal healing
Reduces local inflammation and discomfort

Desired Outcomes (sample)

Client verbalizes relieved or decreased pain after treatment.
Within 48 hours, site is clean without redness, edema, or drainage.

Assessment

Assessment should focus on the following:

Baseline vital signs
Appearance and condition of treatment area
Client and caregiver knowledge of procedure for and benefits of sitz bath
Client inability to remain unattended in bathtub (eg, confusion, weakness)
Status of pain

Outcome Identification and Planning

Key Goals and Sample Goal Criteria
The client will:

Verbalize increased comfort or relief of pain after treatment

Evidence no redness, edema, or discharge from site within 48 hours

Special Considerations

Schedule the procedure when the client can be checked frequently.

If client is confused or unable to remain alone, plan to remain with client or find someone to do so.

Instruct client and family regarding the procedure. Emphasize the importance of a family member's checking on the client frequently if a potential safety hazard (such as falling in tub or on floor) exists.

Geriatric

Vasodilatation from exposure to warm water could cause severe changes in blood pressure and cardiac function in elderly clients with compromised cardiovascular status. Duration and temperature of sitz bath might need to be decreased, and clients must be watched closely for adverse reactions.

 Transcultural

See overview regarding hot/cold conditions.

Discuss therapy with client and relate objections to physician.

IMPLEMENTATION

Action	Rationale
1. Explain procedure to client.	*Promotes relaxation and compliance*
2. Wash hands, organize equipment, and don gloves.	*Reduces microorganism transfer to client or nurse*
	Promotes efficiency
3. Check temperature of water with thermometer (105°F to 110°F [40.5°C to 43°C]); if thermometer is unavailable, test water with your wrist (water should be warm).	*Prevents skin damage from high water temperature*
4. Place rubber ring at bottom of tub and bathmat on floor.	*Prevents accidental falls*
5. Assist client to bathroom.	
6. Close door and assist	*Provides privacy*

Action	Rationale
client with undressing.	
7. Assist client into tub, using footstool if necessary.	*Prevents accidental injury*
8. Seat client on the rubber ring.	
9. Ascertain client stability in the tub alone and assess reaction to the engulfing heat: - Observe facial expressions and body motions for signs of discomfort. - Ask if heat is too warm. - Watch for dizziness, faintness, profuse diaphoresis. - Note any rapid increase in or irregularity of pulse.	*Prevents complications from falling or unusual reaction to therapy*
10. Instruct client to call out if assistance is needed (baby monitor may be used).	*Facilitates client–nurse communication and immediate response to emergency*
11. Recheck client every 5 to 10 minutes.	*Allows assessment of unusual reactions*
12. After 15 to 20 minutes, help client out of the tub.	*Terminates treatment*
13. Assist client with drying and dressing; then place linens in hamper or designated dirty clothes area.	*Prevents chilling*
14. Assist client to room and bed or chair.	*Promotes comfort*
15. Remove equipment and clean tub.	*Reduces microorganism transfer to others using tub*
16. Remove gloves and wash hands.	*Reduces microorganism transfer*

Evaluation

Were desired outcomes achieved?

DOCUMENTATION

The following should be noted on the visit note:

- Appearance of treatment area before and after treatment
- Any unusual reactions to treatment, such as profuse diaphoresis, faintness, dizziness, palpitations, or pulse changes
- Duration of sitz bath
- Status of pain

Sample Documentation

DATE	TIME	
12/3/98	1500	Sitz bath to perineal area for 20 minutes. Client states pain decreased after treatment. No drainage from open perineal wound. No complaints of dizziness.

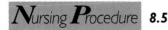

*N*ursing *P*rocedure **8.5**

Tepid Sponge Bath

EQUIPMENT

- Thermometer (oral or rectal)
- Basin of cold water
- Gown
- Plastic-lined pads
- Bath blanket
- Six or seven washcloths
- Two towels
- Nonsterile gloves

Purpose

Provides controlled reduction of body temperature

Desired Outcomes (sample)

Client maintains temperature within normal or acceptable limits (specified by physician).

Client tolerates treatment with no adverse changes in status or vital signs.

Assessment

Assessment should focus on the following:

Doctor's order and client's response to previous treatment
Condition and appearance of skin
Pulse and temperature
Level of consciousness

Outcome Identification and Planning

Key Goals and Sample Goal Criteria

The client will:

Show temperature within normal or acceptable limits for client
Show no untoward reactions to treatment

Special Considerations

If an alcohol bath is ordered, use equal parts of alcohol and water and assess client more frequently. Body temperature is decreased more rapidly by alcohol than by water.

Instruct client and family on the procedure and precautions of the tepid sponge bath and recommend that a thermometer be secured for the home.

Geriatric

The body temperature of elderly clients is less stable than younger adult clients and may require more frequent assessment.

 Transcultural

Note Overview regarding hot/cold conditions.

Adhere to cultural idiosyncracies regarding same-sex or opposite-sex care providers; family member should be instructed on procedure for sponge bath if preferred by client.

IMPLEMENTATION

Action	Rationale
1. Explain procedure to client.	*Reduces anxiety and promotes compliance*
2. Close windows and doors.	*Eliminates drafts, thus preventing chilling*
3. Wash hands and organize equipment.	*Reduces microorganism transfer Promotes efficiency*
4. Undress client, covering body with bath blanket and rolling topsheet to the bottom of bed.	*Prevents chilling and protects privacy*
5. Place washcloths and one towel in basin of water.	*Cools cloths and towel*
6. Place plastic pads under client.	*Prevents linen soilage*
7. Wring washcloths and place one in each of the following areas: - Over forehead - Under armpits - Over groin	*Promotes rapid cooling due to increased vascularity of these regions*
8. Rewet and replace washcloths as they become warm.	*Maintains coolness of cloths*

Action	Rationale
9. Wring the wet towel and place around client's arm (Fig. 8.5).	*Promotes decreased temperature in extremity*
10. Wring a washcloth and sponge the other arm for 3 or 4 minutes. Repeat steps 9 and 10 with the opposite arms.	*Facilitates gradual cooling of extremity*
11. Remove towel from arm and place in basin, dry both arms thoroughly, and replace blanket.	*Prepares towel for future use*
12. Check client's temperature and pulse: - *if temperature is above 100°F (37.7°C)*, proceed with bath. - *If temperature is at or below 100°F (37.7°C)*, terminate the procedure by skipping to step 17. - *If pulse is significantly increased*, terminate procedure for 5 minutes and recheck; if it remains significantly elevated,	*Prevents chilling* *Prevents complications related to overcooling*

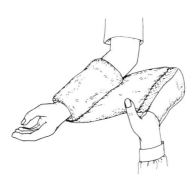

FIGURE 8.5

Action	Rationale
terminate procedure and notify physician.	
13. Continue bath by repeating steps 9 to 11 on arms.	*Facilitates maximum core-temperature reduction by treating greater body surface area*
14. Repeat temperature and pulse check.	*Assesses effectiveness of treatment*
15. Continue by sponging and drying the following areas for 3 to 5 minutes. • chest • left leg • back • abdomen • right leg • buttocks You may use steps 9 to 11 when sponging legs.	*Facilitates cooling by expanding the body surface area being treated*
16. STOP EVERY 10 MINUTES TO REASSESS TEMPERATURE AND PULSE.	*Assesses effectiveness* *Prevents overcooling*
17. Remove all cloths and towels and dry client thoroughly.	*Terminates treatment* *Promotes comfort*
18. Replace gown.	*Restores privacy*
19. Assist client to position of comfort.	*Promotes comfort*
20. Remove and properly discard all washcloths, towels, plastic pads, and wet linens. (If necessary, obtain dry linens and remake bed.)	*Maintains cleanliness of environment*
21. Remove and discard gloves.	*Reduces microorganism transfer*

Evaluation

Were desired outcomes achieved?

DOCUMENTATION

The following should be noted on the visit note:

- Pulse and temperature before and after bath
- Client mentation and general tolerance of the bath
- Untoward reactions to the treatment
- Length of the treatment and percentage of body sponged

Sample Documentation		
DATE	**TIME**	
12/25/98	0100	Tepid sponge bath administered for 20-minute duration because of client's temperature of 104.7°F. Temperature after bath, 102.6°F; pulse, 118 and regular; respirations, 28 and regular; blood pressure, 110/62. Client dozing quietly in bed. Doctor notified of status. Tylenol suppository grains XX given.

Nursing **P**rocedure **8.6**

Transcutaneous Electrical Nerve Stimulation Unit

☒ EQUIPMENT

- Transcutaneous electrical nerve stimulation (TENS) unit
- Lead wires
- Electrodes
- Water (optional)
- Fresh 9-volt battery

Purpose

Controls pain by delivering electrical impulse to nerve endings, which blocks pain message along pathway and prevents brain reception

Reduces amount of pain medication required to maintain comfort

Allows client to remain mentally alert, active, and pain free

Desired Outcomes (sample)

Client ambulates from room to room with minimal complaint of pain.

Client requests pain medication less frequently.

Decreased dosages of medication are needed.

Client and caregiver demonstrate skill in management of TENS unit therapy.

Assessment

Assessment should focus on the following:

Status of pain (location and degree; alleviating and aggravating factors)

Type and location of incision, if applicable

Previous use of and knowledge level regarding TENS unit

Presence of skin irritation, abrasions, or breakage

Outcome Identification and Planning

Key Goal and Sample Goal Criterion

The client will:

Cough and deep breathe 10 times every 1 to 2 hours with minimal or no pain medication.

Special Considerations

Apply electrodes to clean unbroken skin only.

If sensitivity to electrode adhesive is noted, notify doctor before application. If skin irritation is noted during TENS usage, remove electrodes and notify doctor.

Client should be informed that TENS unit may not totally relieve pain but should reduce discomfort.

Physical therapy may be needed in conjunction with TENS use.

Geriatric

Check skin frequently for tenderness and sensitivity.

If client is confused and electrical stimulation increases irritation, decrease or stop stimulation and notify doctor.

IMPLEMENTATION

Action	Rationale
1. Wash hands and organize equipment.	*Reduces microorganism transfer* *Promotes efficiency*
2. Explain procedure to client.	*Promotes relaxation and compliance*
3. Wash, rinse, and dry skin thoroughly.	*Facilitates electrode adhesion*
4. Prepare electrodes as described in package insert.	
5. Place electrodes on body areas directed by doctor or physical therapist (often along incision site or spinal column or both, depending on location of pain).	*Places electrodes in position for optimal results*
6. Plug lead wires into TENS unit (Fig. 8.6).	
7. Turn unit on and regulate for comfort: - Work with one lead (set) at a time.	*Ensures proper stimulation of each area addressed*

Action	Rationale

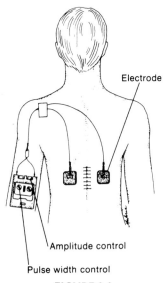

Electrode

Amplitude control

Pulse width control

FIGURE 8.6

- Before beginning, ask client to indicate when stimulation is felt.
- Beginning at 0, increase level of stimulation until client indicates feeling of discomfort (muscle contraction under electrode area).

Achieves maximum stimulation to block pain sensation

- When client indicates discomfort, reduce volume slightly.
- Try to maintain highest tolerable level of stimulation.

Prevents continued contraction of muscles at pain site or around incision

Promotes maximum blockage of pain sensations

Repeat above steps with other lead (set).

Action	Rationale
- Note color of blinking light on unit and change battery, as needed.	*Indicates unit is functional (red light may indicate low battery)*
8. Stabilize unit for client mobility using one of the following methods: - Clamp unit to pajama bottom or gown (may place tape around unit and pin to gown with safety pin). - Place in pants pocket or clip to belt, if client is ambulatory.	
9. Monitor client for comfort level with vital signs assessment; check for increased respiratory rate, pulse, or blood pressure.	*Indicates effectiveness of unit Indicates need to adjust stimulation due to increased discomfort*
10. Be alert for malfunctions and correct them; the following guidelines should be used and taught to client/caregiver for general management of the TENS unit:	*Prevents injury to client and damage to TENS unit*
- Client should remove unit before a shower or bath.	*Prevents shock to client*
- If client complains of increased or sudden pain sensation, check TENS connections and perform general assessment of incision, dressing, and client.	*Verifies function of unit and detects possible causes of increased discomfort*
- TENS unit should be off whenever removing or applying leads; if lead becomes disconnected, TURN UNIT OFF, RECONNECT LEAD, THEN INCREASE STIMULATION LEVEL FROM 0.	*Prevents shocking sensation*

Action	Rationale
- NEVER turn unit on when set at maximum stimulation: always start at 0 and gradually increase level.	*Prevents client discomfort at shocking sensation*
- If client complains of "shocking sensation" or muscle contraction, decrease stimulation level.	*Prevents excessive stimulation*
- Check battery status frequently.	

Evaluation

Were desired outcomes achieved?

DOCUMENTATION

The following should be noted on the visit note:

- Type and location of incision, if applicable
- Time and date of TENS application
- Level of stimulation of each lead (set)
- Area stimulated by each lead (set)
- Pain location, level, aggravating and alleviating factors
- Client teaching done and accuracy with which client repeats instructions

Sample Documentation		
DATE	**TIME**	
1/2/98	1200	TENs unit applied for lumbar back pain. Electrodes applied to lumbar area with setting of 5.5 on lead 1 and 6.0 on lead 2. Client verbalized understanding of unit function and states minimum pain felt at present.

*N*ursing *P*rocedure **8.7**

Patient-Controlled Analgesia and Epidural Pump Therapy

✕ EQUIPMENT

- Patient-controlled analgesia (PCA) infuser
- PCA administration set (pump tubing)
- IV tubing and fluid, as applicable
- PCA infuser key
- PCA flow sheet or appropriate form
- Ordered narcotic analgesic vial or syringe (mixed by pharmacy)
- Vial injector (accompanies vial)
- Client information booklet
- IV start kit (unless venous access is already available)

Purpose

To provide safe, effective, and consistent pain relief
Allows client to control delivery of pain medication in a safe, consistent, effective, and liable manner

Desired Outcomes (sample)

Adequate relief from chronic pain.
Increase in patient activity that is currently limited due to constant pain.

Assessment

Assessment should focus on the following:

Doctor's orders for type of analgesic, loading dosage, concentration of analgesic mixture, *lock-out interval* (minimum time allowed between doses)
Type of illness or surgery
Pain (type, location, character, intensity, aggravating and alleviating factors)
Level of consciousness and orientation
Venous access (patency of IV line, if present; skin status if IV to be started)
Ability to learn and comprehend

Reading ability

If using epidural also include any contraindication for epidural analgesia, ie, allergy to any proposed medication, any coagulopathy due to disease process or administration of systemic anticoagulants; localized infection or inflammation of the area of the epidural catheter, diagnosis of meningitis or CNS injury; history of increased intracranial pressure.

Outcome Identification and Planning

Key Goals and Sample Goal Criteria

The client or significant other will:

Verbalize increased comfort within 2 hours of PCA or epidural initiation

Correctly demonstrate PCA pump usage for continued or intermittent therapy

Participate in increased activities of daily living at greater levels than before the use of epidural analgesia

Demonstrate the care and maintenance activities required to keep the epidural catheter patent

Special Considerations

Pain is very subjective and for pain management to be effective it must meet individual patient needs.

Teach family members how to recognize signs of overdosage.

Naxalone must be readily available and a plan for emergencies must be discussed with the client and their caregiver.

Economic

Portable infusion pumps are not necessarily trouble free or less expensive for the client. The cost-benefit ratio must be considered when discussing this method of controlling pain in the home setting.

Geriatric

The analgesia may have an adverse effect on some elderly clients (eg, change in level of orientation).

HINT

Educate and assist the client in implementing non-pharmacological methods of pain relief as well as administration of medications. Often these techniques have synergistic effects with the medication that increase the home client's tolerance to activities of daily living.

For Epidural Administration

Only preservative free (non-bacterialstatic) opioid solutions or anesthetics are administered through an epidural catheter.

There are many and varied types of pumps for use with pain control in the home. Discuss with the client or their care provider the specific pump applications.

IMPLEMENTATION

Action	Rationale
1. Wash hands and organize equipment.	*Reduces microorganism transfer* *Promotes efficiency*
2. Explain use of system to client and provide written literature; assess accuracy of client's understanding.	*Decreases anxiety* *Promotes compliance*
3. Prepare analgesic for administration:	*Ensures delivery of appropriate medication and dosage*
- Check five rights of drug administration: client, drug, dosage (concentration), route, room.	

For PCA Pump Management

- Connect injector to pre-filled vial or syringe (Fig. 8.7).
- Hold vial vertically and push injector to remove air.
- Connect PCA administration set to vial, prime tubing, and close tubing clamp.
- Plug machine into electrical outlet and use PCA infuser key to open pump door.
- Load vial into machine according to equipment operation booklet.

4. Prepare primary IV fluid and tubing (see Procedure 5.3).

5. Attach primary IV tubing to Y-connector line of PCA tubing.

Provides fluid to keep vein open between medication doses

Action	Rationale

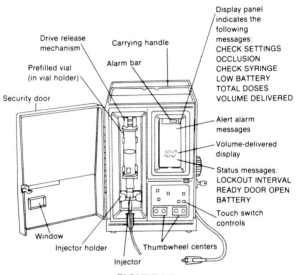

FIGURE 8.7

6. Open primary tubing clamp and prime lower portion of PCA tubing.

Removes air from tubing

7. Close clamp on primary IV.

8. Prepare venous access:
   - Insert IV catheter (see Procedures 5.4, 5.5, and 5.6); or if venous access (heparin lock or central line) is already present, verify patency, and connect PCA tubing directly to IV catheter.
   - Release clamps on PCA and primary tubing.
   - Regulate primary IV to infuse at keep-vein-open (or or-

Maintains patency of vein between medication doses

Action	Rationale

dered) rate (see Procedures 5.7 and 5.8).

9. Administer loading dose, if ordered:
   - Verify ordered dosage.
   - Set lock-out interval on pump at 00 minutes.
   - Set volume to be delivered, using dose-volume thumbwheel control.
   - Press and release loading-dose control switch.

Delivers dose of analgesic to initiate pain relief

10. Set parameters for dosage control:
    - Calculate volume of medication needed to deliver ordered dose (available dose per volume divided by ordered dose equals volume); often vials contain 200 mg per 20-mL vial of Demerol or 30 mg morphine per 30-mL vial.
    - Set *dose volume,* using thumbwheel control for desired volume for each dose.
    - Set *lock-out interval,* using thumbwheel control to set the desired time interval.
    - To set 4-hour limit, push control switch to display current limit; if different limit is desired, depress again and hold switch until desired limit is reached, then release switch.
    - Close and lock security door using infuser key; READY message should appear indicat-

Determines volume that will deliver ordered dose

Delivers 10 mg per 1-mL dose

Delivers 1 mg per 1-mL dose

Sets amount of fluid and medication to be delivered for each dose

Sets minimum time between allotted doses
Prevents medication overdose

Limits total volume to be infused over any consecutive 4-hour period

Action	Rationale
ing PCA infuser is in client-control mode and first dose can be administered.	
- Secure key with designated person or per agency policy.	*Secures narcotic and parameters set into machine*
11. Instruct client and caregiver on administration of dose; inform client of the following information:	
- When pain is experienced, press and release control button.	*Delivers set dose of analgesic*
- Medication will be delivered and infuser will enter a lock-out period during which no additional medication can be delivered.	
- A ready message will appear when next dose can be delivered.	
12. For maintenance of PCA therapy, every home visit:	
- Press TOTAL DOSE switch and note number of client doses administered during past period.	*Allows for monitoring of dosages received by the client*
- Monitor client's respiratory rate, level of sedation (alert to sleeping), and pain level (pain-free to severe pain).	*Monitor for oversedation*
- Document above volumes and observations on flow sheet and calculate total volume on appropriate column.	*Identifies total volume infused and remaining in vial*
- Check volume of medication delivered; if agency pump, open pump door with in-	*Complies with federal narcotic administration laws*

Action	Rationale

fuser key and verify
volume remaining in
analgesic vial (volume
should equal initial
volume minus total
volume infused).

13. Changing PCA vial and
    tubing:
    - Assemble new vial and
      injector.
    - Clear air and close
      tubing clamp.
    - Use infuser key to un-
      lock and open PCA
      pump door.
    - Press on/off switch.
    - Close clamp to old vial
      and primary fluid
      tubing.
    - Remove empty vial (or
      old vial) and adminis-
      tration set from pump
      (see equipment opera-
      tion booklet).
    - Attach new vial and
      injector to PCA admin-
      istration set and prime
      to remove air.
    - Attach primary IV to
      Y-connector of new PCA
      administration set.
    - Insert administration
      set into pump (see
      equipment operation
      booklet).
    - Close and lock pump
      door.
    - Release tubing clamps.
    - Press on/off switch.   *Initiates client-control mode*
    - Record vial change on   *Identifies current volume of*
      PCA flow sheet.   *analgesic in PCA pump*
    - Send previous vial and
      tubing to pharmacy
      (per agency protocol).
14. **To discontinue PCA**

Action	Rationale
therapy, follow step 13, omitting preparation of new vial; remove PCA tubing from IV catheter and replace with primary fluid tubing or infusion plug.	
16. Send vial and tubing to pharmacy (check agency policy).	*Adheres to federal regulations for narcotic control*

For Maintenance of Epidural Pump Therapy

1. Every home visit: - Press Enter button, and record volume remaining. - Instruct caregiver to monitor periodically. - Monitor insertion site for erythema, inflammation or drainage.	*Continuous assessment of infection potential*
- Educate the client and caregiver on the use of a daily diary. Teach them to record temperature, pulse, respirations, pain relief level and any observations. - Check pump function and notify physician of any need for changes in therapy.	*Assessment of adequate control and physical response to medication level; high score requires reassessment. Excessive sedation and any indication of respiratory depression requires pump reprogramming*
2. If you are oncoming home health nurse, check drug infusing, dose volume, and lockout interval with doctor's orders.	*Verifies accuracy of infusion*
3. Change vial and injector if nearly empty per agency policy and per epidural pump operation manual.	*Provides fresh medication*

Evaluation

Were desired outcomes achieved?

DOCUMENTATION

The following should be noted on the visit note:

- Name and dosage of medication being infused
- PCA or epidural parameters (hourly dose, lock-out interval, and 4-hour limit)
- Level of consciousness (on scale of 1 to 5)
- Pain level (on scale of 1 to 5)
- Status of respirations
- Amount of medication (analgesic) used each hour
- Number of client attempts to obtain dose (if agency policy)

For epidural catheters, the following should also be noted on the visit note:

- Condition of insertion site
- Dressing changes
- Client or caregiver education activities

Sample Documentation		
DATE	**TIME**	
1/2/98	1200	Client comfortable after total hip replacement. PCA therapy continued. Dose volume set at 2 mL (2 mg), lock-out interval set at 60 minutes, and 4-hour limit set at 8 mg. Client alert and oriented. States pain measures 2 on a scale of 1 to 5, with 5 indicating severe pain. Return-demonstrated procedure for obtaining dose with 100% accuracy.

Chapter **9**

Hygienic Care

OVERVIEW

▶ Personal interest in hygiene is a key symbol of mental and physical well-being.
▶ Hygiene is usually a private matter; consider the client's preference in timing, family assistance, and toiletries.
▶ Clients should be encouraged to perform as much of hygienic care as they can, within prescribed limitations.
▶ Maintaining good hygiene can promote the following:
  - Healthy skin, by preventing infections and skin breakdown
  - Improved circulation
  - Comfort and rest
  - Nutrition, by improving the appetite
  - Self esteem, by improving the appearance
  - Sense of well-being
▶ Hygiene is frequently determined in part by culture. In some cultures, bathing during an illness is considered detrimental. Be sensitive to the cultural implications of all procedures involving hygienic care.
▶ When performing and instructing in hygienic care, be aware of the availability in the home of adequate supplies of sheets, towels, soap, laundry washing equipment, etc., and individualize instruction accordingly.

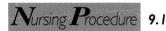

Nursing Procedure **9.1**

Back Care

❌ EQUIPMENT

- Lotion
- Soap
- Towel
- Washcloth
- Warm water

Purpose

Promote comfort
Stimulate circulation
Relieve muscle tension
Facilitate therapeutic interaction

Desired Outcomes (sample)

The client will verbalize comfort, or indicate heightened sense of relaxation after backrub.
The skin integrity of the client will be maintained.

Assessment

Assessment should focus on the following:
Client's desire for backrub
Availability of caregiver in the home to perform the procedure
Skin status and bony prominences
Client's ability to tolerate prone or lateral position
Client allergy to ingredients of lotion

Outcome Identification and Planning

Key Goals and Sample Goal Criteria

The client will:

Verbalize comfort, enhanced relaxation after backrub
Maintain skin integrity

Special Considerations

Geriatric

Assess the skin of the geriatric client carefully. If the skin is very thin and dry, omit the use of soap, and use tepid water. Use very light pressure when applying lotion.

 Transcultural

Touching the client's skin may have special connotations in certain cultures. Be aware of cultural preferences before introducing the procedure.

HINT

Before introducing the procedure, determine if there is a willing, available, and able caregiver to perform the procedure in the absence of home care personnel.

IMPLEMENTATION

Action	Rationale
1. Explain procedure to client and caregiver.	*Promotes relaxation, cooperation, and compliance*
2. Find a quiet, private, restful area in the home in which to perform the procedure.	*Promotes relaxation*
3. Wash hands and organize equipment.	*Reduces microorganism transfer; promotes efficiency*
4. Warm lotion bottle and hands with warm water.	*Cold lotion and hands increase discomfort and cause muscle spasm*
5. Position client in prone or side-lying position, or position most comfortable for client.	*Improves access to back and enhances client comfort*
6. Drape with sheet or blanket.	*Provides warmth and privacy*
7. Wash back gently with soap and water, or with tepid water. Gently dry.	*Cleanses skin; removes dead cells; allows for close inspection of skin*
8. Pour lotion into hands and rub hands together.	*Promotes even distribution of lotion*

Action	Rationale
9. Encourage client to take long, deep breaths as you begin.	*Facilitates relaxation*
10. Place palms of hands on sacrococcygeal area. Once hands have been placed, do not remove from skin until backrub complete.	*Enhances soothing effect by maintaining continuous contact with skin*
11. Make long, gentle strokes up center of back, moving toward shoulders, and back down towards buttocks, covering the lateral areas of the back; repeat several times.	*Stimulates circulation and releases muscle tension* *Gentle strokes enhance circulation without damaging skin*
12. Move hands up center of the back towards the neck and rub nape of neck with fingers; continue rubbing outward toward the shoulders.	*Releases tension in neck and promotes relaxation*
13. Move hands downward to scapula areas and massage in a circular motion over both scapulae for several seconds.	*Stimulates circulation around pressure points*
14. Move hands downward to the buttocks and massage in a figure-8 motion over the buttocks; continue this step for several seconds (Fig. 9.1).	*Stimulates circulation around pressure points*
15. Lightly rub toward neck and shoulders, then back down toward the buttocks for several strokes, using lighter pressure.	*Ends back rub with calming, therapeutic effect*
16. Remove excessive lotion with a towel.	*Excessive moisture may contribute to skin breakdown and bacterial growth*
17. Assist client to comfortable position; assist in dressing if needed.	*Provides comfort*
18. Review procedure with caregiver.	*Reinforces instruction*

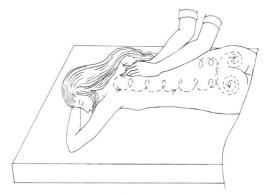

FIGURE 9.1

Evaluation

Were desired outcomes achieved?

DOCUMENTATION
The following should be noted on the visit note:

- Client's response to backrub
- Caregiver's ability to perform procedure
- Condition of skin

Sample Documentation		
DATE	**TIME**	
5/9/99	1200	Procedure for backrub demonstrated to client's spouse. Client skin intact, dry. Very gentle pressure used. Client verbalizes increased comfort after procedure; caregiver verbalizes understanding of procedure and willingness to perform.

Nursing Procedure 9.2

Bed Preparation Techniques

☒ EQUIPMENT

- Bottom sheet
- Top sheet
- Additional top sheet for draw sheet
- Pillow case
- Gloves to remove old linens
- Gown if possible splashing of blood or body fluids

Purpose

Reduce the chance of skin breakdown related to contact with wet, soiled or wrinkled linen

Provide for patient comfort and cleanliness

Desired Outcomes

The client will remain comfortable and be free of skin breakdown.

The significant other or caregiver in the home will demonstrate adequate performance of procedure.

Outcome Identification and Planning

Key Goals and Sample Goal Criteria

The client or significant other will:

Verbalize comfort

Demonstrate no skin breakdown related to soiled linens

Verbalize understanding of washing techniques for soiled linens

Special Considerations

HINT

ECONOMIC: If commercially available bed protectors are not feasible, a large plastic trash bag may be cut along two sides and used as a linen protector under a drawsheet.

HINT

If incontinence or drainage may be a problem, encourage the client or family to purchase a waterproof mattress cover.

Discourage the use of egg-crate mattresses that may have come home with the client at hospital discharge. They absorb perspiration and drainage, are difficult to launder at home, and may promote skin breakdown.

All aspects of this procedure must be taught to someone in the home. Initially the nurse should perform and teach, then periodically observe.

IMPLEMENTATION

Action	Rationale
1. Assist client to chair.	*Allows easy access to bed for changing*
2. Don gloves to remove old linens and place them in a pillow case. Remove gloves and cleanse hands after this is done.	*Reduces microorganism transfer*
3. Examine the mattress. If damp or soiled, spray with household germicidal spray and turn the mattress. If the mattress cannot be turned, cut a plastic bag and secure over the damp or soiled area.	*Provides a clean, dry surface for linens, reduces risk of skin breakdown, microorganism transfer*
4. Apply a clean bottom sheet over the mattress as evenly as possible. Tuck edges under mattress, leaving the surface as wrinklefree as possible. Use pins to secure corners to the mattress if needed.	*Ensures snug fit*
5. If incontinence or drainage is a possibility, place a linen protector on the bottom sheet, or cut two sides of a large plastic bag and lay it flat as a linen protector (Fig. 9.2).	*Reduces number of times bottom sheet must be changed, reduces risk of wet sheet contributing to skin breakdown*

Action	Rationale

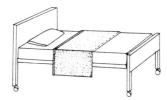

FIGURE 9.2

6. Fold another sheet into thirds and place across the bed so that it will extend from client's hips to shoulders. Be sure plastic or linen protector is covered by sheet.

Assists in repositioning client, prevents shearing of skin if client is pulled up in bed

7. Place a top sheet on the bed, tucking the bottom edge to allow room for free movement of feet.

Increases client comfort

8. If client requests additional blankets on bed, encourage use of washable materials.

Reduces effort of maintaining clean linens

9. Put clean pillowcases on all pillows. If pillows are damp or soiled and no others are available, put pillow in plastic bag before putting on pillowcase.

Increases comfort, reduces microorganism transfer

10. Assist client to bed and adjust covers for comfort.

Promotes client comfort

11. If used linens are soiled with blood and body fluids, instruct caregiver to don gloves when handling linen, rinse first in cold water and wash separately from other clothes, using hot water, any laundry detergent,

Reduces risk of microorganism transfer, reduces caregiver anxiety

Prevents setting of stain prior to removal

Action	Rationale
and liquid bleach. Assure caregiver that there is no risk in using the same washing machine for client linen and family laundry if the linens are washed separately.	

Evaluation

Were desired outcomes achieved?

DOCUMENTATION

The following should be noted on the visit note:

- Instruction to or observation of caregiver performing procedure.
- Caregiver's ability to carry out procedure.
- Client tolerance of move to chair and back to bed.

Sample Documentation

DATE	TIME	
4/13/98	0800	Demonstrated bed preparation techniques to spouse, instructed in linen handling, washing, when linen should be changed. Spouse verbalizes understanding of procedure. Will observe spouse performing procedure next visit; continue instruction if needed.

Nursing **P**rocedure **9.3**

Shampoo for the Bedridden Client

⊠ EQUIPMENT

- Shampoo
- Washcloth
- Two towels
- Nonsterile gloves
- Plastic lined trash can
- Shampoo board or wash basin and plastic trash bag
- Water pitcher
- Hair dryer (safety approved)

Purpose

Improves appearance and self-esteem
Provides opportunity for close examination of scalp
Relaxes client

Desired Outcomes (sample)

Improved client appearance, self-esteem, and comfort.
Improved circulation to scalp.

Assessment

Assessment should focus on the following:
Client need or desire for bed shampoo
Presence of nits or lice
Availability of caregiver when home health personnel not present
Presence of condition that would contraindicate manipulation of the head
Client ability to tolerate procedure
Client allergy to ingredients of shampoo or need for medicated shampoo

Outcome Identification and Planning

Key Goals and Sample Goal Criteria

The client and significant other will:

Verbalize understanding of the procedure
Demonstrate adequate scalp circulation
Demonstrate an increase in comfort and self-esteem by express-
ing interest in grooming

Special Considerations

Some clients require more frequent shampooing than others;
treat each case individually. See basic hair care techniques in
Procedure 9.4 for considerations based on racial diversity.

Geriatric

In the elderly client, skin is often thin and hair brittle. Check
scalp for irritation before shampooing.

HINT

*A shampoo for the bedridden client is usually a procedure as-
signed to the home health aide, or taught to the client's family.
Before assigning or teaching the procedure, the nurse must
examine the client's scalp for irritation, lice, or pressure ulcers and institute treatment.*

IMPLEMENTATION

Action	Rationale
1. Prepare room environment (warm and draft free).	*Avoids discomfort from chills*
2. Obtain physician order for medicated shampoo, if indicated.	*Provides scalp treatment*
3. Explain procedure to client and caregivers.	*Facilitates cooperation*
4. Wash hands and organize equipment.	*Reduces microorganism transfer, promotes efficiency*
5. Remove pillow from under client's head.	*Prevents soiling of pillow*
6. Place linen saver or plastic bag under shoulders and head of client.	*Prevents wetting of linens*

Action	Rationale
7. Place towel on top of linen saver.	*Absorbs water overflow*
8. Place shampoo board under client's neck and head, or place wash basin lined with plastic bag under client's neck and head. Position plastic bag in wash basin so that water flow is directed away from bed linens (Fig. 9.3).	*Facilitates drainage of water*
9. Position plastic-lined trash can in direct line with spout of shampoo board, or with end of plastic bag leading from wash basin.	*Provides reservoir for water*
10. Fill pitcher with warm – water (105°–110°F.); check	*Promotes scalp circulation* *Prevents chilling or skin injury*

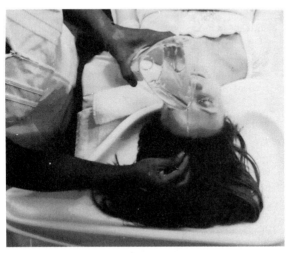

FIGURE 9.3

Action	Rationale
with thermometer or test for comfortable temperature with your inner wrist.	*from excess heat*
11. Ask client to hold washcloth over eyes during procedure.	*Prevents pain from shampoo in eyes*
12. Place bed flat if client can tolerate. Place all supplies within easy reach.	*Facilitates downward flow of water* *Prevents delays in procedure*
13. Pour a small amount of water over hair. Determine if water is flowing into trash can.	*Prevents wetting of linens* *Allows readjustment of shampoo board if necessary*
14. Pour warm water over hair and moisten thoroughly.	*Facilitates action of shampoo*
15. Don gloves and place a small amount of shampoo in palms; massage shampoo into hair at front and back of head, working shampoo into a lather.	*Provides lather for removal of dirt and lather*
16. Massage lather over entire head in a slow, kneading motion.	*Cleans hair and scalp, promotes scalp circulation*
17. Rinse hair by pouring warm water over head several times.	*Removes shampoo and debris*
18. If client can tolerate, repeat application of shampoo and massage hair and scalp vigorously with fingers for a longer period of time.	*Promotes thorough cleansing of hair and scalp*
19. Rinse thoroughly using several pitchers of water.	*Removes remaining residue of shampoo*
20. Support client's head and remove shampoo board or wash basin from bed.	*Clears area for completion of procedure*
21. Position client's head on clean towel and cover head. Briskly massage head with towel.	*Removes water*
22. Replace wet towel with	*Promotes drying of hair*

Action	Rationale
dry one and continue to rub hair.	
23. Leave hair covered with towel until ready to use dryer.	*Prevents chilling, provides for continued absorption of water*
24. Check bed and bed clothes. Change if wet. Remove trash can of water, shampoo board, from area. Ascertain that work area is dry, and client is comfortable. Thoroughly dry hands.	*Promotes safety when using electrical hair dryer* *Prevents chilling*
25. Elevate head.	*Provides access to hair*
26. Turn on dryer to warm setting; feel heat to be sure it is not excessively hot.	*Prevents injury*
27. Blow hair until thoroughly dry; concentrate on one section of hair at a time, moving fingers or comb through hair while drying.	*Facilitates thorough drying of hair; removes tangles and ensures drying of all parts of hair*
28. Brush or comb hair to remove all tangles. Style as per client request.	*Enhances client participation*
29. Straighten room, collect used towels and place in laundry area; dry and store all equipment.	*Provides clean environment*

Evaluation

Were desired outcomes achieved?

DOCUMENTATION

The following should be noted on the visit note:

- Condition of client's scalp
- Client ability to tolerate procedure
- Degree of participation by client or significant other

Sample Documentation

DATE	TIME	
5/21/99	1230	Observed niece performing shampoo procedure. Verbal instruction given in need to be sure area is dry before using hair dryer. Client tolerated procedure well, scalp in good condition. Client and niece comfortable in performance of procedure. No further observation needed.

Nursing **P**rocedure **9.4**

Hair Care Techniques

⊠ EQUIPMENT (varies with hair style desired)

- Comb
- Setting gel and rollers if desired
- Hair dryer (safety approved)
- Brush
- Hair net (optional)
- Moisturizers, oils (optional)
- Rubber bands, hair pins, clamps
- Nonsterile gloves

Purpose

Improves client appearance and self-esteem
Increases client sense of well-being
Stimulates circulation to the scalp
Provides for client relaxation

Desired Outcomes (sample)

Improved client appearance, sense of well-being, self esteem.

Assessment

Assessment should focus on the following:

Presence of lice
Contraindications to excessive movement and lowering and elevating head (eg, skull fractures, neck injury), dizziness
Type of hair care needed
Activity level and level of endurance
Presence in the home of caregiver to perform procedure (or scheduling of home health aide)
Status of hair and scalp
Allergy to ingredients of hair care products

Outcome Identification and Planning

Key Goals and Sample Goal Criteria

The client and significant other will:

Verbalize understanding of the procedure

Demonstrate good circulation to the scalp as evidenced by warm scalp with brisk capillary refill

Evidence no scalp irritation or pressure sores

Demonstrate an increase in self-esteem, as evidenced by initiation of or participation in one or more self-care and grooming activities

Special Considerations

Geriatric

The elderly client's skin is often dry, thin, and fragile, and the hair is brittle. Assess scalp for irritation frequently, and avoid the use of rubber bands and other devices that pull on the hair. Be careful not to scratch scalp with hair pins.

 Transcultural

Clients of different ethnic and cultural origins require shampoos with different frequencies and use different forms of basic hair care. African American clients usually shampoo every 1 to 2 weeks and often add oils or moisturizers; white clients may shampoo daily or every other day to avoid buildup of hair oils. *When in doubt regarding hair practices, consult the client or family members.*

HINT

Hair care is a procedure that is taught to the caregiver in the home, or assigned to the home health aide. It is a nursing responsibility to instruct in the procedure, evaluate the results of the procedure, and periodically reassess the client's need for and ability to tolerate the procedure.

IMPLEMENTATION

Action	Rationale
1. Explain procedure to client or caregiver.	*Increases cooperation and assistance*

Action	Rationale

2. Allow 15–30 minutes uninterrupted time for hair.

Avoids rush and possible injury to client

3. Check and clean comb and brush before beginning.

Prevents risk of passing head lice or infection to client

4. Wash hands and organize equipment.

Reduces microorganism transfer, promotes efficiency

5. Assist client into comfortable position in well-lit area of home, away from food preparation areas.

Allows easier access
Promotes client comfort

6. Don gloves (if broken skin present) and comb hair through with fingers.

Prevents body fluid contact
Assesses degree of tangling

7. Massage scalp and observe status.

Increases circulation

8. Shampoo and dry hair, if needed and allowed (see Procedure 9.3).

Improves appearance of hair

9. Brush hair gently to remove as many tangles as possible. Hold hair with one hand and brush with the other. If hair is coarse or kinky, processed for curls, or naturally curly, a comb may be more effective for removing tangles (Fig. 9.4).

Decreases discomfort from pulling at scalp

10. Divide hair into sections with comb and fingers.

Provides for easier handling

11. Comb one section through at a time:
   - Gently and slowly comb tangles loose from scalp.
   - Hold hair section stable near the scalp with one hand (as when brushing).

Prevents pulling during combing
Decreases pain to client

12. Keep hair loose at the scalp.

Counteracts pulling from comb

13. Instruct in cleaning and storage of equipment used.

Promotes cleanliness in the home

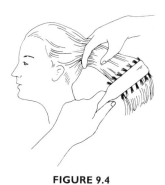

FIGURE 9.4

Evaluation

Were desired outcomes achieved?

DOCUMENTATION

The following should be noted on the visit note:

- Condition of client's scalp
- Client ability to tolerate procedure
- Degree of participation by client or significant other

Sample Documentation		
DATE	**TIME**	
7/11/98	0730	Observed niece performing hair care. Verbal instruction given in avoidance of pulling at scalp. Client tolerated procedure well, shows increasing participation.

*N*ursing *P*rocedures **9.5, 9.6**

Oral Care Techniques (9.5)

Denture Care Techniques (9.6)

❌ EQUIPMENT

- Toothbrush (denture brush)
- Toothpaste
- Large cotton applicators
- Emesis basin
- Nonsterile gloves
- Towel and washcloth
- Cup of warm water
- Mouthwash
- Denture cream
- Denture cup
- Denture cleanser
- Dental floss (optional)
- Bulb syringe for suction

Purpose

Decreases microorganisms in mouth and on teeth and dentures
Decreases cavities and gum disease
Decreases buildup of food residue on teeth and dentures
Improves appetite and taste for food
Facilitates comfort
Stimulates circulation to oral tissues, tongue, and gums
Improves appearance and self-esteem

Desired Outcomes (sample)

Oral tissue intact and free of infection or ulceration.
Increased oral intake.
Oral cavity, teeth, dentures clean.
Improved client appetite, sense of well-being.

Assessment

Assessment should focus on the following:

Client desire and need for oral care
Client or caregiver knowledge of purpose and procedure

Client's ability to understand and follow instructions
Presence of dentures
Status of mouth, tongue, and teeth (eg, presence of lesions, cavities)

Outcome Identification and Planning

Key Goal and Sample Goal Criteria

The client and significant other will:

Demonstrate the correct procedure for oral and/or denture care within 1 week of initiation of instruction

Special Considerations

Clients on anticoagulation therapy or with coagulation defects will require the use of a soft toothbrush or large applicator only.

Clients with oral lesions or sensitive oral tissues may require dilution of mouthwash.

Encourage client and caregiver in the home to perform as much oral care as possible.

HINT

ECONOMIC: For clients who cannot afford toothpaste, toothbrushes, etc., the nurse may need to access local social service agencies or the local dental association for assistance.

HINT

Many home care clients have experienced a recent weight loss due to illness or hospitalization. This will affect the fit of dentures. Every attempt should be made to encourage the client to seek dental care for relining or new dentures.

Oral and denture care is a procedure that is taught to the client and caregiver, or assigned to the home health aide. It is a nursing responsibility to thoroughly assess the client's oral cavity before instructing in or assigning this procedure. Orders should be obtained for the treatment of oral disease or ulcerations. The oral cavity should be reassessed at intervals.

IMPLEMENTATION

Action	Rationale

Procedure 9.5 Oral Care Techniques

1. Wash hands and organize equipment.

   Reduces microorganism transfer, promotes efficiency

2. Provide explanation of procedure to client and caregiver.

   Promotes compliance
   Reduces anxiety

3. Position client in one of the following positions:
   - Supine at an angle greater than 45 degrees, if possible
   - Side lying

   Decreases risk of aspiration

4. If anyone other than client doing procedure, don gloves. Use other appropriate protective equipment if splashing of blood is a possibility.

   Prevents exposure to body fluids

5. If necessary, drape towel under client's neck and assist client to rinse mouth with water.

   Catches secretions
   Facilitates removal of secretions

6. Assist client in brushing teeth:
   - Provide a glass of water, toothbrush, and tooth-paste.
   - Moisten toothbrush with water.
   - Apply toothpaste to brush.
   - Allow client to brush teeth, if able.

   Facilitates self care

7. **If client is unable to per-form own care:**
   - Prepare toothbrush as in step 6.
   - Don gloves.
   - Apply brush to back teeth and brush inside, top and outside of teeth (brush from back to front, using an up and down motion) (Fig. 9.5).

   Permits cleaning back and sides of teeth

Action   **Rationale**

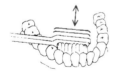   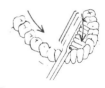

FIGURE 9.5

- Repeat these steps brushing teeth on opposite side of mouth.
- Allow client to expectorate excess secretions, or use bulb syringe to suction.

Removes toothpaste and oral secretions

- Instruct client to clench teeth together, or grasp the mandible and press lower teeth to upper teeth; brush outside of front teeth.

Exposes front teeth for brushing

- Open mouth and brush top and insides of teeth.
- Rinse toothbrush.
- Brush teeth again.

Removes residual toothpaste

- If use of dental floss is desired, provide care at this time.

8. Assist client in cleansing oral cavity:
   - Provide mouthwash soaked large applicator.

Freshens mouth

   - Encourage client to swab inner cheeks, lips, gums, and tongue, or perform these actions for client if needed.

9. **If working with an unconscious client:**
   - Turn client's head to one side.

Decreases possibility of aspiration

   - Don gloves.

Reduces microorganism transfer

Action	**Rationale**

  - Brush teeth with toothbrush and toothpaste,
as in step 7.

  - Irrigate mouth with
small amounts of water,
using bulb syringe to
suction constantly.
Removes water and avoids pooling

  - Swab mouth with large
applicator moistened
with mouthwash.

  - Beginning with inside
of cheek and lips, pro-
ceed to swab tongue
and gums.

  - Suction excess tooth-
paste, mouthwash, and
secretions.

  - Wipe lips with a wet
washcloth.

  - Apply petroleum jelly
or mineral oil to lips.

10. Discard gloves and soiled
materials; assist client or
caregiver in cleaning, and
storing supplies.
Promotes cleanliness of home environment

Procedure 9.6 Denture Care Techniques

1. Wash hands and organize
supplies.
Reduces microorganism transfer, promotes efficiency

2. Explain procedure to
client and encourage par-
ticipation, if able.
Promotes compliance

3. Don gloves.
Prevents body fluid contact

4. Assist client with denture
removal:

  - Half fill denture cup
with cool water.

  - Put denture cleanser
into cup per instruc-
tions.

  - Instruct client to hold
water in mouth and
"float" dentures loose.
Prevents breakage of dentures during removal

  - Allow client to remove
dentures, or gently rock
dentures back and forth
Breaks seal created with dentures

Action	Rationale
until free from gums.	
- Lift bottom dentures up to remove, pull top dentures downward.	*Prevents undue pressure and injury to oral membranes*
- Place dentures in denture cup to soak.	*Facilitates removal of microorganisms*
5. Assist client with cleansing of oral cavity:	*Facilitates removal of microorganisms*
- Provide mouthwash soaked large applicator.	
- Encourage client to swab inner cheeks, lips, tongue, and gums.	
- Instruct client to swirl mouthwash in mouth and expectorate.	
- Follow with water, as desired.	
6. Cleanse dentures:	
- Use same procedure as when brushing teeth (see Procedure 9.5).	
- Thoroughly rinse paste from dentures with cool water.	
7. Reinsert dentures:	*Facilitates intake of solid food*
- Apply denture adhesive to gum side of dentures, if needed.	
- Insert upper plate and press firmly to gums.	
- Repeat with lower plate.	
- Instruct client to swirl mouthwash in mouth, expectorate, and rinse with water.	
8. Apply petroleum jelly or mineral oil to lips.	*Maintains skin integrity of lips*
9. Discard gloves and soiled materials.	
10. Assist client or caregiver in cleaning and storing supplies.	*Maintains clean home environment*

Evaluation

Were desired outcomes achieved?

DOCUMENTATION

The following should be noted on the visit note:

- Condition of client's oral cavity
- Conditions, such as ill-fitting dentures, that could interfere with nutrition
- Amount of care done by client or caregiver
- Client response to procedure

Sample Documentation		
DATE	**TIME**	
11/3/99	1000	Oral care and denture care performed with client cooperation and assistance. Oral cavity with tissue pink, no bleeding, no ulcerations. Caregiver observed procedure and feels able to assist. Client tolerated procedure well. Will instruct and observe caregiver/client performance of procedure next visit.

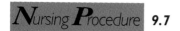

Nursing Procedure **9.7**

Contacts and Artificial Eye Care Techniques

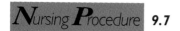 EQUIPMENT

- Container for lenses or prosthesis
- Saline solution
- Nonsterile gloves

Purpose

Prevents corneal damage
If prosthesis, prevents damage to tissue

Desired Outcomes (sample)

Tissues of eye and socket will be maintained.
Caregiver will demonstrate ability to perform procedure.

Assessment

Assessment should focus on the following:

Client/family ability to understand and perform procedure

Outcome Identification and Planning

Key Goals and Sample Goal Criteria

The client and or family will demonstrate correct procedure

The structures of the eye and surrounding tissue will remain free of infection and/or irritation

Special Considerations

HINT

If at all possible, have the client perform the procedure as per the client's routine. If needed, make suggestions as to how to improve technique. This can be a difficult procedure for the nurse to perform in the home setting. If the client and or family is unable to remove a prosthesis or contact lens, and the nurse has any doubt about his or her ability to perform the procedure, every attempt should be made to arrange a rapid referral to an ophthalmologist.

IMPLEMENTATION

Action	Rationale
1. Assemble equipment needed.	*Increases efficiency*
2. Teach, perform, or observe good handwashing techniques.	*Reduces transfer of micro-organisms*
3. If anyone except the client is performing the procedure, don gloves.	*Reduces transmission of microorganisms*
4. If wearing gloves, rinse in saline.	*Removes traces of powder*
5. Position client in recumbent position, stand on right side to remove right contact lens or prosthesis.	*Improves access to eye*
6. Position left thumb on upper eyelid, right thumb on lower eyelid, and gently pull apart.	*Improves visualization*
7. If lens is visible, proceed. If lens cannot be seen, arrange for ophthalmologist to see client.	
8. For hard lens or prosthesis, gently open the eye beyond the edges of the lens or prosthesis, and apply gentle pressure on the eyeball with the right thumb.	*Releases the suction holding the lens or prosthesis in*

Action	Rationale
9. Gently slide the lens or prosthesis out.	
10. If soft lens, perform steps 1 through 7. Once lens is seen, gently pinch between thumb and forefinger and remove.	
11. Inspect the eye tissues for any damage.	
12. Place lenses, prosthesis in appropriate container and perform cleaning.	*Reduces transmission of microorganisms* *Maintains equipment in clean condition*
13. If necessary, repeat steps for left eye.	
14. Dispose of soiled gloves appropriately, wash hands.	*Promotes cleanliness* *Reduces transmission of microorganisms*

Evaluation

Were desired outcomes achieved?

DOCUMENTATION

The following should be noted on the visit note:

- Condition of eye and surrounding tissue
- Ability of client or caregiver to properly perform procedure

Sample Documentation

DATE	TIME	
1/4/99	0900	Observed client removing left eye prosthesis. Instruction given in handwashing before and after procedure, cleaning of eye socket per physician order, storage and cleaning of prosthesis. Client verbalizes understanding but states is forgetful. Will continue observation and instruction next visit.

Chapter 10

Biological Safety Needs

OVERVIEW

► The chain of infection requires that six links be present:
  - An infectious agent in sufficient amount to cause an infection
  - A place for the agent to multiply and grow
  - A point at which the agent can exit the growth area
  - A method of transportation from growth area to other sites
  - An available access or entrance into another site
  - A susceptible host or medium for agent growth
► The aim of all protective procedures (universal precautions as well as disease-specific, category-specific, or body-substance isolation) is to decrease exposure to and the

spread of microorganisms and disease; all actions are aimed at breaking the chain of infection by eliminating the links.

▶ Goggles, gowns, or aprons and masks should be available for use at all times.

▶ Gloves should be worn whenever exposure to body secretions is likely: ALWAYS WEAR GLOVES WHEN EMPTYING DRAINAGE CONTAINERS.

▶ If the sterility of materials, gloves, or gowns is in doubt, treat them as nonsterile.

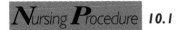

Nursing Procedure 10.1

Infection Control in the Home

✖ EQUIPMENT

- Nonsterile gloves
- Gowns/apron
- Masks
- Face shield or goggles
- 10% bleach solution
- Biohazardous waste containers
- Rigid plastic container (eg, detergent jug)
- Household disinfectant
- Paper towels

Purpose

Prevents transfer of microorganisms from client to others in the home

Prevents contamination of sterile and clean supplies by microorganisms existing in the home

Desired Outcomes (sample)

Transfer of bloodborne or airborne organisms will not occur.

Supplies needed for ongoing client care will be maintained in a clean environment.

Assessment

Assessment should focus on the following:

Client/family ability to understand and perform procedures

General environmental cleanliness

Possibility of insect or rodent infestation

Status of others living in the home

Specific client conditions that could require special infection control technique

Outcome Identification and Planning

Key Goals and Sample Goal Criteria

The client and family will:

Consistently demonstrate good handwashing practices
Demonstrate ability to perform environmental cleaning tasks
Demonstrate correct techniques in special handling of soiled
dressings and used needles, if applicable
Remain free of infection

Special Considerations

Basic infection control practices should be taught to every client
and family as part of instruction in a healthy lifestyle. This is
particularly true in multigenerational families living in one
house.

 Transcultural

Handwashing, environmental cleaning, and laundry may have
cultural implications. If in doubt, contact a resource person
before proceeding with instruction.

HINT

*ECONOMIC: Poor compliance with infection control prac-
tices may be related to insufficient funds with which to purchase soap, laundry detergent, disinfectant, etc. It is a nursing
responsibility to be alert to this possibility and contact social
service agencies and other community resources if necessary.*

HINT

*Insect and/or rodent infestation may be a major obstacle to in-
fection control in the home. If the client and family do not
have adequate resources to eliminate these pests, the nurse
can contact the public health department and other government agencies for advice and assistance.*

IMPLEMENTATION

Action	Rationale

Good Handwashing

1. Explain procedure to
   client and family and
   assemble supplies. — *Reduces anxiety, promotes efficiency*
2. Turn on water. If running

Action	Rationale

water not available, pour
water over hands.

3. Using soap, apply vigorous friction to all skin surfaces for at least 10 seconds. — *Promotes removal of microorganisms*

4. Rinse under running water, or have water poured over hands.

5. Turn off faucet with paper towel. — *Prevents transfer of microorganisms*

6. Dry hands with paper towel, not cloth towel used by others. — *Prevents transfer of microorganisms*

7. Instruct all family members when to perform handwashing:
   - before and after doing client care
   - after using toilet

General Environmental Cleaning

8. Observe/instruct general household cleaning.
   - Bathroom and kitchen with disinfectant and/or bleach solution
   - Surfaces in client area with disinfectant
   - Vacuuming, dusting as needed.

9. Instruct removal of heavy carpet and difficult to clean furniture from client area if possible. — *Promotes ease of use of disinfectant*

10. Instruct all family members to use own towel, washcloth, toothbrush. — *Prevents transfer of microorganisms*

Avoidance of Bloodborne Transmission

11. To wash garments, linens, towels soiled with blood and body fluids: — *Prevents transmission of microorganisms*
    - Wear gloves.
    - Rinse all items in cold water. — *Prevents setting of stain*

Action	Rationale
- Wash separately from family laundry in washer with hot water and bleach.	
12. To dispose of used dressing soiled with blood or body fluids:	*Prevents transfer of microorganisms* *Protects the environment*
- Wear gloves.	
- Wear other personal protective equipment if splashing is anticipated.	
- Place soiled dressings in an approved biohazardous waste container.	
- **Nurse must arrange for pick-up of biohazardous waste containers from home.**	
13. If needles are being used, instruct in use of sharps container or heavy plastic jug with lid:	*Prevents transfer of microorganisms* *Reduces risk of needlestick to other family members* *Protects environment*
- Place small amount of bleach solution in jug.	
- Place all used sharps in jug and replace lid each time.	
- Discard when two-thirds full.	
- **If sharps container exchange program is available in the community, instruct in how to access.**	
14. All family members and caregivers must be instructed in standard precautions if they are going to be exposed to blood or body fluids.	*Reduces transfer of microorganisms*

Maintenance of Supplies

15. If sterile or clean supplies are to be left in the home for client use:	*Promotes efficiency, reduces transfer of microorganisms*
- Assist client to locate	

Action	Rationale

clean, protected storage
area that may be used
for supplies only.
- Cover supplies with
clean plastic or towel.

Evaluation

Were desired outcomes achieved?

DOCUMENTATION

The following should be noted on the visit note:

- Infection control instructions given.
- Special circumstances in the home.

Sample Documentation

DATE	TIME	
11/3/99	1032	Client and family instructed in handwashing, environmental cleaning, laundry precautions. Written instructions given in disposal of used needles, sharps. Multiple family caregivers in home; will continue instruction, observation of techniques each visit.

*N*ursing *P*rocedure *10.2*

Disposal of Biohazardous Waste (By Nurse)

☒ EQUIPMENT

- Approved sharps container
- Approved rigid biohazardous waste container
- Approved biohazardous waste bags
- Spill kit or spill cloth
- Nonsterile gloves
- Gowns
- Goggles
- Masks
- Handwashing supplies

Purpose

Provides for safe disposal of contaminated items in accordance with safety, laws, and regulations.

Desired Outcomes (sample)

Biohazardous waste will be collected, transported, and disposed of safely, in compliance with agency guidelines and applicable laws and regulations.

Assessment

Assessment should focus on the following:

Determination of what items are considered biohazardous waste
Requirements for safe disposal of biohazardous waste
Method of disposal of biohazardous waste (agency and community specific)

Outcome Identification and Planning

Key Goals and Sample Goal Criteria

The nurse will:

Appropriately identify items that meet the definition of biohazardous waste.

Safely and appropriately package, transport, and dispose of all items.

Special Considerations

 Transcultural

Some cultures consider blood and body fluids to be a vital part of the individual. Explain disposal procedures and regulatory requirements carefully to avoid misunderstandings.

HINT

> *Disposal requirements for biohazardous waste vary by state and by agency. Know the policy of the agency, and the laws of the state.*
>
> *This procedure is for the disposal of biohazardous waste by the nurse. Handling and disposal of biohazardous waste by the client is covered in "Infection Control in the Home" (Procedure 10.1).*

IMPLEMENTATION

Action	Rationale
1. Have all equipment readily available for use at all times.	*Allows for safe disposal of waste even if not anticipated prior to the visit*
2. If using needles, lancets, or other devices classified as sharps, bring the sharps container into the home.	*Permits disposal of contaminated sharp at point of use, reducing risk of injury or contamination*
3. When exposure to blood and body fluids is a possibility, use personal protective equipment. If the possibility of splashing exists, use gloves, gown, mask, and goggles as appropriate.	*Reduces risk of contamination*
4. When use of sharps is anticipated, wear gloves to do the procedure, and until all sharps are safely in a	*Reduces risk of contamination or injury*

Action	Rationale
container. Hands must be washed before and after gloves are worn.	
5. Use a sharps container only until it is two-thirds full.	*Reduces risk of needlestick when putting additional sharp in the container*
6. When container is two-thirds full, close securely, label, and date according to agency policy and applicable local law.	*Complies with local regulation of biohazardous waste disposal*
7. If transporting closed sharps containers in the car, designate an area in the car for this purpose. Use a second rigid-walled container to hold the sharps container and transport to final destination for disposal, *ie,* agency office, as soon as possible.	*Prevents contamination of supplies in the car*
8. Follow agency policy regarding logging in sharps containers for disposal.	*Complies with agency policy, regulatory requirements*
9. For non-sharps biohazardous waste, know the agency and legal definition in the state in which you are practicing.	*Complies with law, regulation and policy*
10. Have all necessary biohazardous waste disposal bags and containers available.	*Reduces the risk of contamination by disposing of waste at the point of use*
11. Wear gloves throughout the procedure. Wash hands before and after using gloves.	*Reduces risk of contamination*
12. Place contaminated items, *ie,* dressing materials, in an approved biohazardous waste bag, and close. Then place the bag in a rigid-walled biohazardous waste container.	*Eliminates the possibility of the bag tearing and contaminating other surfaces*

Action	Rationale
13. Place properly closed, labeled waste containers in a designated area of the car for transport, segregated from other supplies, and contained in a second rigid-walled container.	*Eliminates risk of contamination of clean supplies*
14. Transport to end destination for disposal as soon as possible. Follow agency policy regarding logging in.	
15. If a spill of blood or body fluids occurs in the home, use spill kit or spill cloth.	*Reduces contamination, as packaged kits and cloths contain antibacterial and antiviral components*

Evaluation

Were desired outcomes achieved?

DOCUMENTATION

Documentation of biohazardous waste disposal varies from agency to agency. Check policy.

Nursing **P**rocedure **10.3**

🖑 *Obtaining A Blood Specimen*

✖ EQUIPMENT

Both:
- Appropriately colored test tube or vacutainer (consult agency laboratory manual):
  - striped (red/black, green/black, or other), used for chemical or drug studies and containing a preservative
  - solid red, used for blood bank
  - purple, used for complete blood count
  - blue or lavender, used for coagulation
- Blood culture bottle(s) (optional)
- Appropriate labels

Peripheral venipuncture
- Nonsterile gloves
- Alcohol pads
- Tourniquet (or blood-pressure cuff)
- Povidone-iodine (Betadine) pad (optional)

Syringe method
Peripheral Venipuncture:
- Sterile needles
  - 20 or 21 gauge
    or
  - scalp vein (butterfly) catheter
- Sterile syringe of appropriate size
Peripheral Venipuncture: Vacutainer method
- Blood-collecting device or vacutainer holder with double-point needle

Central line aspiration
- Alcohol and Povidone-iodine pads (per agency policy)
- Normal saline flush
- Heparin lock solution (per agency policy)
- Gloves
- Eye protective glasses (optional)
Central Catheter: Vacutainer method
- Vacutainer holder with multiple luer adapters

Central Catheter:
- 10 mL syringes number appropriate for the amount of blood to be drawn (see Table 10.3)
- 10 mL syringe with normal saline flush
- 10 mL syringe with heparin locking solution (agency-specific policy)

Purpose

Provides blood specimen for analysis

Desired Outcomes (sample)
Blood is drawn with minimal discomfort to client.
Blood is placed in appropriate tubes and sent to lab.
Intravenous access and blood specimen are not contaminated during the procedure.

Assessment

Assessment should focus on the following:

Type of lab test ordered
Time for which test is ordered
Adequacy of client preparation (*eg*, fasting state, medication withheld or given)
Client's ability to cooperate

Outcome Identification and Planning

Key Goals and Sample Goal Criteria
The client will:

Experience no injury to vein or extreme pain during procedure
Receive therapy based on correct test results

Special Considerations
For peripheral venipuncture, a blood pressure cuff may be used instead of a tourniquet (maintain a pressure greater than the client's diastolic pressure).

Geriatric
The elderly often have veins that appear large and dilated. Use a blood pressure cuff instead of a tourniquet to prevent excessive stress on the vessel and subsequent collapse or rupture.

HINT

- *To obtain uncontaminated blood specimens, it is necessary to turn off all infusions before drawing a blood specimen.*
- *To assist in collecting a quality sample, clamp all lumens of the catheter before obtaining the specimen.*
- *To reduce the risk of contaminating the central line, the Vacutainer method for obtaining a blood specimen is preferred.*
- *Heparin flush may range from 10 m/mL to 100 m/mL concentrations.*

Safety

- *Use a 10 mL syringe for all flushing and heparin locking. This assists in keeping the PSI syringe pressures below most manufacturers recommendations.*
- *Use the lowest possible concentrations of heparin locking solution. This helps to prevent untoward bleeding complications that have been associated with frequent lumen.*

IMPLEMENTATION

Action	Rationale
1. Wash hands and organize equipment; explain procedure and cooperation required to client.	*Reduces microorganism transfer* *Promotes efficiency* *Promotes relaxation and compliance*
2. Assist client into a semi-Fowler's position; raise bed to high position if electric bed is used.	*Provides easier access to veins* *Promotes comfort during procedure* *Facilitates good body mechanics*
3. Open several alcohol and Betadine pads	*Provides fast access to cleaning supplies*
4. Turn off all IVs, including those infusing into other lumens, and clamp the catheter.	*Assists in eliminating specimen contamination*

Peripheral Venipuncture

5. Screw needle into blood collection device, if used (Fig. 10.3.1) or into syringe.	
6. Place towel under extremity.	*Prevents soiling of linens*
7. Locate largest, most distal vein (see Procedure 5.2); place tourniquet on ex-	*If insertion attempt fails, vein can be entered at a higher point*

Action	Rationale

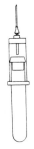

FIGURE 10.3.1

tremity 2 to 6 inches (5 to 15 cm) above venipuncture site or inflate blood pressure cuff.

Restricts blood flow, distending vein

8. Don gloves.

Reduces microorganism transfer

9. Clean vein area, beginning at the vein and circling outward to a 2-inch diameter.

Maintains asepsis

10. Encourage client to take slow, deep breaths as you begin.

Facilitates relaxation

11. Remove cap from needle and hold skin taut with one hand while holding syringe or vacutainer holder with other hand (with butterfly catheter, pinch "wings" together).

Stabilizes vein and prevents skin from moving during insertion

Decreases pain during needle insertion

12. Maintaining needle sterility, insert needle, bevel up, into the straightest section of vein; puncture skin at a 15- to 30-degree angle.

Provides clear area for puncture

Provides for downward movement toward vein

13. When needle has entered skin, lower needle until almost parallel with skin.

Decreases risk of penetration of both walls of the vein

14. Following path of vein,

Action	Rationale

insert needle into wall
of vein.

15. Watch for backflow of
    blood (not noted with
    vacutainer); push needle
    slightly further into vein.
    Indicates needle has pierced vein wall

16. Gently pull back syringe
    plunger until adequate
    amount of blood is
    obtained.

17. If using blood collection
    device, put tube or blood
    culture bottle into device
    and push in until needle
    punctures rubber stopper
    and blood is pulled into
    tube by vacuum; keep
    tube in device until it is
    three-fourths full or until
    culture medium is blood-
    colored; remove tube and
    replace with new tube, if
    additional specimens are
    needed.
    Connects needle with tube
    Allows suction in tube to pull blood into tube

18. Place alcohol pad or cot-
    ton ball over needle inser-
    tion site and remove
    needle from vein while
    applying pressure with
    pad or cotton ball.
    Facilitates sealing of vein
    Decreases bleeding from site

19. Hold pressure for 2 to 3
    minutes (5 to 10 minutes
    if client is on anticoagu-
    lant therapy); check for
    bleeding and apply pres-
    sure until bleeding has
    stopped.
    Facilitates clotting

20. Proceed to Finishing
    Steps (p. 499)

Central Catheter Syringe Method

1. Cleanse connection or injection port with alcohol or
   betadine swab (Table 10.3).
   Reduces introduction of micro-organisms into the internal lumens

2. Remove Luer-lock con-
   nector or IV tubing from

Action	Rationale

TABLE 10.3 **Obtaining Blood Specimens**

Infusion Device	Technique
Implanted ports	• Pre-flush with 5 mL NS • Withdraw and discard 5 mL of blood • Obtain required specimens • Heparin lock maintaining positive pressure Vacutainer method may be used
Hickman catheter	• Discard 3 mL of blood • Obtain required specimens • Heparin lock maintaining positive pressure Vacutainer method may be used
PICC	• Withdraw and discard 5 mL of blood • Obtain required specimens • Heparin lock maintaining positive pressure Check for specific manufacturer recommendations regarding the use of vacutainers
CVC line	• Clamp off lumens that are not being used for blood withdraw • Withdraw and discard 5 mL of blood via the proximal lumen • Obtain required specimens • Flush lumen with 5 mL NS • Heparin lock maintaining positive pressure Vacutainer method may be used
Groshong catheter	• Pre-flush with 5 mL NS • Withdraw and discard 5 mL of blood • Obtain required specimens • Flush lumen with 20 mL NS • Heparin lock maintaining positive pressure DO NOT USE VACUTAINER METHOD

NS, normal saline

Action	Rationale

the catheter and connect
an empty 10-mL syringe to
the hub.

3. Release the catheter clamp.

4. Aspirate 3–5 mL of blood   *Assists in obtaining accurate*
   to clear the lumen, reclamp   *and uncontaminated speci-*
   the catheter and discard   *mens*
   this syringe.

5. Attach a new 10-mL
   syringe, and aspirate the
   amount of blood needed
   for the specimen.

6. Reclamp the line and remove the specimen
   syringe.

7. Cleanse the hub with an
   alcohol or betadine swab,   *Keeps the lumens from occluding*
   flush the lumen with NS,
   attach a new sterile injection port and heparin lock
   or restart all IV fluids.

8. Transfer the blood into the
   specimen tubes.

9. Proceed to Finishing Steps.

Central Catheter Aspiration Vacutainer Method

1. Cleanse the connection
   with alcohol or betadine   *Reduces introduction of micro-*
   swab.   *organisms into the internal*
   lumens

2. Remove Luer-lock con-
   nector or IV tubing from
   the catheter and connect
   the vacutainer holder to
   catheter hub.

3. Release catheter clamp,
   insert vacutainer tube, discard.

4. Collect discard sample   *Assists in obtaining accurate*
   and then obtain appro-   *and uncontaminated speci-*
   priate lab specimens by   *mens*
   inserting appropriately
   topped vacutainer tubes.

5. Reclamp the line and remove the vacutainer holder.

6. Cleanse the hub with an
   alcohol or betadine swab.

Action	Rationale
7. Flush the lumen with NS, attach a new sterile injection port and heparin lock, or restart all IV fluids.	*Keeps the lumens from occluding*
8. Proceed to Finishing Steps.	

Finishing Steps

1. Assist client to position of comfort.	*Promotes comfort and communication*
2. Attach properly completed identification label to each tube, affix requisition.	*Tests should be performed properly* *Incorrect labeling can cause diagnostic error*
3. Dispose of and store equipment properly.	*Maintains clean and organized environment*
4. Remove gloves and wash hands.	*Reduces microorganism transfer*
5. Store appropriately and transport specimen to appropriate laboratory (see Procedure 10.4).	*Protects specimen from breakage and temperature damage, maintaining integrity of specimen until nurse reaches laboratory*

Evaluation

Were desired outcomes achieved?

DOCUMENTATION

The following should be noted on the visit note:

- Date and time blood is drawn
- Site used and method used
- Test to be run on specimen
- Amount of discarded blood
- Client's tolerance to procedure
- Status of skin (eg, bruising, excessive bleeding)
- Laboratory that sample was sent to for processing

Sample Documentation

DATE	TIME	
9/15/98	1330	CBC and electrolytes obtained using a vacutainer method from the proximal lumen. Specimens labeled with patient name, registration number, and date. Sent to ABC Laboratory for processing. Results to be faxed to primary physician.

Nursing Procedure **10.4**

Handling and Transport of Specimens

⊠ EQUIPMENT

- Sterile and nonsterile gloves
- Gowns
- Masks
- Goggles
- Sterile specimen containers
- Equipment for collection of blood specimens:
  - Vacuum tubes
  - Blood drawing devices and needles
  - Syringes
  - Small vein infusion sets
  - Specimen bags
- Biohazardous waste containers
- Laboratory requisitions
- Small cooler for transport of specimens

Purpose

Provides safe collection of specimens
Ensures proper handling during transport
Ensures the integrity of the specimen received at the laboratory

Desired Outcomes (sample)

Specimen is successfully collected.
Handling and transport of specimen is appropriate.
Integrity of specimen is maintained, and ordered tests are done.

Assessment

Assessment should focus on the following:

Specimen needed
Specific requirements of the laboratory which will process the
  specimen
Equipment needed to ensure safe collection and transport

Outcome Identification and Planning

Key Goals and Sample Goal Criteria

The nurse will:

Collect the ordered specimen in the appropriate container
Transport the specimen safely to the laboratory in a timely fashion
Complete all needed documentation that accompanies the specimen

Special Considerations

 Transcultural

There may be cultural implications in the collection of body fluids. Know the cultural factors involved for any particular client and be prepared to work within any restrictions to the extent possible.

HINT

Carry a list of contact people at each laboratory who can answer questions on the proper collection, handling, and transport of specimens. Keep a list of which physicians routinely use which laboratories. Keep a list of preferred laboratories for specific insurance companies and managed care organizations. Ask the lab to send a copy of the report to the agency for inclusion on the client chart.

IMPLEMENTATION

Action	Rationale
1. Review chart or obtain verbal order for specimen to be collected or test to be run. Be sure any verbal order is documented in writing and signed by a physician.	*Ensures compliance with standards that require a written physician order, assists in payment for ordered tests by third-party payors*
2. Determine what is to be collected, what laboratory will do the test, what con-	*Reduces the chance that the specimen will be unacceptable and have to be recollected*

Action	Rationale
tainer is to be used, what information is needed on the lab requisition, and if any client preparation is needed.	
3. Notify the client of the procedure to be done, and instruct in any special preparation.	*Includes client in plan of care, prepares client for specimen collection*
4. Assemble all needed equipment, check expiration dates of containers, complete demographic information on requisition.	*Increases efficiency*
5. At time of visit, explain procedure of collection to client.	*Reduces client anxiety, increases client cooperation*
6. Wear gloves for all specimen collection, use gown, goggles, mask if splashing of body fluids is possible.	*Prevents potential transmission of pathogens*
7. *Sputum*—Early morning specimens are usually easier for the client to produce. Always position the client in a well-ventilated area when obtaining a sputum specimen. If tuberculosis is a possibility, wear the appropriate protective mask.	*Increases chance of obtaining acceptable specimen if early AM visit is made. Ventilation and appropriate protective mask for the nurse reduces the risk of transmission of airborne pathogens*
8. *Blood*—If a venipuncture is needed, take time to examine both of the client's arms carefully to determine the best site. If central or peripheral line is present, assess the policy and procedure for obtaining specimen from existing line (see Procedure 10.3).	*Increases chance of successful venipuncture. Recently hospitalized clients may have damage to commonly used veins, such as those in the antecubital area. Careful examination will allow the nurse to choose the most suitable area*
9. *Wound culture*—If using a sterile swab, take care to	*Reduces chance of contamination from skin bacteria*

Action	Rationale
obtain the culture from the center of the wound, not the skin edges.	
10. *Stool*—Instruct client thoroughly in proper collection of specimen (varies with type of test ordered; consult laboratory). If multiple containers are to be used, label each. Instruct client in storage of specimens until next visit.	*Increases chance of successful specimen collection*
11. Examine all specimen containers. If any blood or body fluid is on the outside of the container, wipe clean with a solution of 10% bleach.	*Prevents risk of transmission of organisms to others handling specimens*
12. Dispose of all contaminated gloves, needles, etc. in a biohazardous waste container at the point of use.	*Prevents contamination of client environment*
13. Label each container with all required information.	*Ensures proper identification of specimen*
14. Package each container in the manner requested by the laboratory.	*Ensures acceptance of specimen by the laboratory*
15. Check that each requisition is complete and accompanies the appropriate specimen.	*Promotes efficient handling of specimen by laboratory*
16. Place specimens in cooler for transport to lab. Avoid direct contact between specimen container and ice or chemical coolant (Fig. 10.4). Take specimens to the laboratory immediately.	*Maintains integrity of specimen and ensures accurate test results*

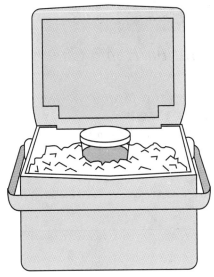

FIGURE 10.4

Evaluation

Were desired outcomes achieved?

DOCUMENTATION

The following should be noted on the visit note:

- Type of specimen
- Method of collection
- Specific body area from which specimen was collected
- Laboratory used
- Tests to be done on specimen

Sample Documentation		
DATE	TIME	
6/26/99	1100	Wound culture obtained lower left abdominal wound, using packaged culture swab. Specimen to City Laboratory for culture and sensitivity.

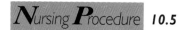

*N*ursing *P*rocedure *10.5*

Coagulation/Hema Check Testing

☒ EQUIPMENT

- Appropriate diagnostic testing machine
- Appropriate teststrips for machine
- Disposable gloves
- Alcohol wipe pads
- Cotton balls
- Lancet (and lancet holding device, if available)
- Paper towel
- Needle disposal unit

Purpose

Obtains specimen for testing of blood coagulation time or hemoglobin level.

Desired Outcomes (sample)

Blood is drawn with minimal discomfort to client.
Accurate results are obtained.

Assessment

Assessment should focus on the following:

Physician's order for type and frequency of test
Time and results of previous test(s)

Outcome Identification and Planning

Key Goals and Sample Goal Criteria

The client will:

Experience no injury or undue pain during procedure.
Receive therapy or teaching based on test results.

Special Considerations

It may be easier to obtain blood sample if fingers are warmed with washcloth prior to finger puncture.

IMPLEMENTATION

Action	Rationale
1. Calibrate machine per manual.	*Verifies accuracy of machine reading*
2. Wash hands.	*Reduces microorganisms*
3. Explain procedure to client.	*Reduces anxiety*
4. Don gloves.	*Prevents nurse exposure to blood*
5. Cleanse finger with alcohol wipe.	*Reduces microorganisms*
6. Gently squeeze finger near area to be punctured.	*Entraps blood for obtaining of adequate specimen size*
7. Puncture finger with lancet.	*Obtains blood*
8. Touch blood to test pad area and place on paper towel.	*Covers test pad area with specimen*
9. Wipe finger with alcohol (or cotton ball may be used).	*Removes blood from finger*
10. Quickly place specimen in machine as per manufacturer's directions.	*Begins process for obtaining machine reading*
11. Wait appropriate number of seconds, then note numerical value on display screen.	*Obtains calculated results for coagulation time or hemoglobin level*
12. Turn machine off.	
13. Reposition client.	*Provides for comfort*
14. Clean, restore, or discard equipment appropriately.	*Disposes and restores equipment*
15. Wash hands.	*Prevents microorganism transfer*
16. Perform necessary teaching and/ or notify physician, as indicated by results.	*Provides appropriate follow-up based on results*

Evaluation

Were desired outcomes achieved?

DOCUMENTATION

The following should be noted on the visit note:

- Specimen type and time obtained
- Results of test
- Complaints of client discomfort
- Signs or symptoms of indicators of abnormal test results
- Follow-up teaching
- Physician notification if indicated

Sample Documentation

DATE	TIME	
2/20/99	1800	Fingerstick puncture for hematest check. Hemoglobin reading 9.0. States has been very tired lately, but no other complaints. Skin pale, capillary refill time 4 seconds, skin cool. Instructed to avoid excessive activity at this time and given list of foods rich in iron. Dr. Walker notified of test results. Client scheduled for office visit on 2/24.

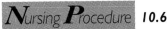

*N*ursing *P*rocedure **10.6**

Blood Glucose Testing

☒ EQUIPMENT

- Blood glucose machine (optional)
- Chemical strips for blood glucose with color chart (on container or insert)
- Nonsterile gloves
- Lancets
- Autoclix or lancet injector (optional)
- Cotton balls
- Alcohol pads (or bottle of alcohol)
- Watch with second hand or kitchen timer
- Needle disposal unit

Purpose

Determine level of glucose in blood
Promotes stricter blood glucose regulation

Desired Outcomes (sample)

Blood glucose elevation is noted and treated promptly per sliding scale.
Blood glucose is maintained within acceptable range.
Client demonstrates consistent ability to perform all tasks, take appropriate action, and record results accurately.
Client maintains and stores equipment and supplies safely and appropriately.

Assessment

Assessment should focus on the following:

Doctor's order for frequency and type of glucose testing, and sliding scale for insulin coverage
Client's knowledge of procedure and diabetic self care
Response to previous testing
Client's previous experience in learning techniques
Client's vision status, cognitive status, and manual dexterity
Family member or significant other's reliability to assist with procedure

Outcome Identification and Planning

Key Goals and Sample Goal Criteria

The client and/or significant other will:

Demonstrate consistent ability to perform procedure, record results, and take appropriate action prior to discharge
Demonstrate early detection of blood glucose elevations
Demonstrate ability to safely store, use, and dispose of used supplies

Special Considerations

If client has a personal blood glucose monitor, be sure monitor has been calibrated properly before using.

Geriatric

If a blood glucose meter is used, the type should be the easiest for the client to use, based on assessment of the client's cognitive status, vision status, and manual dexterity.

HINT

ECONOMIC: If finances are a factor, use community resources and national organizations to assist with the purchase of the meter and supplies.

HINT

If there is no community program for safe disposal of biomedical waste, the client may use a rigid container, such as an empty laundry container jug. A small amount of dilute bleach solution may be poured into the jug, and used needles and contaminated lancets may be put into the jug. Emphasis should be placed on storing the container in a safe place, and being sure that it is tightly closed and secured when it is discarded.

An egg timer may be used to time the reaction of the blood-glucose testing procedure.

IMPLEMENTATION

Action	Rationale
1. Assist client in determining clean area for storage	*Promotes efficiency*

Action	Rationale

of equipment and supplies.
2. Wash hands and organize equipment.

Reduces microorganism transfer

3. Explain procedure to client and inquire as to preference of finger and use of lancet injector.

Facilitates cooperation and promotes sense of involvement in, and control of own care

4. Perform, teach, observe calibration of glucose meter, if used:
   - Turn machine on.
   - Compare number on machine or strip in machine with number on bottle of chemical strips (Fig. 10.6.1).
   - Perform, observe, teach procedures to ready machine for operation;

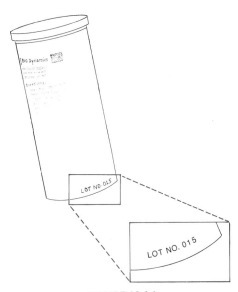

FIGURE 10.6.1

Action	Rationale
consult user's manual for steps and readiness indicator.	
- Machine calibration should be done per manufacturer's instruction/agency policy, with high and low glucose solutions to ensure accuracy. The client should maintain a calibration record.	
5. Remove chemical strip from container; client should place face up where it is most accessible.	*Prevents delay* *Allows client to concentrate on fingerstick task*
6. Load lancet in injector, if used, set trigger, prepare alcohol sponge and cottonball for use.	*Prepares injector to push lancet into finger*
7. If nurse performing procedure, gloves should be worn. If client is performing procedure, hands should be clean.	*Use of gloves prevents blood exposure. As there is no risk in a client's exposure to his/her own blood, gloves are not necessary and their use could make procedure more difficult.*
8. Hold chosen finger downward and squeeze gently from lower digits to fingertip, or wrap finger in warm wet cloth for 30 seconds or longer.	*Facilitates flow of blood to finger for easy sampling*
9. Wipe intended puncture site with alcohol pad.	*Removes dirt and skin oils* *Decreases microorganisms*
10. Place injector against side of finger, (where there are fewer nerve endings) and release trigger; or stick side of finger with lancet using a darting motion.	*Obtains a large drop of blood with minimal pain stimulation*
11. Hold chemical strip under puncture site and squeeze gently until drop of blood is large enough to drop onto strip	*Ensures that indicator squares are covered with blood* *Prevents uneven exposure of indicators*

Action	Rationale
and cover indicator square.	
12. Push timer button on machine as soon as blood has covered indicator squares, or note position on watch or kitchen timer.	*Determines time to remove excess blood from strip and when to read color change*
13. Apply pressure to puncture site until bleeding stops, or have client do it, and place lancet in needle disposal unit.	
14. When timer or watch indicates 60 seconds or designated time (per machine user's manual) has passed, wipe excess blood from strip.	*Removes blood cells*
15. Place into machine, if used, with indicator patch facing reading window (consult user's manual). After an additional 60 seconds have passed, read results from the machine.	*Determines blood glucose level after timed chemical reaction*
16. Or compare colors on strip with those in chart on chemical strip container or insert after the additional 60 seconds (Fig. 10.6.2).	
17. Discard soiled materials and gloves in proper container.	*Prevents exposure to blood soiled materials*
18. Assist client with recording results on glucose flow sheet, and administering insulin, if indicated.	*Maintains record of glucose levels and insulin coverage*
19. Assist client in cleaning equipment and storing in a safe, clean, secure area.	*Promotes efficiency and maintenance of cleanliness, avoids possibility of use by others in the home*

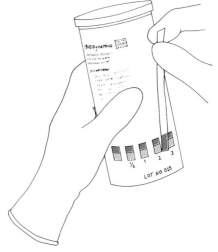

FIGURE 10.6.2

Evaluation

Were desired outcomes achieved?

Are additional services needed? (eg, social worker for assistance with finances; occupational therapy to assist with increase in manual dexterity)

DOCUMENTATION

The following should be noted on the visit note:

- Method of glucose testing
- Level of glucose
- Insulin coverage provided and route
- Teaching done
- Client's response to teaching
- Functional limitations that interfere with client performance of procedure
- Plan for future visits
- Discharge planning

Sample Documentation

DATE	TIME	
1/2/99	1200	Observed client performing finger-stick with no assistance needed. Observed client performing glucose meter use with moderate difficulty. Verbal instructions and physical assistance needed with application of blood to strip and reading of result. Glucose level 124, recorded appropriately by client. Client demonstrates eagerness and ability to learn techniques, but has difficulty with use of this meter due to poor vision. Expresses concerns regarding buying chemical strips. PLAN: Will contact MD re: possible use of other meter, need for social worker to assist with financial concerns impacting care; continue to instruct in glucose monitoring technique, insulin administration. Discharge when able to demonstrate self-care.

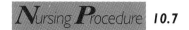

Nursing Procedure 10.7

▓ *Principles of Medical Asepsis*

▓ EQUIPMENT

- Soap and warm running water
- Nonsterile gloves
- Clean gown
- Mask, as needed
- Waste disposal materials: trash can, bags (isolation bags optional)
- Linen bags (pillowcases and plastic bags)
- Specimen bags, if agency policy

Purpose

Prevents the growth and spread of pathogenic microorganisms to one individual from another individual or the environment

Desired Outcomes (sample)

Client shows no signs of infection or of additional infection.
Medical procedures are performed with no evidence of exposure to microorganisms.

Assessment

Assessment should focus on the following:

Data from medical history and physical or diagnostic studies indicating susceptibility to, or presence of, infection (fever, cloudy urine, positive culture, decreased white blood count, history of immunosuppression or steroid intake)
Client or nurse's allergy to soap or bacteriostatic solutions
Number of persons in the home and in contact with client
Client and family knowledge of principles of asepsis
Ability of client to cooperate and not contaminate sterile field

Outcome Identification and Planning

Key Goals and Sample Goal Criteria

The client will:

Demonstrate no signs of infection within 3 weeks of therapy
Demonstrate no signs of infection during postoperative recovery period

Special Considerations

Keep your fingernails short and filed. Dirt and secretions that lodge under fingernails contain microorganisms. Long fingernails can scratch client's skin.

Restrict pets from the room in which a medical procedure is being performed.

Most procedures are performed with clean, rather than sterile, technique.

If a client is disoriented and restless, restrain the client during procedures that require maintenance of sterile or clean materials. Be sure to explain to family and client importance of restraints if needed during procedures (see Procedure 10.10).

IMPLEMENTATION

Action	Rationale

Hand Washing—Medical

1. Perform 2- to 4-minute hand washing:

- Remove rings (often may retain wedding band) and chipped nail polish; move watch to position high on wrist.

- Wet hands from wrist to fingertips under flowing water.

- Keep hands and forearms lower than elbows during washing.

- Place soap, preferably bacteriostatic, on hands and rub vigorously for 15 to 30 seconds, massaging all skin areas, joints, fingernails, between fin-

Reduces microorganisms from hands

Removes sources that harbor and promote growth of microorganisms

Cleans from least to most dirty
Aids in removal of microorganisms
Hands are the most contaminated parts to be washed
Cleans from least to most contaminated area

Creates friction to remove organisms

Action	Rationale
gers, and so forth; slide ring up and down while rubbing fingers (if unable to remove).	*Permits cleaning around and under ring*
- Rinse hands from fingers to wrist under flow of water.	*Washes dirt and organisms from cleanest to least clean area*
- Repeat soaping, rubbing, and rinsing until hands are clean.	
- Dry hands with paper towel moving from fingers to wrist to forearm.	*Dries hands from clean to least clean area*
- Turn off faucet with paper towel.	*Prevents recontamination of hand*
2. **Management of contaminated materials:**	
- Don gloves when contact with body fluids or infected area is possible.	*Prevents contamination of hands* *Prevents contact with secretions*
- Don mask if organism can be transmitted by airborne route through contact with mucous membranes. Keep room door closed.	*Prevents exposure to airborne microorganisms or projectile body fluids*
- Don gown if contact with body secretions or contaminated area is likely, if client has highly contagious condition, or if client is immunosuppressed.	*Avoids contact with potentially infectious material* *Avoids spread of infection* *Protects client from exposure to microorganisms*
- Place disposable contaminated materials in bag before leaving; place in designated disposal area in the home.	*Provides added protection to client and family against exposure to body fluids or infectious materials*
- Reusable items should be bagged separately and cleaned or stored appropriately before leaving the home.	*Decreases spread of microorganisms on used medical equipment*
- Linens should be placed in linen bags before leaving and placed in appro-	

Action	Rationale
priate utility area for client to clean appropriately.	
- Clean stethoscope between use with different clients with soap and water and wipe with alcohol swab (if used in an infected area or with infected client, a thorough disassembly and cleaning may be needed); use a separate stethoscope for an infected client, if possible.	*Decreases spread of microorganisms on stethoscope* *Limits exposure to infection*
- Sphygmomanometers, thermometers, or similar daily-use items should be sprayed or wiped with a bacteriostatic substance between use with different clients.	*Decreases exposure to potentially infectious medium* *These items provide a good medium for organism growth*
- Used syringes and needles, scalpels and other sharp disposables should be placed in appropriately marked container. DO NOT REPLACE CAPS ON NEEDLES.	*Prevents accidental stick and contact with client's blood* *Prevents accidental sticks during attempts to recap needle*
- Discard gown, gloves, and mask before leaving client's room.	*Prevents spread of infection*

3. **Handling of personal effects of patients with infection:**
   - Instruct client and family on the following: NEVER SHARE PERSONAL-CARE ITEMS, such as toothbrushes, toothpaste, towels, eating utensils, cups, soap, roll-on deodorant.
   - If papers, books, or other items become soiled with infectious material, items

Action	Rationale

should be discarded un-
less sterilization is possible and desired.

4. **Sleeping arrangements:**
   - An isolated area of the
     home may be indicated if
     client has highly infec-
     tious disorder.
   - A semiprivate room may
     be used when the micro-
     organism is limited to
     one body area; however,
     good medical asepsis
     must be maintained by
     staff, client, family, and
     others to prevent
     spread of infection.

5. **Room cleaning:**
   - Instruct family that   *Reduces microorganisms in the*
     room should be cleaned   *environment*
     with disinfectant daily.
   - If soiled materials spill
     on floor, clean area with
     disinfectant or bacteri-
     ocidal agent specific to
     organism, if known.
   - If client dies,
     room should be cleaned
     and disinfected thor-   *Promotes thorough removal of*
     oughly and allowed to   *microorganisms*
     remain vacant 12 to 24
     hours if possible (see
     Procedure 12.3 for post-
     mortem care if indicated).

Evaluation

Were desired outcomes achieved?

DOCUMENTATION

The following should be noted on the visit note:

- Status of source of infection/potential infection (wound, dressing, breath sounds, secretions)
- Procedure performed
- Protective garments used
- Client and family teaching completed
- Disposition of items disposed

Sample Documentation		
DATE	**TIME**	
1/2/99	1200	Abdominal abscess site dressed. Site clean and without redness. Drains intact. Client tolerated procedure without complaint of unusual discomfort. States understands dressing change process and would like to change dressing in morning. Family and client able to verbalize instructions on maintaining clean home environment and preventing contamination with others.

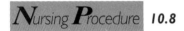

Principles of Surgical Asepsis (Aseptic Technique)

⬛ EQUIPMENT

- Bacteriocidal or antimicrobial soap
- Sink
- Surgical scrub brush
- Sterile gloves
- Sterile gown
- Mask
- Hair covering and booties (optional)
- Sterile materials (dressing, instruments)
- Sterile sheets or towels as needed
- Waste disposal materials: trash can, bags (isolation bags optional)
- Bedside (or overbed) table

Purpose

Avoids the introduction of microorganisms onto a designated field

Desired Outcomes (sample)

Client shows no signs of infection or of additional infection.
Procedures are performed with no evidence of exposure to microorganisms.

Assessment

Assessment should focus on the following:

Data from medical history and physical or diagnostic studies indicating susceptibility to infection (decreased leukocyte count, history of immunosuppression, or steroid intake)
Doctor's orders or agency policy regarding dressing changes and isolation procedures
Client or nurse's allergy to soap or bacteriostatic solutions

Date of expiration and sterility indicator on sterile supplies and solutions

Client and family knowledge of principles of asepsis

Client's ability to cooperate and not contaminate sterile field

Agency policy regarding surgical scrub procedure

Outcome Identification and Planning

Key Goals and Sample Goal Criteria

The client will:

Demonstrate no signs of infection throughout TPN therapy and central line maintenance

Demonstrate no signs of infection during postoperative recovery period

Special Considerations

Variations in sterile technique—eg, the omission of some protective coverings (hair cover, booties, mask)—may be used in performing some procedures. CONTINUE TO USE ASEPTIC PRINCIPLES TO GOVERN ACTIONS DURING A PROCEDURE.

Restrict pets from the room in which a sterile or clean procedure is being performed. Most procedures are performed with clean, rather than sterile, technique. Enlist and instruct a family member to serve as an assistant.

IF UNSURE OF STERILITY OF MATERIAL, GLOVE, OR FIELD, CONSIDER IT CONTAMINATED.

If a client is disoriented and restless, restrain the client during procedures requiring maintenance of sterile materials. Enlist family assistance for manual restraint of the client or use mechanical restraints (see Procedure 10.10). Be sure to explain to client and family the importance of using restraints during procedure (see Procedure 10.10).

IMPLEMENTATION

Action	Rationale
1. A private room is preferable for performance of a sterile procedure.	*Minimizes microorganisms in environment*
Hand Washing—Surgical	
2. Don mask, hair cover, and booties, if required.	*Prevents introduction of contaminants from mouth, hair or shoes into environment*

Action	Rationale
3. Perform 5- to 10-minute surgical scrub using counted brush stroke method:	*Reduces organisms on hands* *Counted brush method places emphasis on detail to specific areas and ensures that all skin surfaces are exposed to sufficient friction*
- Remove rings (often must remove wedding band), chipped nail polish, and watch.	*Removes sources that harbor and promote growth of microorganisms*
- Wet hands and arms from elbows to fingertips under flowing water.	*Cleans from least to most dirty* *Aids in removal of microorganisms*
- Place soap, preferably antimicrobial/bacteriostatic, on hands and rub vigorously for 15 to 30 seconds; use scrub brush gently—do not abrade skin.	*Creates friction to remove organisms*
- Using circular motion scrub all skin areas, joints, fingernails, between fingers, and so forth (on all sides and 2 inches above elbows); slide ring, if present, up and down while rubbing fingers.	*Permits cleaning around and under ring*
- Continue scrub for 5 to 10 minutes or per agency policy.	
- Rinse hands from fingers to elbows under flow of water.	*Washes dirt and organisms from cleanest to least clean area*
- Repeat soaping, rubbing, and rinsing until hands and arms are clean.	
- Pat hands dry with sterile towel moving from fingers to wrist.	*Dries hands from clean to least clean area*
- Turn off faucet with towel.	*Prevents recontamination of hand*

Sterile Field
4. To create a sterile field:
   - Arrange sterile supplies

Action	Rationale
on overbed table or closest available dresser, table, or chair.	
- Never use opened items or items of questionable sterility.	
- Open packages to reveal supplies, using insides of packages to form sterile field; open package's outer flap away from you, open side flaps next, and then pull inner flap toward you (Fig. 10.8.1); spread edges of package cover over table with fingertips.	*Prevents reaching over exposed materials* *Edges are considered unsterile*
5. To add items to sterile field:	
- Drop sterile items onto field, keeping packaging between items and hands (Fig. 10.8.2); *use sterile forceps or tongs* to remove items from package, if unable to do so with sterile technique; if unable to remove item from package without contamination, wait until sterile garb is applied, then place items on sterile field.	*Prevents contamination of supplies*

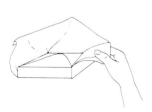

FIGURE 10.8.1

Action	Rationale

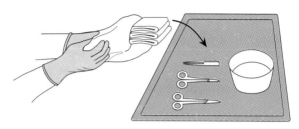

FIGURE 10.8.2

- Use sterile gloves or *sterile tongs* to remove sterile towel and cover field and supplies if not beginning procedure immediately.

DO NOT REACH OVER OPEN STERILE FIELD.

- Don sterile gown and sterile gloves (see procedures for gown and glove application at end of this procedure).

- Begin procedure with hands held above waist.

6. To maintain a sterile environment:

- Drape sterile sheets or towels over area surrounding site being treated.

- Use tongs or forceps to clean site thoroughly with bacteriocidal agent.

- Discard *tongs* from sterile field.

- Pour liquids into a sterile basin held by an assistant in sterile garb or by holding bottle over 1-inch outer parameter of field;

Sterility will be lost if field is exposed to air for extended period of time

Exposes field to contamination

Prevents exposure of sterile field to hands or clothing

Area below waist considered nonsterile

Decreases chance of exposure to nonsterile sites

Maintains sterility of gloves
Reduces microorganisms

Prevents field contamination

Prevents reaching over sterile field

Action	Rationale

avoid splashing on field.
IF FIELD BECOMES
WET, CONSIDER IT
CONTAMINATED.

Water conducts microorganisms from nonsterile area to sterile field

Maintain Asepsis During Procedure

7. As procedure is performed:
   - Remove soiled equipment from area or sterile field; drop trash in bag or receptacle.
   - Avoid touching nonsterile surfaces.
   - When procedure is complete and dressing is intact, label dressing with date, time, and your initials.

Indicates when next dressing change is due

Sterile Gown Application

1. Wash hands and organize equipment; apply mask, if needed; enlist assistant to tie gown.

Reduces microorganism transfer
Promotes efficiency

2. Remove sterile gown package from outer cover and open inner covering to expose sterile gown; place on bedside table, touching only outsides of covering, and spread covering over table; open outer glove package and slide inside glove cover onto sterile field.

Maintains sterility of gown

Provides sterile field
Places gloves in convenient location and on sterile field

3. Remove gown from field, grasping inside of gown and gently shaking to loosen folds; hold gown with inside facing you (Fig. 10.8.3).

Prepares gown for application

4. Place both arms inside gown at the same time and stretch outward until hands reach edge of sleeves; don sterile gloves.

Preserves sterility of gown

Action	Rationale

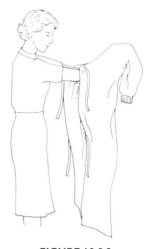

FIGURE 10.8.3

5. Have assistant pull tie from back of gown and fasten to inside tie; have assistant pull outside tie around with sterile tongs or sterile gloves. Grasp tie, pull around to front of gown, and secure to front tie.

Secures gown without contamination of outer portion

Secures gown

Sterile Glove Application

1. Don gown, if needed; otherwise, open glove package, place on bedside table, and remove inner glove covering; open inner package, using sterile technique, and expose gloves.
2. Pick up one glove by cuff and slip fingers of other hand into glove (keep

Action	Rationale
gown sleeve inside glove if applicable); pull glove over hand and sleeve.	
3. Place gloved hand inside cuff of remaining glove and lift slightly; slide other hand into glove and pull cuff over hand and wrist and sleeve of gown, if applicable (Fig. 10.8.4). DO NOT TOUCH SKIN WITH GLOVED HAND.	*Facilitates placing glove on hand without contaminating glove or gloved hand* *Stabilizes gown sleeve and creates continuous sterile hand-to-arm connection*
4. Pull gloves securely over fingers and adjust for fit using one hand to fix the other.	*Places fingers deeply into gloves while maintaining sterility*
5. Proceed to sterile field, maintaining hands above waist; do not touch non-sterile items. IF GLOVE OR GOWN BECOMES CONTAMINATED, DISCARD AND REPLACE WITH STERILE GARB.	*Prevents contamination of gloves*

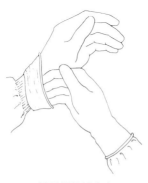

FIGURE 10.8.4

Evaluation

Were desired outcomes achieved?

DOCUMENTATION

The following should be noted on the visit note:

- Sterile procedure performed
- Sterile garments used
- Client teaching done regarding maintenance of dressing and sterile protective environment and verbalized understanding by client

Sample Documentation

DATE	TIME	
1/2/99	1200	Wet-to-dry abdominal dressing change with sterile technique used. Client tolerated procedure with no reports of unusual discomfort. Client and wife state understanding of dressing change process and need for sterility.

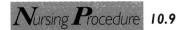

*N*ursing *P*rocedure *10.9*

🖐 *Pre- and Postoperative Care*

⊠ EQUIPMENT

- Pre- and postoperative physicians orders
- Assessment equipment (eg, blood pressure cuff, stethoscope, pen light)
- Scale
- Teaching materials (films, booklet, sample equipment)
- Preoperative checklist
- Shave and preparation kit (razor, soap, sponge, tray for water) (optional). Check agency policy.
- Procedure (hospital) gown
- Fingernail polish remover
- Denture cup (optional)
- Nonsterile gloves
- Other equipment as indicated by type of surgery

Purpose

Preoperative

Prepares client physically and emotionally for impending surgery

Postoperative

Promotes return to state of physical and emotional well-being
Detects complications related to postsurgical status
Prevents postoperative complications
Facilitates wound healing

Desired Outcomes (sample)

Preoperative

Client verbalizes purpose of postoperative regimen.
Client correctly demonstrates pulmonary and cardiovascular exercise regimens.

Postoperative

Client verbalizes purpose of postoperative regimen.
Client correctly demonstrates pulmonary and cardiovascular exercise regimen.

Assessment

Assessment should focus on the following:

Type of surgery
Preparatory regimen for type of surgery (per doctor's order or agency policy)
Perceptions of previous surgical experiences
History and physical for factors increasing risks of surgery or recovery (eg, age, chronic or acute illness, depression, fluid and electrolyte imbalance)
Learning or comprehension ability
Reading ability
Language barriers
Family support
Physician's preoperative and postoperative orders
Tubes, drains, dressings

Outcome Identification and Planning

Key Goals and Sample Goal Criteria

Preoperative
The client will:

Verbalize purpose of surgery and the general surgical procedure before day of surgery
Demonstrate understanding of postoperative pulmonary and circulatory regimen

Postoperative
The client will:
Verbalize understanding of postoperative instructions
Attain and maintain clear breath sounds after surgery
Verbalize decreased discomfort within 30 minutes of complaint of pain
Perform postoperative pulmonary and circulatory exercises every 1 to 2 hours

Special Considerations

Assess the client's readiness to learn and, if preoperative teaching time is limited, gear teaching toward essential items of concern.
Prior understanding of postoperative procedures, staff, and regimen often decreases the client's anxiety and promotes co-operation postoperatively.

Geriatric

Fear of death may be particularly profound in some elderly clients, especially if this is a first hospitalization or first surgery. Supply clear and thorough explanations of all procedures. Encourage the client to participate in preoperative preparations.

IMPLEMENTATION

Action	Rationale
1. Wash hands and organize supplies.	*Reduces microorganism transfer* *Promotes efficiency*
2. Assess client's knowledge of impending surgery; reinforce information and correct errors in understanding. *Note,* it is the physician's responsibility initially to inform client about surgery, options, and risks.	*Determines client's teaching needs* *Clarifies misinformation*
3. Show films and provide booklets regarding surgery and postoperative care; encourage questions; answer questions clearly.	*Reduces anxiety* *Imparts knowledge*
4. Verify that operative permit has been signed. *Note,* it is the physician's responsibility to obtain proper informed consent.	*Avoids error in sending client to surgery without written consent*
5. Verify that ordered lab work and diagnostic studies (x-ray films, EKGs) have been done; check results of diagnostic studies and include results on preoperative checklist; alert doctor to abnormal values	*Assesses client preparation and readiness for surgery* *Determines if treatment of abnormalities is needed or if surgery must be postponed*
6. Check to be certain preoperative medications have been obtained.	*Avoids delays for client and surgical team on day of surgery*
7. Obtain client's height and weight; perform head-to-toe assessment with in-	*Provides baseline data*

Action	Rationale
depth assessment of areas related to surgery (see Procedures 1.5 and 1.8).	
8. Instruct client about procedures or equipment that will be used to provide adequate oxygenation:	
- Demonstrate use of oxygen mask/cannula, or of endotracheal tube and ventilator	*Prepares client for postoperative regimen*
- Explain related noises and sensations.	*Decreases anxiety produced by postoperative regimen*
- Demonstrate turning, coughing, and deep-breathing exercises, demonstrating use of pillow to splint incision site.	
- Explain techniques of chest physiotherapy, if applicable.	
- Stress the importance of pulmonary toilet in prevention of secretion buildup.	
9. Discuss and demonstrate, if applicable, techniques for maintaining adequate circulation and pain control:	
- Demonstrate range-of-motion and leg exercises, and check client's technique.	*Maintains circulation while client is bedridden*
- If transcutaneous electrical stimulation (TENS) unit is to be used, explain procedure to client.	*Prepares client for use of TENS unit postoperatively*
- Arrange for physical therapist to visit client.	*Facilitates postoperative relationship and cooperation*
10. Discuss with client and family the postoperative unit or environment; if	*Reduces anxiety about unfamiliar setting and caregivers*

Action	Rationale
applicable; review tentative timetable of surgery and recovery room period; instruct family on agency's methods of communicating status updates during and after surgery.	
11. **On the night before surgery** (client/family instructions)	
- Shave designated body areas.	*Prevents postoperative infection*
- Shower with povidone solution, if ordered or agency policy.	
- Take laxative or other medications, if ordered.	*Helps flush bowel to prevent contamination of sterile field*
- Perform enema and check results.	*Evacuates bowel to prevent sterile field contamination*
- Withhold foods and fluids after midnight the night before surgery (clear fluids may often be administered up to 3 to 4 hours before surgery, particularly if no IV fluids are infusing); consult agency policy.	*Prevents sterile field contamination* *Prevents bowel and bladder puncture because of distended organs*
- Discuss which, if any, medications are to be given (permit sips of water) and at what time.	*Delivers drugs client needs to maintain therapeutic levels during surgery while eliminating those that may cause compatibility problems with drugs given in surgery*
12. **On day before or morning of surgery, prepare client** (client/family instructions)	
- Remove jewelry (may retain wedding ring—wrap with tape); ask client to leave valuables and jewelry home with family	*Prevents loss during surgery* *Secures valuables and belongings*
- Remove nail polish.	*Allows for good visualization*

Action	Rationale
	of nail beds to monitor oxygenation status
- Remove and label glasses, contact lenses, or other prostheses.	*Prevents loss*
- Remove full or partial dentures and label container (place with family).	*Prevents loss*
- Void before leaving home.	*Prevents sterile field contamination and/or accidental bladder puncture during surgery*

Postoperative Care

1. On client visits:
   - Assess respiratory, neurological and neurovascular status, vital signs, apical pulse, bowel status, and other parameters pertaining to specific body systems affected by surgery.

   Provides baseline data on postoperative status

   - Assess incisional dressings and surgical-wound drainage systems.
   - Note urine output and output from drainage systems as well as diaphoresis, emesis, and diarrhea.

   Enables early detection of fluid imbalances or systemic changes

   - Monitor surgical dressing and change or reinforce as needed and permitted. MANY DOCTORS PREFER TO REMOVE INITIAL DRESSING.

   Promotes sense of well-being
   Increases self-esteem and sense of self-control

2. Instruct client/family on the following (observe demonstration during visit)
   - Turn, deep breathe, and cough/suction client every 2 hours.
   - Instruct client in use of

   Facilitates lung expansion

Action	Rationale
incentive spirometry equipment and encourage use every hour.	*Mobilizes secretions*
- Range-of-motion and leg exercises as well as chest physiotherapy, if applicable; if transcutaneous electrical nerve stimulation (TENS) unit is to be used, how to apply and turn on (see Procedure 8.6).	*Maintains circulation while client is bedridden* *Facilitates removal of accumulated secretions* *Promotes comfort by blocking pain reception of nerves*
- Signs and symptoms of infection, care of dressings, drains, or wounds, as indicated.	

Evaluation

Were desired outcomes achieved?

DOCUMENTATION

The following should be noted on the visit note:

Preoperative Teaching and Assessment

- Verbalization of signed consent form
- Preoperative teaching done and client response
- Preparation procedures performed (eg, enema, shave)
- Vital signs and other clinical data
- Preoperative medications teaching
- Completed preoperative checklist or areas pending completion
- Abnormal test results and time doctor was notified of these
- Further teaching or preparation needed

Postoperative

- Assessment with emphasis on abnormal findings
- Status of operative dressings, tubes, drains, and incisions
- Support equipment initiated
- Procedures performed
- Client tolerance to therapy
- Abnormal test results noted and time doctor is notified
- Medications administered
- Client and family concerns
- Teaching needs noted

Sample Documentation

DATE	TIME	
1/2/99	1200	Preoperative and anticipatory postoperative teaching done with instructions on importance of pulmonary toilet, range-of-motion and calf exercises. Client verbalizes understanding. Preoperative checklist completed.

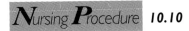

Nursing Procedure **10.10**

Use of Limb and Body Restraints

EQUIPMENT

- Restraint appropriate for limb or body area (ie, wrist, ankle, vest or waist restraint)
- Wash cloths for each limb restraint
- Lotion and powder (optional)
- Kerlix gauze (3- or 4-inch roll)
- 2-inch tape

Purpose

Prevents injury to client from falls, wound contamination, and tube dislodgment

Prevents injury to others from disoriented or hostile client when other methods of control have been ineffective

Desired Outcomes (sample)

Client experiences no falls or injury while under nurse's care.

Skin remains intact at site of restraint.

Assessment

Assessment should focus on the following:

Doctor's order (obtain if not on chart)
Agency policy regarding use of restraints
Client's orientation and level of consciousness
Skin status in areas requiring restraint
Effectiveness of other safety controls and precautions
Availability of staff or family members to sit with client

Outcome Identification and Planning

Key Goal and Sample Goal Criterion

The client will:

Experience no physical injury related to falls.

Special Considerations

A doctor's order should be obtained before applying restraints. Learn standing orders or agency policy regarding use of restraints.

Some agencies require that restraints be used in certain situations.

Sheets may be used to tie client securely to a bed or chair to prevent falls. Socks or other soft pieces of cloth may be fashioned into wrist restraints and mittens may be used to prevent pulling of tubes.

Geriatric

The skin of elderly clients is often very sensitive, and the blood vessels are easily collapsed. Restrain such clients loosely with linen or soft restraints and check the circulation frequently. Remove restraints frequently to check the skin beneath them.

IMPLEMENTATION

Action	Rationale
1. Wash hands and organize equipment.	*Prevents microorganism transfer* *Promotes efficiency*
2. Explain procedure to client and state why restraints are needed.	*Promotes cooperation* *Reduces anxiety*
3. Place client in a comfortable position with good body alignment.	
4. Wash and dry area to which restraint will be applied; massage area and apply lotion if skin is dry; apply powder, if desired.	*Facilitates circulation to skin* *Decreases friction on skin from dirt and dead skin cells*
5. To apply wrist or ankle restraints: - Use 10-inch strip of Kerlix gauze folded to 2-inch width; wrap strip in a figure eight (Fig. 10.10) and fold the circles of the figure over one another; slip wrist or ankle through loop	

Action	Rationale

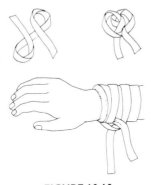

FIGURE 10.10

- To use commercial re-
  straints, wrap padded
  portion of restraint
  around wrist or ankle,
  thread tie through slit in   *Holds restraint intact around*
  restraint, and fasten to   *wrist/ankle*
  second tie with secure
  knot
- Secure ends of ties to   *Prevents accidental pull on*
  bed frame. DO NOT   *limb with movement of bed*
  SECURE TO BED RAILS,   *rail*
  if present (with some two-
  part restraints, the wrist
  section snaps into a   *Allows removal of restraint for*
  separate section that is   *skin care without removal of*
  secured to bed frame)   *portion secured to bed*

6. Vest restraint: *Prevents client from getting out*
   - Place vest on client with   *of bed without restricting arm*
     opening in front.   *and hand mobility*
   - Pull tie on end of vest
     flap across chest and slip
     through slit in opposite
     side of vest.
   - Wrap other end of flap   *Secures vest to client*
     across client and around
     chair or upper portion
     of bed frame.

Action	Rationale
- Fasten ends of ties together behind chair or to sides of bed frame.	
- Check respiratory status for distress related to restriction from vest.	
- Reposition client for minimal pressure on chest.	
7. Waist restraint:	
- Wrap restraint around waist.	*Prevents client from getting out of bed without binding chest*
- Slip end of one tie through slit in restraint.	
- Secure ends of ties to bed frame.	
- Monitor for complaints of nausea or abdominal distress.	*Indicates possible restriction on abdomen*
8. Hand mittens:	*Prevents pulling of tubes*
- Wrap Kerlix gauze around hand until totally covered.	*Allows mobility of limb*
- Fold hand into fist and continue to wrap fist.	
- Put tape around fist to secure gauze; cover with sock or stocking.	*Minimizes pulling of gauze and disruption of mitt*
9. When a client is in restraints instruct caregiver to:	
- Remove restraint every 4 to 8 hours.	*Decreases continuous pressure on skin*
- Massage skin beneath restraint and apply lotion or powder; wrap folded washcloth around limb and place restraint on top of cloth.	*Increases circulation to skin* *Decreases friction and skin irritation*
- Monitor the extremity distal to the restraint every 1 to 2 hours for color and temperature.	*Determines adequacy of circulation below restraint* *Identifies need for removal*
- Monitor for skin irritation.	

Action	Rationale
- Check every 1 to 2 hours for added pull on restraints and limb, tangled ties, or pressure points from knots; remove and adjust restraint to eliminate problem.	*Prevents loss of skin integrity due to excessive pressure*
10. Continually assess client's orientation and continued need for restraints and remove as soon as safe to do so.	*Decreases risk of disruption of skin integrity* *Restores sense of self-control*

Evaluation

Were desired outcomes achieved?

DOCUMENTATION

The following should be noted on the visit note:

- Reason for restraint application
- Time doctor's order obtained
- Type of restraint applied
- Client's response to restraints
- Periodic removal of restraints
- Skin care performed

Sample Documentation

DATE	TIME	
1/2/99	1200	Admission history reveals frequent falls and pulling of tubes during recent stay at nursing home. Client diagnosed with senile dementia, anorexia, and severe dehydration. IV and feeding tube inserted. Bilateral wrist restraints applied loosely with waist restraint secured to bed. Family instructed on care and observations of restraints.

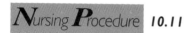

*N*ursing *P*rocedure **10.11**

Pressure Ulcer Management

EQUIPMENT

- Dressing change materials (see Procedure 10.12); use multi-pack gauze in plastic container
- Nonsterile gloves and sterile gloves
- Towel or linen saver pad
- Sterile irrigation saline
- Povidone-iodine (Betadine) solution or peroxide, as ordered
- Povidone-iodine (Betadine) swabs, as ordered
- Topical-care agents (may vary from agency to agency, case to case):
  - Karaya Gum patches (Duraderm)
  - gelatin sponge
  - Silvadene cream (Duraprep)
  - zinc oxide
  - granulated sugar
  - topical antibiotics (when infection has been confirmed)
  - antacid (eg, Maalox, Riopan)
- Moist wound barrier/transparent wound dressing (Duoderm)
- Overbed table or bedside stand
- Paper bag, trash bag
- Pressure relief pad:
  - sheepskin mattress
  - egg crate mattress
  - water mattress
  - gel flotation pads

Purpose

Removes accumulated secretions and dead tissue from wound or incision
Decreases microorganism growth on wounds or incision site
Promotes wound healing

Desired Outcomes (sample)

Client regains skin integrity within 3 weeks.
Client demonstrates no signs of infection or of further infection.

Assessment

Assessment should focus on the following:

Doctor's order regarding type of dressing change, procedure, and frequency of change

Type and location of the pressure ulcer (Fig. 10.11).

Client factors contributing to development of the pressure ulcer (eg, prolonged immobility, poor circulation, nutritional status, incontinence, seepage of wound drainage onto skin)

Time of last pain medication

Allergies to iodine (ie, shellfish or seafood) or tape

Protective bed cover (sheepskin, egg crate, flotation mattress)

Client's activity regimen (frequency of turning, getting out of bed)

Client and family knowledge regarding factors contributing to development of a pressure ulcer

Risk assessment for development of the pressure ulcer

Potential complications (eg, sinus tract or abscess)

Outcome Identification and Planning

Key Goals and Sample Goal Criteria

The client will:

Regain skin integrity within 3 weeks

Demonstrate no signs of infection or further infection during confinement

Special Considerations

Pressure ulcer care is often painful. Assess the client's pain needs. May need to phone ahead and instruct client to take medication 30 minutes before beginning the procedure if procedure is painful.

A clean, instead of sterile, dressing change is often permitted.

Pressure ulcer care tends to vary among agencies; consult the agency manual for guidelines.

Newspaper should be used to cover the table surface during a dressing change and animals in the home should be restricted from the area during the procedure.

Geriatric

Debilitation and decreased activity often accompany advanced age. Family members should be informed of the importance of preventing pressure to certain skin areas for extended periods of time.

Sample pressure ulcer assessment guide

Patient Name: _____ Date: _____ Time: _____

Ulcer 1:
Site _____
Stage^a_____
Size (cm)
    Length_____
    Width _____
    Depth _____   No   Yes

Sinus Tract
Tunneling
Undermining
Necrotic Tissue
    Slough
    Eschar
Exudate
    Serous
    Serosanguineous
    Purulent
Granulation
Epithelialization
Pain
Surrounding Skin:
Erythema
Maceration
Induration
Descripton of Ulcers(s):

Ulcer 2:
Site _____
Stage^a_____
Size (cm)
    Length_____
    Width _____
    Depth _____   No   Yes

Sinus Tract
Tunneling
Undermining
Necrotic Tissue
    Slough
    Eschar
Exudate
    Serous
    Serosanguineous
    Purulent
Granulation
Epithelialization
Pain

Erythema
Maceration
Induration

Indicate Ulcer Sites:

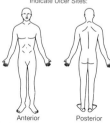

Anterior   Posterior

(Attach a color photo of the pressure ulcer(s) [Optional])

^aClassification of pressure ulcers:

Stage I: Nonblanchable erythema of intact skin, the heralding lesion of skin ulceration. In individuals with darker skin, discoloration of the skin, warmth, edema, induration, or hardness may also be indicators.

Stage II: Partial thickness skin loss involving epidermis, dermis, or both.

Stage II: Full thickness skin loss involving damage to or necrosis of subcutaneous tissue that may extend down to, but not through, underlying fascia. The ulcer presents clinically as a deep crater with or without undermining adjacent tissue.

Stage IV: Full thickness skin loss with extensive destruction, tissue necrosis, or damage to muscle, bone, or supporting structures (e.g., tendon or joint capsule).

FIGURE 10.11

IMPLEMENTATION

Action	Rationale
1. Wash hands and organize equipment.	*Reduces microorganism transfer* *Promotes efficiency*
2. Explain procedure and assistance needed from client.	*Promotes cooperation*
3. Assess pain level; deliver medication, if needed, and allow time for medication to take effect before beginning dressing removal.	*Decreases discomfort of dressing change*
4. Place bedside table close to area being dressed and prepare supplies: - Place supplies on bedside table.	*Facilitates management of sterile field and supplies*
- Tape paper bag or trash bag to side of table.	*Facilitates easy disposal of contaminated waste*
- Open sterile gloves and use inside of glove package as sterile field.	*Promotes use of supplies without contamination and prepares work field*
- Open gauze-pad packages and drop several onto sterile field (leave remaining gauze pads in plastic container).	
- Open dressing tray.	
- Open liquids and pour normal saline on two gauze pads and Betadine on four gauze pads (or more if wet-to-dry dressing change).	
- Open Betadine swabs, if used, to expose end of plastic stick.	
- Place several sterile cotton-tip swabs and cotton balls on sterile field.	
5. Don nonsterile gloves.	*Prevents exposure to damage*
6. Place towel or pad under wound area.	
7. Loosen tape by pulling toward the pressure ulcer and remove soiled dressing; note appearance of	*Exposes site for cleaning* *Permits assessment of site*

Action	Rationale
dressing and wound. SOAK DRESSING WITH NORMAL SALINE IF IT ADHERES TO WOUND AND THEN GENTLY PULL FREE.	
8. Place soiled dressing in paper bag.	*Prevents spread of organisms*
9. Discard gloves and wash hands.	
10. Don sterile gloves.	
11. Pick up normal saline-soaked dressing pad with forceps and form a large swab.	
12. Cleanse away debris and drainage from the pressure ulcer, moving from center outward; use a new pad for each area cleaned, discarding the old pads.	*Prevents contamination of wound from organisms on skin surface* *Maintains sterility of supplies*
13. Wipe the pressure ulcer with povidone-soaked pads moving from center of wound outward using a circular motion; use a dry pad to dry the wound and surrounding skin and a skin prep or tincture of benzoin on the surrounding skin; discard forceps. DO NOT ALLOW TINCTURE OF BENZOIN TO TOUCH BROKEN SKIN AREAS.	*Decreases microorganisms* *Facilitates adherence of dressings/pads* *Sometimes causes painful tissue erosion*
14. Place ordered topical agent onto or into the pressure ulcer; may place povidone pads in the pressure ulcer and allow to remain until dry.	*Provides antiinfective agent*
15. Dress the pressure ulcer by covering with a single 4 × 4-inch gauze pad or a transparent wound	*Allows air to reach wound but removes drainage*

Action	Rationale
	dressing; secure dressing with tape.
16. Write date and time of dressing change on a strip of tape and place tape across top of dressing.	*Indicates last dressing change and need for next change within 24 to 48 hours*
17. Dispose of gloves and materials and store supplies appropriately.	*Decreases spread of microorganisms*
18. Position client for comfort.	*Promotes comfort and communication*
19. Wash hands.	*Decreases spread of microorganisms*

Evaluation

Were desired outcomes achieved?

DOCUMENTATION

The following should be noted in the visit note:

- Materials and procedure used for the pressure ulcer management
- Location, size, and type of wound or incision
- Status of the pressure ulcer site and stage of healing
- Status of previous dressing
- Solution and medications applied to wound
- Frequency of turning and repositioning client
- Client teaching done and additional learning needs
- Client tolerance to procedure

Sample Documentation

DATE	TIME	
1/2/99	1100	Pressure ulcer site cleaned with saline and povidone swabs. Sacral pressure ulcer approximately 5 cm in diameter, pink, with slightly granulated edges; no drainage or foul odor noted. Povidone pads placed into and over wound. Wound covered with 4 × 4-inch pad. Client turned to side with pillow at back. Tolerated pressure ulcer care with minimal discomfort.

Nursing Procedure 10.12

🖐 *Wound Care and Dressing Change*

❎ **EQUIPMENT**

- Sterile dressing tray (forceps, scissors, gauze pads [optional])
- Sterile gauze dressing pads (2 × 2-inch, 4 × 4-inch, or surgical [ABD] pads, depending on drainage and size of area to be covered), or transparent dressing
- Sterile bowl
- 2-inch tape or Montgomery straps (paper tape, if allergic to others)
- Sterile gloves
- Nonsterile gloves
- Towel or linen-saver pad
- Cotton balls and cotton-tip swabs (optional)
- Sterile irrigation saline or sterile water
- Povidone-iodone (Betadine) solution or peroxide, as ordered
- Povidone-iodine (Betadine) swabs
- Bacteriostatic ointment
- Overbed table or bedside stand
- Paper bag, trash bag

Purpose

Removes accumulated secretions and dead tissue from wound or incision site
Decreases microorganism growth on wound or incision site
Promotes wound healing

Desired Outcome (sample)

Wound healing noted with no signs of infection.

Assessment

Assessment should focus on the following:

Doctor's orders regarding type of dressing change, procedure, and frequency of change
Type and location of wound or incision

Time of last pain medication
Allergies to iodine (shellfish or seafood) or tape

Outcome Identification and Planning

Key Goals and Sample Goal Criteria
The client will:

Regain skin integrity
Demonstrate no signs of infection

Special Considerations
Newspaper should be used to cover the table surface before arranging the work field. Animals in the home should be restricted from the area during the procedure.

Dressing changes are often painful; assess pain needs. If necessary, phone ahead and have client or family medicate client 30 minutes before beginning the procedure.

Many clients are immunosuppressed and have decreased resistance; strict asepsis is needed to minimize exposure to microorganisms.

IMPLEMENTATION

Action	Rationale
1. Wash hands and organize equipment.	*Reduces microorganism transfer* *Promotes efficiency*
2. Explain procedure and assistance needed to client.	*Decreases anxiety* *Promotes cooperation*
3. Assess client's pain level and wait for medication to take effect before beginning.	*Decreases discomfort of dressing change*
4. Place bedside table close to area being dressed.	*Facilitates management of sterile field and supplies*
5. Prepare supplies:	
- Place supplies on bedside table.	*Promotes swift dressing change*
- Tape paper bag or trash bag to side of table.	*Facilitates easy disposal of contaminated waste*
- Open sterile gloves and use inside of glove package as sterile field.	*Facilitates use of supplies without contamination*
- Open gauze-pad packages and drop several	

Action	Rationale
onto sterile field; leave some pads in open packages if in plastic container (if not, place some pads into sterile bowl).	*Permits wetting of some pads*
- Open dressing tray and bowl.	
- Open liquids and pour saline on two gauze pads and povidone on four gauze pads (more if wet-to-dry dressing).	*Prevents transmission of organisms from table to supplies*
- Open povidone swabs, if used, to expose plastic stick end.	
- Place several sterile cotton-tip swabs and cotton balls on sterile field (use gauze instead if staples are present because cotton may catch on edges of staples).	
6. Don nonsterile gloves.	
7. Place towel or pad under wound area.	
8. Loosen tape by pulling toward the wound and remove soiled dressing (note appearance of dressing, wound, and drainage). SOAK DRESSING WITH SALINE IF IT ADHERES TO WOUND, THEN GENTLY PULL FREE.	*Permits observation of site and exposes site for cleaning*
9. Place dressing in paper bag.	
10. Discard gloves and wash hands.	

Sterile Dressing Change

11. Don sterile gloves and face mask (optional).
12. Pick up saline-soaked

Action	Rationale

dressing pad with forceps and form a large swab.

13. Cleanse away debris and drainage from wound, moving from center outward and using a new pad for each area cleaned (Fig. 10.12.1); discard old pads away from sterile supplies.

Prevents contamination of wound from organisms on skin surface
Maintains sterility of supplies

14. Wipe wound with povidone-soaked pads, moving from center of wound outward; discard forceps.

Reduces microorganism transfer
Avoids cross contamination

15. Assess need for frequent dressing changes and effect of tape on skin. Apply Montgomery straps to hold dressing, if a deeper wound or wound with heavy drainage.
    - Place 8-inch strip of tape on table with sticky side up and cover with 4-inch strip of tape, sticky side down.
    - Place sticky side of tape

Prevents infection due to soiled dressings
Prevents skin injury

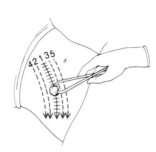

FIGURE 10.12.1

Action	Rationale

on client with nonsticky
end reaching across half
of wound area.
- Repeat process on other
side of wound; if
wound is long, apply
straps to upper and
lower portion.
- Place dressings (step 16)
over wound and secure
by pinning, banding or
tying Montgomery
straps together (The
tying method may be
used when frequent
dressing changes are an-
ticipated.) (Fig. 10.12.2).

16. Dress the wound or incision in the following
manner:

*Prevents contamination of
dressing or wound*

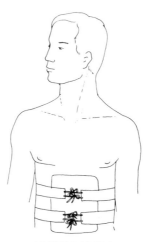

FIGURE 10.12.2

Action	Rationale
- Pick up dressing pads by edge (Betadine- or saline-soaked, if wet-to-dry dressing).	
- Place pads over wound or incision site until site is totally covered.	*Allows air to reach wound*
- Cover with surgical pad (if wet-to-dry).	
- Secure dressing with tape along edges or use Montgomery straps.	*Indicates last dressing change and need for next change within 24 to 48 hours*
17. Write the date and time of dressing change on a strip of tape and place tape across dressing.	*Decreases spread of micro-organisms*
18. Dispose of gloves and materials and store supplies appropriately.	*Maintains organized environment*
19. Position client for comfort.	*Facilitates comfort and communication*
20. Wash hands.	*Decreases spread of micro-organisms*

Nonsterile/Clean Dressing Change

21. Follow steps 11 to 19 but forceps and gloves need not be sterile.	*Allows handling of dressing without sterile instruments*

Evaluation

Were desired outcomes achieved?

DOCUMENTATION

The following should be noted on the visit note:

- Location and type of wound or incision
- Status of previous dressing
- Status of the wound/incision site
- Solution and medications applied to wound
- Client teaching done
- Client's tolerance of procedure

Sample Documentation

DATE	TIME	
1/12/99	1000	Abdominal wound dressing saturated with serous drainage. Area surrounding wound is red. Site cleansed with saline and wiped with Betadine swabs. Gauze pads (4 × 4 inches) moistened with saline applied and covered with dry dressings. Client turned to side with pillow at back. Tolerated dressing change with minimal discomfort. Client and family instructed on signs and symptoms of infection and to phone if drainage becomes any heavier.

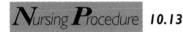

*N*ursing *P*rocedure *10.13*

🖐 *Wound Irrigation*

❎ EQUIPMENT

- Irrigation solution
- Sterile irrigation set, including sterile syringe with sterile tubing (or catheter) attached
- Sterile basin
- Gauze pads
- Materials for dressing change, if applicable (see Procedure 10.12)
- Linen saver
- Large towel
- Waste receptacle
- Sterile gloves

Purpose

Facilitates removal of secretions and microorganisms from wound

Desired Outcomes (sample)
Client regains skin integrity within 1 month.
Client demonstrates no signs of infection.

Assessment

Assessment should focus on the following:

Doctor's order for irrigation orders
Type and location of wound
Irrigant (type of medication added, if applicable)
Pain status and time of last pain medication

Outcome Identification and Planning

Key Goals and Sample Goal Criteria
The client will:

Regain skin integrity within 1 month
Demonstrate no signs of infection during confinement

Special Considerations

Wound irrigation can be painful; instruct caregiver to medicate
  client 30 minutes before beginning the procedure.

Newspaper should be used to cover the table surface during
  wound irrigation and animals in the home should be restricted from the area during the procedure.

IMPLEMENTATION

Action	Rationale
1. Assess pain level; deliver medication, if needed, and wait for medication to take effect.	*Decreases discomfort during procedure*
2. Wash hands and organize supplies.	*Reduces microorganism transfer* *Promotes efficiency*
3. Explain procedure and assistance needed from client; provide privacy.	*Facilitates cooperation* *Decreases anxiety*
4. Place bedside table near wound area and open supplies (arrange for dressing change in addition to wound irrigation).	*Permits replacement of dressing after wound irrigation*
5. Don nonsterile gloves and remove dressing.	
6. Place linen saver and towel under wound.	*Catches overflow of irrigant*
7. Discard nonsterile gloves, wash hands, and don sterile gloves.	*Maintains sterility of process*
8. Place basin beside wound and tilt client to side toward basin.	*Facilitates drainage of irrigation into basin*
9. Irrigate wound:	
- Insert irrigation tubing into upper portion of wound (or above cleanest portion of wound so that fluid flows from cleanest to dirtiest portion of wound; Fig. 10.13).	*Flushes debris and contaminants from wound*
- Attach syringe to tubing or catheter and pour in irrigant; continue to pour irrigant until wound de-	

Action	Rationale

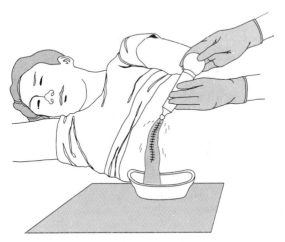

FIGURE 10.13

bris and drainage are washed into basin.

- Move catheter to different part of wound and repeat irrigation until total wound area has been irrigated and all irrigant has been used.

10. Use sterile pads, if needed, to remove additional debris; pack wound with gauze pads, if ordered; apply sterile dressing.

11. Write the date and time of dressing change on a strip of tape and place tape across dressing.

Indicates last dressing change and need for next change within 24 to 48 hours

12. Dispose of gloves and materials and store supplies appropriately.

Decreases spread of microorganisms

Action	Rationale
13. Position client for comfort.	*Promotes comfort and communication*
14. Wash hands.	*Decreases spread of microorganisms*

Evaluation

Were desired outcomes achieved?

DOCUMENTATION

The following should be noted on the visit note:

- Location, appearance, and type of wound or incision
- Status of previous dressing
- Solution and medications applied to wound
- Client and caregiver teaching done
- Client tolerance to procedure

Sample Documentation

DATE	TIME	
1/12/99	0600	Gaping abdominal incisional wound irrigated with sterile saline. Incision about 8 inches in length and gapes open at 2 cm crosswise along entire length of incision. No purulent drainage from wound. Open area pink with whitish yellow edges. Wound packed with moist saline gauze. Client turned to side with pillow at back. Tolerated procedure with minimal discomfort.

*N*ursing *P*rocedure 10.14

🖐 *Wound Drain Management*

✖ EQUIPMENT

- Graduated container
- Sterile dressing tray (forceps, scissors, gauze pads [optional])
- Sterile gauze dressing pads (2 × 2-inch, 4 × 4-inch, or surgical [ABD] pads, depending on drainage and size of area to be covered), or transparent dressing
- Sterile bowl
- 2-inch tape or Montgomery straps (paper tape, if allergic to others)
- Sterile gloves
- Nonsterile gloves
- Towel or linen-saver pad
- Cotton balls and cotton-tip swabs (optional)
- Sterile irrigation saline or sterile water
- Povidone-iodine (Betadine) solution or peroxide, as ordered
- Povidone-iodine (Betadine) swabs
- Bacteriostatic ointment
- Bedside table
- Paper bag, trash bag
- Additional gauze pads

Purpose

Removes accumulated secretions and dead tissue from wound or incision

Decreases microorganism growth on wounds or incision site

Promotes wound healing

Desired Outcomes (sample)

Client regains skin integrity within 3 weeks.

Client demonstrates no signs of infection in wound.

Assessment

Assessment should focus on the following:

Type of drain

Doctor's order or agency policy regarding frequency of drainage measurement

Type, appearance, and location of wound or incision
Time of last pain medication
Client allergies to iodine (shellfish or seafood) or tape
Client and family knowledge of managing drains and assessing
  status of drainage and wound

Outcome Identification and Planning

Key Goals and Sample Goal Criteria

The client will:

Regain skin integrity within 3 weeks
Demonstrate no signs of infection in the wound, such as redness, pain, purulent drainage, or foul odor

Special Considerations

Newspaper should be used to cover the table surface before arranging a sterile field. Animals in the home should be restricted from the area during the procedure.
Dressing changes and drain manipulation are often painful. Assess client's pain needs and medicate, if needed, 30 minutes
  before beginning procedure.

IMPLEMENTATION

Action	Rationale
1. Wash hands and organize equipment.	*Reduces microorganism transfer* *Promotes efficiency*
2. Explain procedure and assistance needed from client; provide privacy.	*Promotes cooperation* *Avoids embarrassment*
3. Assess pain level, wait for medication to take effect before beginning.	*Decreases discomfort of dressing change*
4. Place bedside table close to area being dressed.	*Facilitates management of sterile field and supplies*
5. Place towel or pad under wound area.	*Eliminates drainage onto surrounding skin*
6. Perform dressing change (see Procedure 10.12); during wound cleaning, note condition of drain-insertion site (intactness of sutures, presence of redness or purulent drainage).	

Action	Rationale
7. Clean wound with Betadine-soaked pads or swabs, moving from drain outward in a circular motion; place gauze dressing around drain-insertion site (Fig. 10.14.1).	*Prevents contamination of wound with microorganisms* *Decreases skin irritation from drainage*
8. Check that tubings are not kinked, twisted, or dislodged.	
9. Continue procedure by performing steps appropriate for type of drain used; then proceed to steps 20 through 22 for completion of procedure.	

Penrose Drains

10. Place extra 4 × 4-inch pads over drain.	*Facilitates absorption of drainage*
11. Cover with one or two surgical pads and tape securely.	

Hemovac

12. Apply and secure dressing; note drainage color and amount; empty if half-full or more by opening pouring spout, holding it inverted over	*Assesses drainage* *Empties drain to prevent overfilling and applying tension on suture areas*

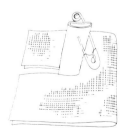

FIGURE 10.14.1

Action	Rationale
graduated container, and squeezing hemovac gently.	*Facilitates flow of clots and drainage*
13. Compress evacuator after emptying: - Place palm of hand on top of evacuator and press flat with top of spout open. - Replace stopper to spout while holding evacuator flat (Fig. 10.14.2). - Remove hand from evacuator and check that it remains flat.	*Activates suction needed to maintain drainage evacuation*
14. When assessing wound, drainage, and drain, check to be sure evacuator is still compressed; if not, empty drain and re-compress.	*Maintains suction pressure*

Jackson-Pratt (Bulb Drain)

15. Apply and secure dressing; note drainage color and amount; empty if half-full or more by opening pouring spout, inverting over graduated container, and squeezing bulb.	*Assesses drainage* *Prevents overfilling and tension pull on suture line* *Releases contents from the bulb drain*

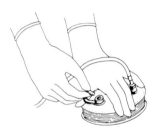

FIGURE 10.14.2

Action	Rationale
16. After emptying, recompress bulb by squeezing bulb in palm of hand with top of spout open, then closing spout and releasing bulb.	*Initiates suction needed for drainage evacuation*
17. When assessing wound, drainage, and drain, check to be sure evacuator is still compressed; if not, empty drain and recompress.	*Maintains suction pressure*

T-tube

18. Apply and secure dressing; hang bag off trunk of body.	*Facilitates use of gravity for drainage*
19. To empty, open pouring spout, tilt to side with spout positioned over graduated container, pour, and recap spout.	*Prevents overfill of tube and tension on suture line*
20. Dispose of gloves and materials and store supplies appropriately.	*Decreases spread of microorganisms*
21. Position client for comfort.	*Promotes comfort and communication*
22. Wash hands.	*Decreases spread of microorganisms*

Evaluation

Were desired outcomes achieved?

DOCUMENTATION

The following should be noted in the visit note:

- Location and type of wound or incision and drain insertion site(s)
- Status of previous dressing
- Status of the wound or incision site and drain
- Type and amount of drainage
- Solution and medications applied to wound

- Client teaching done
- Client's tolerance to procedure

Sample Documentation

DATE	TIME	
1/12/99	0600	Abdominal-wound dressing saturated with serous drainage. Dressing removed, Penrose drain intact with moderate drainage. Area surrounding drain intact without redness. Site cleaned and wiped with Betadine swabs. Dressing change performed. Client tolerated dressing change with minimal discomfort.

*C*hapter *11*

Medication Management

OVERVIEW

▶ Assisting a client with medication management is the most crucial responsibility of the home health nurse. Ultimately, the client or family will be responsible for the ongoing management and administration of all medications. The ability to do this successfully is dependent on the nurse's skill in teaching all areas of medication management. Assessment and evaluation of medication management should be a part of every visit made to a client.

▶ The ability of a client to successfully manage medications is influenced by the client's:
  - acceptance of the benefits of the medication
  - ability to obtain the medication
  - ability to schedule and take all doses

- knowledge of side effects and interactions
- understanding of methods of storage and disposal

▶ It is the responsibility of the home health nurse to constantly instruct, assess, and evaluate the client's performance in all of these areas.

▶ Administration of medication in the home setting and instruction in medication management requires that the nurse be completely proficient in medication administration techniques, and be absolutely certain of the individual client's medication profile. All home health nurses should carry a current drug guide at all times. All clients should be assessed for the appropriateness of their drug therapy, and if questions arise, the physician and/or pharmacist should be consulted. During a home visit, there is no other health care professional in the home to check dosages and administration techniques. It is the home health nurse's responsibility to resolve any questions or uncertainties before administering a medication, or providing instruction to a client or caregiver in preparation and administration techniques.

▶ Clients at home frequently have prescriptions from multiple physicians. When reviewing medications with a client, it is the nurse's responsibility to be sure that the attending physician is aware of all medications that the client is taking.

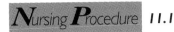
Nursing Procedure **11.1**

Principles of Medication Management, Storage, Disposal

☒ EQUIPMENT

- Ordered client medications

Purpose

Increases client and caregiver understanding of general medication principles

Assures client use of current medications only

Assures proper disposal of discontinued or expired medications

Desired Outcomes (sample)

The client or caregiver will administer medications as ordered.

The client or caregiver will store medications in a safe and secure area.

The client or caregiver will administer only current medications, and demonstrate appropriate disposal techniques for outdated medications.

Assessment

Assessment should focus on the following:

Previous client/caregiver understanding of medications

Client/caregiver ability to understand and retain information

Functional limitations that might interfere with medication administration

Client/caregiver literacy level

Ability of client/caregiver to obtain ordered medications

Outcome Identification and Planning

Key Goals and Sample Goal Criteria

The client/caregiver will:

Demonstrate understanding of importance of medication management in treatment

Demonstrate correct procedures for storage and disposal of medications

Consistently administer medications as ordered

Special Considerations

An assessment of functional limitations is essential to medication management. The nurse must assess the client or caregiver's manual dexterity, vision, memory, and ability to read and understand labels. An individual plan for each client must include all of these factors.

Economic

It is not unusual in the home health setting to see clients who are unable to purchase ordered medications. This information is not readily volunteered to the nurse. It is a vital nursing responsibility to assess the client's ability to purchase each drug that is ordered. If there is a problem, there are resources that may be accessed. Many local health departments have programs or the client's physician may be approached for samples. Many drug manufacturers have assistance programs for clients who are unable to pay for medications.

HINT

Many clients are very reluctant to discard unused medication. If a client refuses to dispose of unused or outdated medications, the nurse should make every attempt to have the client package and store these medications away from current medications in a safe and secure area.

IMPLEMENTATION

Action	Rationale
1. Ask client/caregiver to assemble all current medications, including over-the-counter medications.	*Allows evaluation of scope of medication usage*
2. Check client medication bottles against ordered medications.	*Determines discrepancies between medications ordered, and those actually being taken*
3. Observe client medication storage habits: - Multiple pills in one bottle	*Determines need for instruction in storage*

Action	Rationale
- Unlabeled bottles	
4. Ask client how he or she takes specific medications.	*Assesses client ability to follow label instructions*
5. Interview client concerning how he or she feels about taking medication. Determine if client feels medications are helpful and important, or a burden.	*Allows client to ventilate feelings* *Provides nurse with information needed to formulate teaching plan*
6. Inquire as to how medications are obtained. - Mail order pharmacy - Local pharmacy - Are medications delivered? - Economic problems?	*Provides information concerning possible barriers to compliance with medication administration*
7. Explain to client and caregiver that you will be working with them to make them comfortable in all aspects of medication management.	*Enhances client participation* *Reduces anxiety* *Promotes cooperation*
8. Instruct in safe storage of medications: - In original labeled containers. - If refrigeration needed, away from food items. - In a safe area with limited access. - Current medications grouped together.	*Allows for easy identification* *Reduces potential for transmission of microorganisms* *Prevents accidental use or ingestion by other family members* *Increases efficiency of administration*
9. Instruct in disposal of outdated drugs: - How to determine expiration date. - Danger of confusing old drugs with new. - Flush old pills down toilet and discard bottle.	*Promotes safety* *Reduces confusion*
10. If client resistant to disposing of old drugs, explain expiration dates, possibility of taking	*Promotes understanding and compliance*

Action	Rationale

wrong drug, possibility of accidental use by another family member.

11. If client interview reveals incorrect medication administration, proceed immediately with specific medication teaching.

Promotes proper medication administration

Evaluation

Were desired outcomes achieved?

DOCUMENTATION

The following should be documented on the visit note:

- Client ability to procure medications
- Assessment of need for client instruction in medication management
- Instructions in management, storage, and disposal of medications
- Client or caregiver response

Sample Documentation

DATE	TIME	
8/01/99	1035	Instructions begun in medication administration, storage, and disposal. Client confused by multiple medications, has difficulty reading labels, appears frustrated by inability to remember medication times and dosages. Storage of current medications and disposal of old medications done with client agreement and assistance. Client and caregiver eager to learn medication schedule. Will need continued instruction in all aspects of medication administration.

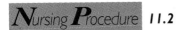

Nursing Procedure 11.2

Scheduling of Medication Administration

EQUIPMENT

- Client medications in original prescription bottles, verified with current orders
- Paper
- Pen
- Seven-day medication box (optional)
- 9" × 12" cardboard and tape (optional)
- Calendar (optional)

Purpose

Contributes to accurate administration of all medications
Contributes to client understanding of drug labels, refill information, interactions

Desired Outcomes (sample)

The client and/or caregiver will understand and adhere to a medication schedule.
The client and/or caregiver will demonstrate awareness of need for medication refills.
The client and/or caregiver will demonstrate understanding of drug/drug and drug/food interactions.

Assessment

Assessment should focus on the following:

Client and/or caregiver ability to understand and follow procedure
Usual client sleeping and eating habits
Possible need for visual charts or medication boxes to enhance compliance

Outcome Identification and Planning

Key Goals and Sample Goal Criteria

The client/caregiver will:

Consistently adhere to the established medication schedule
Maintain an adequate supply of each ordered medication
Verbalize awareness of applicable drug/drug and drug/food
  interactions

Special Considerations

A medication schedule must fit the individual client. Careful scheduling of medications around already established client habits of sleeping and eating may enhance compliance. Visual cues may be needed. A schedule posted on the refrigerator may remind the client of medication administration times. Single pills taped to a piece of cardboard may increase client recognition and understanding of each medication and its appropriate administration. A color code or notation on each pill bottle may be helpful. Highlighting the number of refills on a prescription bottle with a marker may assist the client in timely re-ordering of medication. A seven-day pill box, with areas for specific times, may be helpful in allowing the client to focus on setting up medication only once a week.

HINT

If the nurse is working with a client to use a medication box that is set up once a week, it is imperative that a family member or caregiver be found who can continue to set up the medication box after the client has been discharged from nursing services. While some insurance companies and state Medicaid programs permit nursing visits for the sole purpose of filling a medication box, many do not.

IMPLEMENTATION

Action	Rationale
1. Review each prescription bottle label with the client, pointing out: - The location of the name of the drug. - The administration instructions.	*Enhances client understanding* *Increases client independence in medication re-ordering*

Action	Rationale
- Where to look for the number of refills.	
- Where the prescription number is.	
- Where the phone number of the pharmacy is.	
2. Instruct client or caregiver in the importance of refilling prescriptions in a timely manner. Provide written calendar if indicated.	*Prevents interruption in medication administration*
3. Determine client's normal sleeping patterns, mealtimes, activities.	*Allows scheduling of medication in conjunction with already established patterns*
4. With the client's assistance, look at each prescription bottle and write a preliminary list of each drug and the circumstances, eg, time between doses, with food, fasting.	*Promotes client participation*
5. If two prescribed drugs may interact, or if specific drugs have specific interactions with food, explain to client that those drugs may need to be scheduled at different times (Appendices C and D).	*Increases client understanding* *Promotes client cooperation*
6. Prepare a written schedule, listing all medications and the times they are to be taken.	*Provides a baseline schedule*
7. Adjust the schedule, where possible, to match the client's sleeping patterns and mealtimes.	*Enhances client participation*
8. If possible, have the client or caregiver participate in writing out the schedule. Where possible, allow the client the choice of using specific times, or relating medications to meals.	*Enhances client participation* *Improves compliance*

Action	Rationale
9. Review the completed schedule with the client. Note the number of pills to be taken at each specified time. Explain that some medications must be taken at certain time intervals.	*Promotes client understanding* *Allows client to review number of pills to be taken*
10. If the finished schedule is unworkable for the client, (ie, client must be awakened several times during night for medication), consider contacting the physician for possible alternative medications. If no alternatives are possible, stress to the client the importance of adhering to the schedule.	*Allows client to see that all efforts are being made to create a workable schedule* *Increases compliance*
11. Review the schedule each visit, and with each change in medication.	*Reinforces instruction* *Evaluates ongoing compliance*
12. Post the schedule in the home in a place of the client's choosing.	*Recognizes client participation*

Evaluation

Were desired outcomes achieved?

DOCUMENTATION

The following should be documented on the visit note:

- Instruction given in medication labeling, procurement of refills
- Instruction given in medication interactions
- Development of medication schedule
- In addition, a copy of the medication schedule should be retained in the client's agency chart.

Sample Documentation

DATE	TIME	
01/05/99	1610	Instructed in need to refill digoxin and furosemide. Instructed in label reading, how to determine refills remaining, need to refill 1 week before using last pill. Instructed to take tetracycline only until bottle empty, avoid taking with milk products. Medication schedule prepared and left in home. Client verbalizes understanding of schedule, will keep on refrigerator. Nurse to evaluate compliance with schedule each visit, review and revise as needed.

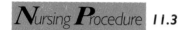

Nursing Procedure 11.3

Medication Teaching

☒ EQUIPMENT

- Current client medication schedule
- Medication bottles

Purpose

Contributes to client understanding of medication effects and
   side effects

Increases client compliance with medication administration

Desired Outcomes (sample)

The client/caregiver will verbalize recognition of each medication and its effects.

The client/caregiver will administer each medication appropriately.

The client/caregiver will verbalize understanding of side effects and actions to take.

Assessment

Assessment should focus on the following:

Client/caregiver ability to understand and retain instruction

Client/caregiver functional limitations that might interfere
   with appropriate use of medication (eg, poor memory, poor
   vision, limited manual dexterity)

Outcome Identification and Planning

Key Goals and Sample Goal Criteria

The client/caregiver will:

Recognize and state the reason for each medication

Verbalize major side effects of each medication, and the actions
   to take if a side effect occurs

Verbalize understanding of the reasons why each medication
   must be taken as scheduled

Special Considerations

HINT

Use visual aids to assist the client in recognizing each medication. Prepare a simple chart listing the medication name, the reason for it (in layman's language), and the most common side effects. Highlight those side effects that the client should report immediately to the physician.

Medication teaching is an ongoing process. At each visit, review the medication list and instruct as necessary in each medication.

For medications that require labwork for monitoring, the nurse must be responsible for verifying who is to do the labwork and when it is to be done.

IMPLEMENTATION

Action	Rationale
1. Assemble medications, medication list.	*Promotes efficiency*
2. For oral medications, show the client the pill.	*Promotes understanding of instruction if visual aid is used*
3. Explain the action of the medication in language that can be understood by the client. Emphasize what the medication will do for the client in concrete, understandable terms (eg, explain warfarin as a "blood thinner" that will "prevent blood clots that could lead to another stroke").	*Allows the client to understand what the medication can do to improve his or her health*
4. Write down the brand and generic name of the medication for the client.	*Prevents confusion if prescriptions are filled under the generic name*
5. Explain the reason why the medication needs to be taken at a specific time, or on a specific schedule.	*Enhances compliance with the schedule by increasing client understanding*
6. Explain major side effects in language that the client can understand.	
7. For each side effect, ex-	*Increases client control and*

Action	Rationale
plain to the client the action that is to be taken (eg, if taking warfarin and stools turn dark, call physician immediately).	*associates each side effect with a specific action*
8. Make a chart for the client to keep that reflects all teaching. List generic and brand names for the medication, the reason for its use, the major side effects, the action to take, and food or drug interactions (Appendices C and D).	*Reinforces instruction*
9. If visit limitations permit, instruct in only one or two medications at a visit.	*Prevents information overload*
10. Conclude instruction by asking client to explain the medication to you.	*Assesses client understanding*

Evaluation

Were desired outcomes achieved?

DOCUMENTATION

The following should be noted on the visit note:

- The name of the medication
- The specific instructions given
- The client's response to the instruction

Sample Documentation
Instructed client in newly prescribed warfarin. Instructed in brand and generic names, use as "blood thinner," need for labwork every week to be done by home health nurse. Instructed to watch for dark stools, excessive bruising, bleeding gums, report any occurrence to physician immediately. Written instructions left in home. Client verbalizes full understanding of instructions. Will reassess next visit, continue instruction in additional medications.

*N*ursing *P*rocedure **11.4**

Preparation of Injectable Medication

☒ EQUIPMENT

- Medication ampule or vial clearly labeled by pharmacist
- Appropriate syringe and needle
- Extra needle if indicated
- Alcohol sponges
- Sharps container or rigid plastic jug used as sharps container
- Sterile 2" × 2" gauze if using ampule

Purpose

Obtains medication from a vial or ampule, using aseptic technique, for parenteral administration

Desired Outcomes (sample)

The client/caregiver will demonstrate correct procedure for medication preparation.
The client/caregiver will dispose of used sharps appropriately.

Assessment

Assessment should focus on the following:

Client/caregiver manual dexterity, memory, vision
Client/caregiver ability to understand and follow all steps of procedure

Outcome Identification and Planning

Key Goals and Sample Goal Criteria

The client/caregiver will demonstrate correct technique
Correct amount and type of drug is prepared

Special Considerations

Preparing injectable medications is a very basic nursing procedure, yet it is a difficult procedure to teach. Before instructing
a client in this skill, the nurse should perform the procedure
and note all of the separate hand motions that are involved.

Geriatric

Carefully assess client's vision and ability to see markings on
the syringe. Assess arthritic changes or loss of manual dexterity that may interfere with management of syringe and vial or
ampule.

Economic

Assess client's ability to afford medication and syringes. Use
community resources as needed.

HINT

> *Before beginning demonstration or instruction, have client or
> caregiver handle syringe (Fig. 11.4.1) to become familiar with
> the feel of the material, the amount of effort needed to move
> the plunger, etc.*

IMPLEMENTATION

Action	Rationale
1. Assess home and perform procedure in a clean, well-lit area of the home.	*Provides optimal performance of procedure*
2. Wash hands and assemble equipment.	*Promotes efficiency*
3. Demonstrate, observe, or instruct in reading pre-scription label on vial or	*Ensures accuracy of medication Prevents client injury from wrong drug or dosage*

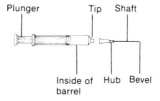

FIGURE 11.4.1

Action	Rationale

ampule and matching against written medication order on client medication schedule.

4. Demonstrate, observe, or instruct in checking vial or ampule for clarity, sediment, and expiration date.

5. Demonstrate, observe, or instruct in removal of syringe from packaging.

   Separates procedure into small, more easily learned tasks

6. Demonstrate, observe, or instruct in removal of cap from vial and swabbing with alcohol swab, or breaking of ampule (Fig. 11.4.2). You may suggest using a 2 × 2 gauze to protect fingers.

7. Demonstrate, observe, or instruct in removal of needle cap:

   Prevents accidental needlestick, contamination of needle

   - Hold syringe in non-dominant hand with needle end pointed away from body.
   - With dominant hand, pull needle cap straight off, away from body.

8. Demonstrate, observe, instruct in inserting needle into center of rubber cap on vial, or into ampule (Fig. 11.4.3).

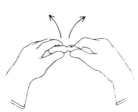

FIGURE 11.4.2

Action	Rationale
9. If using a vial, demonstrate, observe, instruct in keeping needle above fluid level and using plunger to insert air into vial.	*Increases ease of withdrawing medication repeatedly from multi-dose vial*
10. Demonstrate, observe, instruct in placing needle into fluid and preparing to withdraw medication: - If vial, demonstrate, observe, instruct in holding syringe in dominant hand and holding vial upside down in nondominant hand. - If ampule, demonstrate, observe, instruct in steadying ampule with nondominant hand, holding syringe in dominant hand.	
11. Demonstrate, observe, instruct in withdrawing the ordered amount of medication.	*Ensures accuracy of dosage*

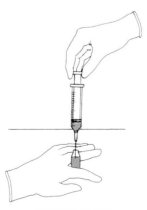

FIGURE 11.4.3

Action	Rationale
12. Demonstrate, observe, instruct in clearing air from syringe (Fig. 11.4.4).	*Ensures accuracy of medication dosage*
13. Demonstrate, observe, instruct in removing needle from vial or ampule carefully, avoiding contact with outside of vial or ampule.	*Prevents contamination of needle*
14. Demonstrate, observe, instruct in avoidance of needle contamination once needle is out of vial or ampule.	*Reduces microorganism transfer*
15. Demonstrate, observe, instruct in needle recapping.	*Maintains sterility until administration*
16. If needle must be changed, demonstrate, observe, instruct in technique of recapping, removal and application of new needle.	
17. Demonstrate, observe, instruct in proper disposal of used needles, ampules, etc.	*Maintains cleanliness and efficiency of procedure*
18. Have client/caregiver write down in his or her	*Enhances understanding and client confidence in ability*

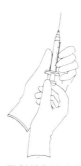

FIGURE 11.4.4

Action	Rationale
own words how the procedure is to be done, and the steps to be followed. Assist as necessary.	

Evaluation

Were desired outcomes achieved?

DOCUMENTATION

The following should be noted on the visit note:

- The specific instructions given
- The client's progress toward performance of the procedure

Sample Documentation

DATE	TIME	
7/11/99	1130	Instructions begun in preparation of medication for injection. Caregiver performed assembly of materials, checking of label, checking of medication for clarity and expiration date without assistance. Nurse demonstrated insertion of needle into vial, insertion of air, and withdrawal of medication. Caregiver wrote procedure during demonstration. Next visit caregiver will attempt entire procedure with nurse observing.

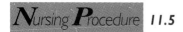

Nursing Procedure 11.5

Intramuscular Injection

EQUIPMENT

- Disposable gloves (if anyone but client giving injection)
- Alcohol swabs
- Prepared medication to be administered
- Sharps container or rigid plastic jug for sharps disposal

Purpose

Delivers ordered medication into muscle tissue

Desired Outcomes (sample)

The client will receive the ordered medication in a safe and effective manner.
The client/caregiver will demonstrate appropriate technique for injection administration.

Assessment

Assessment should focus on the following:

Ability of client/caregiver to learn and follow procedure
Client allergies, response to previous injections
Condition of client skin, amount of muscle tissue
Factors that determine appropriate size and gauge of needle (client size and age, site of injection, viscosity, and residual effects of medication)

Outcome Identification and Planning

Key Goals and Sample Goal Criteria

The client/caregiver will:

State the major purpose of the injection before receiving it
Tolerate the procedure with minimal discomfort
Demonstrate correct procedure for administration
Store and dispose of all materials in an appropriate manner

Special Considerations

Before any procedure involving an injectable, verify the medication order with the physician. If the client has not previously received the medication in a more supervised setting, check agency policy. Many agencies do not administer the first dose of any injectable in the home. Other agencies have specific protocols and emergency drugs that must be available if a first dose of any drug is to be given in the home.

Administration of an intramuscular injection is a skill that is frequently taught to clients and caregivers. Throughout the procedure, the nurse may be demonstrating, giving verbal instruction, or observing the client or caregiver performing the procedure.

Geriatric

Because of loss of muscle mass with aging, most geriatric clients should receive intramuscular injections with a 1-inch needle. The nurse is responsible for evaluating the needed size of needle, and being sure that supplies are available.

HINT

Most agencies supply syringes, alcohol swabs, and gloves while the client is receiving home health services. If you are preparing to discharge, and the client will continue to give injections of medications, be sure that an alternate source of these supplies has been arranged.

IMPLEMENTATION

Action	Rationale
1. Wash hands.	*Reduces microorganism transfer*
2. Refer to Procedure 11.4, "Preparation of Injectable Medication."	*Prepares drug correctly for administration*
3. Again verify client allergies if necessary.	
4. If anyone but client giving injection, put on gloves.	*Reduces risk of contact with body fluids*
5. Select site appropriate for client size, muscle mass, and age.	*Ensures appropriate site for adequate absorption of medication from muscle tissue*
- The client may use the thigh muscle for injection. However, if re-	*Prevents overuse of a single site*

Action	Rationale

peated injections are ordered, other sites must be used, and a caregiver or nurse must administer those injections.
(See Figure 11.5.1 for injection sites located by anatomical landmarks.)

6. Assist client into position for comfort and easy visibility of injection site.

7. Clean site with alcohol. — *Maintains asepsis*

8. Remove needle cap.

9. Pull skin taut at insertion site by using the following sequence: — *Facilitates smooth and complete insertion of needle into muscle*
   - Place thumb and index finger of nondominant hand over injection site (taking care not to touch cleaned area) to form a V.
   - Pull thumb and index finger in opposing directions, spreading fingers about 3 inches apart.

10. Quickly insert needle at a 90-degree angle with dominant hand (as if throwing a dart). — *Minimizes pain from needle insertion*

11. Move thumb and first finger of nondominant hand from skin to support barrel of syringe; fingers should be placed on barrel so that when you aspirate, you can see the barrel clearly (Fig. 11.5.2). — *Maintains steady position of needle and prevents tearing of tissue*

12. Pull back on plunger and observe for possible blood return in the syringe (Fig. 11.5.3). — *Determines if needle is in a blood vessel rather than in muscle*

Action   **Rationale**

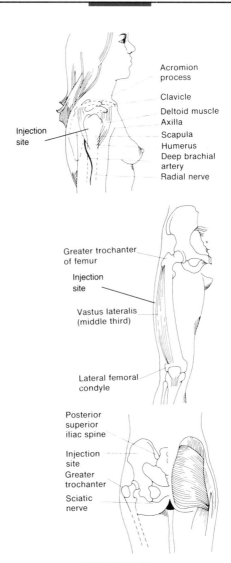

Acromion process

Clavicle

Deltoid muscle

Axilla

Scapula

Humerus

Deep brachial artery

Radial nerve

Injection site

Greater trochanter of femur

Injection site

Vastus lateralis (middle third)

Lateral femoral condyle

Posterior superior iliac spine

Injection site

Greater trochanter

Sciatic nerve

FIGURE 11.5.1

Action	Rationale

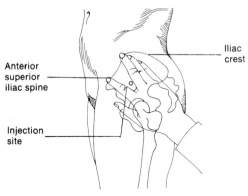

FIGURE 11.5.1 (cont.)

13. If blood does return when aspirating, pull the needle out, discard the syringe, prepare new medication, and repeat steps 5 through 12.

   Prevents inadvertent intravenous injection

14. If no blood return, push plunger down slowly and smoothly.

   Delivers medication

15. Remove needle at same angle as angle of insertion.

   Prevents tissue tearing

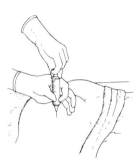

FIGURE 11.5.2

Action	Rationale

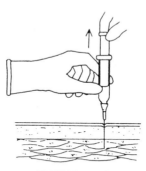

FIGURE 11.5.3

16. Apply firm pressure to site with an alcohol wipe.

Cleans area
Prevents escape of medication into subcutaneous tissue

17. Place used syringe with needle into sharps container.

Prevents accidental needlestick

18. Remove gloves.
19. Assist client to position of comfort.
20. Dispose of all used supplies; store medication, syringes, and supplies in a clean, secure, covered area.

Maintains safety

21. Instruct in site rotation, client to keep a chart of injection sites used.

Prevents muscle damage

Evaluation

Were desired outcomes achieved?

DOCUMENTATION

The following should be noted on the visit note:

- The medication injected
- The injection site
- The client's tolerance of the procedure
- The extent of the participation of the client and/or caregiver
- The plan for continued instruction or observation

Sample Documentation

DATE	TIME	
12/6/99	1210	60-mg gentamycin administered IM left gluteal muscle by spouse. Nurse observed procedure, verbal reminders given. Spouse noted injection site on chart, disposed of used supplies properly. Needs additional visit for observation of technique; expect that spouse will become independent in procedure rapidly. Client tolerated procedure well.

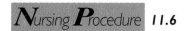

Nursing Procedure **11.6**

Z-Track Injection

☒ EQUIPMENT

- Medication to be administered
- Disposable gloves
- Alcohol swabs
- 3-mL syringe with 2–3-inch needle (20–22 gauge)
- Sharps container or rigid plastic container for disposal of used sharps

Purpose

Delivers irritating or caustic medications deep into muscle tissue to prevent seepage

Desired Outcomes (sample)

Skin remains intact without bruising or hematoma after injection.

Client offers no complaint of severe pain after injection.

Caregiver consistently demonstrates correct procedure for injection and disposal of used sharps.

Assessment

Assessment should focus on the following:

Complete medication order

Frequency of medication and duration of administration (determines whether caregiver in the home must be taught technique)

Intended injection site (presence of bruising, tenderness, skin breaks, nodules, or edema)

Site of last injection, allergies, and client response to previous injections

Factors that determine size and gauge of needle (client size and age, site of injection, viscosity and residual effects of medication)

Outcome Identification and Planning

Key Goals and Sample Goal Criteria

The client will:

Verbalize no extreme discomfort after the injection.
Experience no tissue damage from leakage of medication into subcutaneous tissue.

If applicable, the caregiver will:

Consistently demonstrate correct injection procedure.

Special Considerations

If the medication ordered is to be administered frequently, or over a long period of time, the nurse may need to teach a caregiver in the home to perform the procedure. For all of the steps of the procedure, the nurse may be demonstrating, instructing, observing, or performing the procedure.

HINT

If there is no caregiver in the home, and the medication is expected to be needed for a long period of time, the nurse must immediately begin planning for how the client will get the injection on an ongoing basis if the client will need the injection yet no longer meets criteria for home health services.

IMPLEMENTATION

Action	Rationale
1. Wash hands.	*Reduces microorganism transfer*
2. If first injection, or new caregiver, explain purpose of drug, need for special injection technique. Verify correct medication and client allergies.	*Reduces anxiety, provides information*
3. Prepare syringe with medication. See Procedure 11.4.	*Prepares drug properly*
4. Change needle after drug has been drawn up. Dispose of used needle.	*Prevents staining of skin and subcutaneous tissue when needle is inserted in skin*
5. Pull plunger back another 0.3 mL.	*Creates air lock in syringe*

Action	Rationale
6. Provide privacy.	*Decreases client embarrassment*
7. Don gloves.	*Prevents exposure to body fluids*
8. Assist client to prone position with toes pointed inward, if possible.	*Promotes comfort by relaxing gluteal muscles*
9. Outline dorsogluteal site by identifying appropriate landmarks (may also use ventrogluteal and vastus lateralis areas); leave illustration in the home for caregiver use.	*Prevents sciatic nerve damage*
10. Clean site with alcohol swab.	*Maintains asepsis*
11. Remove needle cap.	
12. Hold syringe with needle pointed downward and observe for air bubble to rise to top (away from needle).	*Ensures that air clears needle after drug so drug can be "sealed" into muscle tissue*
13. Using fingers of non-dominant hand, pull skin laterally (away from midline) about 1 inch and downward (Fig. 11.6.1).	*Retracts skin and subcutaneous tissue from muscle*
14. While maintaining skin retraction, rest heel of nondominant hand on skin below fingers.	*Allows nurse to maintain retraction and stability of needle while aspirating or if client suddenly moves*
15. Warn client of impending needlestick.	*Prevents jerking response*

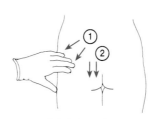

FIGURE 11.6.1

Action	Rationale

16. With dominant hand, quickly insert needle at a 90-degree angle (as if throwing a dart). — *Minimizes pain from insertion*
Ensures needle enters muscle mass

17. Pull plunger back and aspirate for blood return. — *Determines if accidental insertion into blood vessel has occurred*

18. If blood returns, remove needle, clean site with alcohol swab, assess site, apply adhesive bandage, and begin at step 1.

19. If no blood returns, inject drug slowly and hold needle in place for 10 seconds. — *Prevents leakage into subcutaneous tissue*
Gives adequate absorption time

20. Remove needle at same angle as angle of insertion while releasing skin at same time (Fig. 11.6.2). — *Prevents needless tearing of tissue*
Avoids direct track between muscle and surface of skin

21. Place alcohol swab over insertion area, but DO NOT MASSAGE. — *Avoids displacing drug into tissues and causing irritation and pain*

22. Place syringe and needle immediately into sharps container. — *Prevents accidental needlestick*

23. Make client comfortable.

24. Dispose of all used supplies, return sharps con- — *Maintains safety*

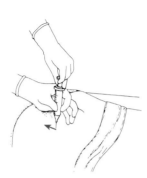

FIGURE 11.6.2

Action	Rationale

tainer, supplies to safe,
secure storage area.

25. Wash hands.   *Reduces microorganism transfer*

26. Recheck site 15–30   *Verifies that no medication seep-*
    minutes later.   *age has occurred*

Evaluation

Were desired outcomes achieved?

DOCUMENTATION

The following should be noted on the visit note:

- The medication and dosage
- The client's tolerance of the procedure
- Who administered the injection
- The specific instructions given
- Caregiver progress toward performance of the procedure
- Plan for future care

Sample Documentation

DATE	TIME	
03/21/99	0840	2-mL multivitamin administered IM via Z-Track technique left gluteal area. Client tolerated procedure well. Due to arthritis in both hands, spouse unable to perform procedure. Will contact physician re: need for ongoing injections, attempt to locate caregiver who can be instructed in technique.

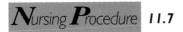

Intermittent Intravenous Medication

✖ EQUIPMENT

- Mixed medication, labeled by pharmacist
- Disposable gloves
- Alcohol swabs
- Infusion pump
- Appropriate tubing for infusion pump being used
- Small roll of tape
- Flush solution (may be saline and heparin solution in prepackaged syringes, or vials of heparin solution and saline and 3-mL syringes)
- Sharps container

Purpose

Intermittently delivers medication through intravenous (IV) route for various therapeutic effects, most frequently for the treatment of infections.

Desired Outcomes (sample)

The client will receive the ordered medication at the appropriate times without adverse incident.

The client/caregiver will consistently perform the procedure correctly.

The client/caregiver will verbalize when to call the nurse for assistance.

The client/caregiver will demonstrate correct storage and disposal of supplies.

Assessment

Assessment should focus on the following:

Client/caregiver ability to learn and follow procedures

Suitable areas in the home for storage and administration of medication (adequate refrigeration, lighting, and electrical power)
Condition of IV site (patency, discoloration, edema, pain)
Appearance of premixed medication (discoloration, sediment)
Expiration date of medication

Outcome Identification and Planning

Key Goals and Sample Goal Criteria

The client will receive the ordered medication at the ordered times.
The client/caregiver will demonstrate correct procedures for storage, administration, disposal of used supplies.
The client/caregiver will verbalize understanding of circumstances which indicate a need to call the nurse for assistance.

Special Considerations

The majority of IV medications delivered in the home setting are administered via infusion pump through a heparin lock or needleless access in a peripheral site, PICC, or central line. While in some circumstances it is acceptable for the nurse to go to the home to administer every dose, the majority of payor sources are increasingly insisting that a caregiver in the home be instructed in the technique, with periodic nursing visits for assessment.

When instructing clients and caregivers in this procedure, the nurse should break the procedure into small tasks, in an organized and sequential manner. It may be helpful to have the client or caregiver write down each step in their own words to use as a reference.

When accepting a client who is to receive intermittent IV medication, the nurse must assess the household carefully for adequate lighting, refrigeration, electrical power, and a method for reaching help in an emergency.

Check agency policy regarding IV medications before proceeding. Most agencies do not permit the administration of a first dose of any antibiotic in the home setting.

For all steps of the procedure, the nurse may be demonstrating, instructing, observing, or performing the procedure.

Geriatric

Carefully assess vision and manual dexterity. Simplify the procedure as much as possible.

HINT

Many different infusion pumps are used in the home setting. It is a nursing responsibility to be familiar with the type of pump being used in each situation.

For the duration of care, the nurse must maintain close communication with the infusion company. The agency nurse and the infusion company must be in agreement on policies regarding flush protocols, tubing changes, timing of supply deliveries, etc. All orders must be written and verified by the ordering physician. If emergency drugs are to be left in the home in case of an anaphylactic reaction, the nurse must document the procedure for use of those drugs, and instruct the client and caregiver accordingly.

IMPLEMENTATION

Action	Rationale
1. Instruct in storage of supplies and medications.	*Promotes organization and efficiency*
2. Instruct in reading label on mixed medication, verification of expiration date.	*Ensures proper medication being administered*
3. Instruct in removal of medication from refrigerator 30–60 minutes prior to administration.	*Promotes client comfort during administration*
4. Assist client to a well-lit area in the home, where there is space for the nurse or caregiver to work.	*Promotes safety and efficiency*
5. Assemble equipment and supplies: - gloves - alcohol swabs - medication - tubing and needle, or needleless connector - infusion pump - flush solutions and syringes	*Promotes efficiency*
6. Wash hands.	*Reduces microorganism transfer*

Action	Rationale
7. Assess site. Examine for redness, edema, pain, drainage.	*Identifies possible site infection*
8. Verify label on medication.	*Ensures correct medication*
9. Attach tubing to medication bag and fill tubing with fluid.	
10. Attach medication bag and tubing to pump. Remove air bubbles per pump instructions.	*Ensures sterile, fluid-filled path way*
11. Set pump controls for the flow rate according to physician order and pump manufacturer instructions.	*Ensures correct administration rate*
12. Prepare flush solutions according to physician order and agency/infusion company policy.	
13. Position client in a comfortable position.	*Promotes client comfort throughout infusion*
14. Don gloves. (Optional if client performing procedure and has washed hands thoroughly.)	*Reduces exposure to blood and body fluids*
15. Wipe heparin lock cap with alcohol sponge. If needleless system, remove protector cap.	*Maintains asepsis*
16. Stabilize with nondominant hand and insert needle of syringe with saline flush, or needleless syringe if needleless system.	
17. Pull back slightly on plunger and check for blood return (SMALL GAUGE CATHETERS IN PERIPHERAL SITES MAY BE PATENT EVEN IF A BLOOD RETURN IS NOT PRESENT).	*Checks patency*

Action	Rationale
18. Slowly inject the saline. Stop if resistance is met, or pain or edema at site (Fig. 11.7).	*Checks patency* *Flushes catheter*
19. If pain or edema at site, and saline will not inject, stop procedure. If peripheral site, discontinue and start new site. If PICC or central line, have client change position and begin procedure again. If still unable to flush, contact physician.	
20. Remove syringe and immediately drop in sharps container.	*Prevents accidental needlestick*
21. Wipe heparin lock cap or needleless system connector with alcohol swab.	*Promotes asepsis*
22. Attach infusion pump tubing to site. Tape to secure if needed.	*Prevents accidental dislodgment of tubing from site*
23. Turn pump on and observe for several minutes.	*Ensures that medication is being delivered*
24. At conclusion of infusion, wash hands and don gloves.	*Maintains asepsis*

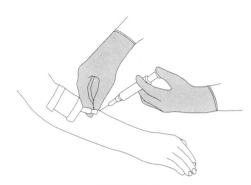

FIGURE 11.7

Action	Rationale
25. Turn pump off and carefully remove tubing from site. If tubing is to be reused, cover site end with sterile needle and cap. If tubing to be discarded, discard appropriately.	*Maintains sterility of tubing to be reused*
26. Clean heparin lock or needleless cap with alcohol.	*Maintains asepsis*
27. Insert syringe with saline flush and inject. Follow with ordered heparin solution flush.	*Clears medication from catheter* *Maintains patency*
28. Discard all used supplies appropriately. Remove gloves, wash hands.	*Prevents accidental needlestick*
29. Return pump and other supplies to clean area for storage.	
30. Instruct client/caregiver in recognition of phlebitis, infection at site, or occlusion, and leave written instructions on when to call nurse.	*Promotes client participation*
31. Post agency phone number and infusion company phone number in a prominent area in the home.	*Assists in rapid communication*

Evaluation

Were desired outcomes achieved?

DOCUMENTATION

The following should be noted on the visit note:

- Appearance of site
- Medication administered, diluent used, time of administration
- Flush solutions used
- Client tolerance of procedure

- Client/caregiver participation in procedure
- Plan for future visits

Sample Documentation

DATE	TIME	
7/06/99	0930	Observed spouse administering 1 g Rocephin in 100 mL D_5W over 1 hour via infusion pump. PICC R arm patent, no evidence of complication. Flushed with 3 mL saline before and after med, final flush of 3 mL heparin solution 100 u/mL. Spouse demonstrates proficiency in all areas of procedure, needed some verbal instruction in assembling tubing to infusion pump. Client tolerated procedure well. Will need additional nursing visit for observation of procedure, instruction in recognition of site complications.

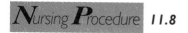
*N*ursing *P*rocedure 11.8

Administration of Subcutaneous Medications

⊠ EQUIPMENT

- Medication to be administered
- Alcohol swabs
- Disposable gloves
- Insulin syringe, or syringe with ½–⅞ inch needle (25, 26, 27 gauge)

Purpose

Delivers medication into subcutaneous tissue for absorption

Desired Outcomes (sample)

The client/caregiver will demonstrate correct procedure for subcutaneous injection.
No scars, craters, or lumps are noted in skin tissue.
The client/caregiver demonstrates correct procedure for disposing of used syringes.

Assessment

Assessment should focus on the following:

Condition of skin at all intended injection sites (presence of tearing, abrasions, lesions, and scars)
Client/caregiver ability to learn and retain information related to procedure
Client/caregiver functional limitations, (vision, manual dexterity limitations) that may interfere with procedure

Outcome Identification and Planning

Key Goals and Sample Goal Criteria

The client/caregiver will consistently demonstrate correct procedure
The client/caregiver will consistently demonstrate correct disposal of used syringes

Special Considerations

Check agency procedure and policy prior to procedure. Many agencies do not recommend that aspiration after needle insertion be performed with heparin administration.

Subcutaneous injection is a procedure commonly taught to clients who will be receiving long-term heparin therapy, or insulin therapy. When initiating care for a client needing this procedure, the nurse must be working toward turning over the procedure to the client or caregiver. If there is no caregiver, and the client cannot perform the procedure, the nurse must actively work with other community resources that can assist when home health nursing is no longer indicated.

For each step of the procedure, the nurse may be demonstrating, instructing, or observing.

Geriatric

Elderly clients often experience a loss of subcutaneous fat tissue. Choose needle length carefully to avoid painful injections and trauma to underlying bone.

Economic

The cost of insulin and syringes may be very difficult for some clients to afford, and they may try to reuse syringes to save money. This problem must be assessed early in care, and community resources used to assist clients with the purchase of insulin and syringes.

HINT

> *Begin instruction in this procedure with the clear goal of turning it over to the client as soon as possible. Give the client all available information on sharps disposal in the community, or assist the client in setting up a rigid plastic container for sharps disposal at the initial visit.*

IMPLEMENTATION

Action	Rationale
1. Assemble all supplies.	*Promotes efficiency*
2. Perform procedure in a well-lit area of the home, where there is room for supplies to be spread out.	*Enhances client learning*
3. Wash hands.	*Reduces microorganism transfer*
4. Prepare medication (see Procedure 11.4).	

Action	Rationale
5. Explain procedure and purpose of drug.	*Reduces anxiety*
6. Don gloves (optional if client learning to self-administer).	*Reduces exposure to body fluids*
7. Select injection site on upper arm, lateral thigh, or abdomen. (Note: heparin should be injected in abdomen.) Use one of the following alternative sites if these three areas are not available, because of tissue irritation, scarring, tubes, or dressings: upper chest, scapular areas. Sites should be rotated (Fig. 11.8.1).	*Prevents repeated and permanent tissue damage*
8. Position client for site selected.	*Accesses injection area*
9. Cleanse site with alcohol swab.	*Reduces microorganism transfer*
10. Remove needle cap.	
11. Grasp about 1 inch of skin and fatty tissue between thumb and fingers.	*Prevents trauma to tissue*

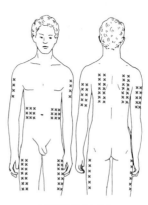

FIGURE 11.8.1

Action	Rationale

(Note: for heparin injection, hold skin gently; do not pinch.)

12. With dominant hand, insert needle at a 45-degree angle quickly and smoothly; for a larger person, insert at a 90-degree angle (Fig. 11.8.2).

Facilitates injection into subcutaneous tissue (a large person has a thicker layer of subcutaneous tissue)

13. Quickly release skin fold with nondominant hand.

Facilitates spread of medication

14. Aspirate with plunger and observe barrel of syringe for blood return.

Determines if needle is in a blood vessel

15. If blood does not return, inject drug slowly and smoothly.

Delivers the medication

16. If blood returns:
    - Withdraw needle from skin.
    - Apply pressure to site for about 2 minutes.
    - Observe for hematoma or bruising.
    - Apply adhesive bandage if needed.
    - Prepare new medication, begin procedure again.

Prevents injection into blood vessels

17. Remove needle at same angle at which it was inserted.

Prevents tissue damage

18. Cleanse injection site with alcohol swab and

Promotes comfort
Prevents bruising and tissue

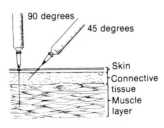

FIGURE 11.8.2

Action	Rationale
lightly massage. DO NOT massage after heparin injection.	*damage*
19. Apply adhesive bandage if needed.	*Contains residual bleeding*
20. Place used syringe in sharps container.	*Prevents accidental needlestick*
21. Discard and store all supplies appropriately.	*Promotes cleanliness*
22. Wash hands.	*Reduces microorganism transfer*

Evaluation

Were desired outcomes achieved?

DOCUMENTATION

The following should be noted on the visit note:

- Name, dosage, route of medication
- Site of injection
- Client/caregiver participation in procedure
- Client tolerance of procedure
- Plan for future visits

Sample Documentation

DATE	TIME	
8/15/99	0830	5 units regular insulin administered sc upper right quad of abdomen by client. Client performed procedure with verbal reminders concerning site selection, disposal of syringe. Tolerated procedure well. Anticipate client will be independent in procedure after one to two additional nursing visits. Written site rotation chart left in home.

*N*ursing *P*rocedure **11.9**

Administration of Rectal and Vaginal Medications

⊠ EQUIPMENT

- Suppository to be administered
- Disposable gloves
- Water-soluble lubricant and/or water

Purpose

Delivers medication for absorption through mucous membranes of rectum or vagina

Desired Outcomes (sample)
Client/caregiver will demonstrate correct administration technique.

Assessment

Assessment should focus on the following:

Client/caregiver ability to learn and retain information on procedure
Client/caregiver functional limitations that could impact on ability to perform procedure
Condition of tissue surrounding rectum or vagina

Outcome Identification and Planning

Key Goals and Sample Goal Criteria
The client/caregiver will demonstrate correct procedure
The client/caregiver will administer medication correctly, as ordered by physician

Special Considerations
This procedure is always taught to the client or caregiver, unless recent surgery or other pathological conditions exist that require the skills of a nurse to perform the procedure.

If mobility limitations exist, the client may not be able to perform this procedure.

Vaginal medications may be delivered in cream form via an applicator. The principles of the procedure remain the same.

 Transcultural

In some cultures, touching the rectal or vaginal area is a significant act that may only be done by certain family members. Before proceeding, check with a reference person at the agency who knows the customs of the specific culture.

IMPLEMENTATION

Action	Rationale
1. Explain the purpose of the medication and when it is to be administered.	*Relieves anxiety*
2. Wash hands.	*Reduces microorganism transfer*
3. Don gloves.	*Reduces exposure to secretions*
4. Position client.	*Provides access to area*
- For rectal suppository, client in side-lying position. If client is self-administering, use position of comfort.	
- For vaginal suppository, supine with knees bent. If client self-administering, use position of comfort.	
5. Remove suppository from wrapper and inspect tip.	*Detects sharp tip*
6. If possible, gently rub tip to reduce sharpness.	*Promotes comfort*
7. Lubricate suppository by using small amount of water-soluble lubricant or by moistening with water.	*Decreases tissue tearing*
8. If rectal suppository, gently spread buttocks with nondominant hand. If vaginal suppository, gently spread labia with nondominant hand.	*Exposes area of insertion*

Action	Rationale

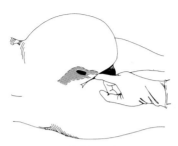

FIGURE 11.9.1

9. Instruct client to take slow deep breaths through mouth and avoid bearing down.

   Relaxes muscles, facilitating insertion

10. For rectal suppository, insert until closure of anal ring is felt (Fig. 11.9.1). For vaginal suppository, using applicator when indicated, insert gently 2½–3 inches (Fig. 11.9.2).

11. Remove finger, wipe excess lubricant from area (if lubricant has been used).

   Promotes client comfort

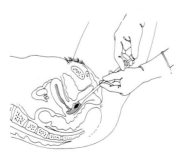

FIGURE 11.9.2

Action	Rationale
12. Advise client to remain in side-lying or supine position for 15 minutes.	*Decreases urge to expel suppository* *Promotes absorption of vaginal medication by reducing gravity effect*
13. Remove and discard gloves.	*Maintains clean environment*
14. Wash hands.	*Reduces microorganism transfer*
15. Instruct in proper storage of suppositories (ie, refrigeration).	*Reduces melting*

Evaluation

Were desired outcomes achieved?

DOCUMENTATION

The following should be documented on the visit note:

- Medication given
- Client tolerance of procedure
- Progress of client or caregiver toward independent administration
- Plan for future visits

Sample Documentation

DATE	TIME	
9/16/99	1210	Acetominophen rectal suppository administered by spouse with client in side-lying position. Client tolerated well; spouse independent in administration, verbalizes understanding of use of suppository. Will recheck spouse technique as needed.

Nursing **P**rocedure **11.10**

Topical Administration of Medication

⬛ EQUIPMENT

- Medication to be administered (creams, ointments, patches)

For creams, gels, lotions, ointments:
- Disposable gloves (unless client is administering)
- Tongue blade if multidose container used
- Mild soap
- Small towel
- Warm water

For sterile application to open skin area or incision:
- Sterile gloves, if sterile technique ordered
- Sterile gauze
- Sterile cleansing solution
- Sterile tongue blade if multidose container used

Purpose

Delivers medication to skin for local or systemic effects, such as lubrication and reduction of inflammation.

Desired Outcomes (sample)

Client/caregiver will demonstrate correct administration technique.

Client/caregiver will verbalize understanding of signs of irritation or inflammation.

Assessment

Assessment should focus on the following:

Client/caregiver ability to learn and perform procedure correctly

Condition of last treatment area and intended site of this application

Outcome Identification and Planning

Key Goals and Sample Goal Criteria

Client/caregiver will demonstrate correct application of medication

Client/caregiver will verbalize understanding of signs of inflammation, adverse reaction to medication

Special Considerations

All clients must be instructed in signs and symptoms of local inflammation, and must be instructed in the importance of rotating sites, if using patches.

Application of topical medications, unless part of sterile wound care, is a skill that is always taught to the client or caregiver. For all steps of the procedure, the nurse may be demonstrating, instructing, or observing.

HINT

If patches are being applied, observe the client opening the package. Some packages are very difficult to open and the client may need assistance.

Clients may not view topical applications as medication. Reinforce the importance of applying as ordered, like any other medication.

For clients using medication patches, instruction in removal and disposal is vital. Forgetting to remove a patch before applying a new one may lead to excess medication absorption, and improper disposal may expose other family members to the medication.

IMPLEMENTATION

Action	Rationale
1. Wash hands.	*Reduces microorganism transfer*
2. Explain procedure and purpose of drug.	*Decreases anxiety*
	Promotes cooperation
3. Verify medication order.	*Assures correct medication is being applied*
4. Don disposable gloves if applying gel, cream, ointment, or lotion; use sterile gloves if applying to open wound and use sterile	*Decreases exposure to body secretions*
	Protects nurse or caregiver from receiving effects from the drug

Action	Rationale

technique throughout procedure.

5. Wash intended application site with warm, soapy water, rinse and pat dry (unless contraindicated); if applying drug to open skin area, use sterile cleaning solution and gauze for cleaning.

Removes surface debris
Facilitates absorption

6. Wash hands and change gloves.

Maintains asepsis

7. Apply drug to treatment area, using appropriate application method:

Ointments, creams, lotions, gels

- Pour or squeeze ordered amount onto palmar surface of fingers; or use tongue blade if using multidose container.

Removes drug from container

- Lightly spread with fingers of other hand.

Thins texture of the substance
Warms cold gels and creams

- Gently apply to treatment area, lightly massaging until absorbed or as per package instructions.

Spreads drug for intended effect

Nitroglycerin ointment
(Special preparation and application)

- Remove previous ointment pad and wash area.

Prevents adverse reactions from dose greater than ordered dose

- Squeeze ordered number of inches of drug onto paper measuring rule supplied with ointment.

Obtains ordered amount of drug

- Place on skin surface that is less hairy than other areas (such as upper chest, upper arm); DO NOT apply to areas where there is a heavy skinfold (abdomen) or heavy muscle mass

Facilitates optimal absorption for dilation of coronary vessels

Action	Rationale
(gluteal muscles), or heavy fat tissue, or to the axilla or groin.	
- Secure with tape.	*Prevents accidental or premature removal of pad*
Medication patches	
- Remove outer package.	
- Carefully remove backing.	*Obtains patch containing premeasured drug*
- Place patch on skin surface that is less hairy than other areas (such as upper chest, upper arm); DO NOT apply to areas where there is a heavy skinfold (abdomen) or heavy muscle mass (gluteal muscles) or heavy fat tissue, or to the axilla or groin.	*Facilitates optimal absorption of drug*
- Gently press around edges with fingers.	*Provides for stability during long-term use*
- Instruct in removal of old patch, cleansing of residual medication from skin.	*Prevents excessive medication absorption*
Sprays	
- Instruct client to close eyes or turn head if spray is being applied to upper chest and above.	*Protects against inhaling aerosol particles*
- Apply a light coat of spray onto treatment area (usually 2–10 seconds, depending on size of treatment area).	
8. Discard and store all supplies appropriately.	*Promotes cleanliness*
9. Wash hands.	*Prevents spread of infection*

Evaluation

Were desired outcomes achieved?

DOCUMENTATION

The following should be documented on the visit note:

- Client ability to perform procedure
- Appearance of application site
- Efficacy of medication
- Plan for future visits

Sample Documentation

DATE	TIME	
11/10/99	1015	Observed client removing clonidine patch, preparing and applying new patch. Client independent in procedure, verbalizes understanding of signs and symptoms of inflammation. Will reassess periodically.

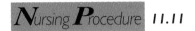

*N*ursing *P*rocedure **11.11**

Home Preparation of Solutions

✖ EQUIPMENT

- Glass containers with tight-fitting lids (pint, quart, or larger for acetic acid)
- Large saucepan
- Tongs or oven mitts
- Salt
- White distilled vinegar
- Bleach

Purpose

Prepares solutions for use in care

Desired Outcomes (sample)

Client/caregiver will demonstrate correct technique in preparation of solution.

Assessment

Assessment should focus on the following:

Economic need to prepare solutions at home instead of purchasing already prepared solutions
Client/caregiver ability to learn and perform procedure

Outcome Identification and Planning

Key Goals and Sample Goal Criteria

The client/caregiver will demonstrate correct preparation of ordered solution

Special Considerations

Before instructing in this procedure, the nurse must assess the capability of the client or caregiver to consistently carry out all steps of the procedure. If sterile saline, Dakins, or acetic acid solution is ordered for a client, check with the physician to determine if home preparation is acceptable. In some instances, it may be necessary to use purchased solutions, and the nurse should access community resources if cost to the client is a factor.

IMPLEMENTATION

Action	Rationale
1. Wash hands.	*Reduces microorganism transfer*
2. Assemble equipment— glass jars with metal lids, clean saucepan large enough to hold jar, tongs or oven mitts, measuring spoons.	*Promotes efficiency*
3. Clean all equipment with warm, soapy water and rinse thoroughly.	*Reduces microorganism transfer*
4. Prepare container:	*Sterilizes container for use*
- Lay jar on its side in the saucepan.	
- Place lid in saucepan.	
- Fill saucepan with water, be sure jar is filled, as well.	
- Cover pan, bring water to boil.	
- Boil for 20 minutes.	
- Remove from heat.	
- Using tongs or oven mitt, and handling only the outside of the jar and lid, remove the jar, and stand it, empty, in a clean area.	
- Remove the lid, handling only the outside. Place the lid loosely on the jar.	
5. *Sterile water*	
- Prepare jar as in step 4.	
- Boil 6 cups of water for 20 minutes in a clean saucepan.	*Removes microorganisms*
- Slowly pour water into jar until almost full.	
- Place lid on jar.	
- Allow to cool.	
- Tighten lid and label.	

Action	Rationale
- Prepare new solution every day.	*Prevents growth of microorganisms*
6. *Sterile saline 0.9%*	
- Prepare jar as in step 4.	
- Boil 6 cups of water as above.	
- Pour 4 cups of sterile water into sterile jar.	
- Using a clean teaspoon, add 2 teaspoons of table salt.	*Creates proper percentage solution*
- Put lid on jar and shake well.	
- Label with contents and date.	
- Allow to cool before use.	
- Prepare new solution every day.	*Prevents growth of microorganisms*
7. *Acetic acid 0.25%*	
- Prepare jar as in step 4.	
- Boil 6 cups of water for 20 minutes.	
- Pour 5 cups of water into prepared jar.	
- Let cool.	
- Using a clean measuring spoon, add 4 tablespoons of white distilled vinegar.	*Creates proper percentage solution*
- Close lid and shake to mix.	
- Label with contents and date.	
- Prepare new solution every day.	*Prevents growth of microorganisms*
8. *Dakins solution*	
- Prepare pint jar as in step 4.	
- Boil water for 20 minutes.	
- For ½ strength Dakins, put 25 mL of bleach in the pint jar and fill to top with prepared, cooled, sterile water.	
- For full strength Dakins, put 50 mL of bleach in the jar and fill to top with	

Action	Rationale

   prepared, cooled, sterile
   water.
- Place lid on jar.
- Label contents and date.
- Prepare new solution at
  least weekly.

Evaluation

Were desired outcomes achieved?

DOCUMENTATION

The following should be noted on the visit note:

- Solution prepared
- Client/caregiver ability to prepare solution
- Order from physician for home preparation

Sample Documentation

DATE	TIME	
10/11/99	1200	MD order received for instruction in home-prepared sterile saline. Observed caregiver preparing sterile container, sterile water, proper measurement of salt to create 0.9% solution of sterile saline. Instructed in labeling, need to prepare daily. Caregiver demonstrates competence in procedure.

*C*hapter *12*

Special Procedures

OVERVIEW

▶ The implantable cardiac defibrillator is a life-saving device. This device also presents a risk for great physical and emotional injury to the client if the device is improperly used or the client is inadequately prepared for the sensation associated with the device. Appropriate use of this device requires that the client, family members, and the nurse be fully educated regarding the use of and maintenance of the device before an incident requiring intervention by the AICD to reverse a life-threatening dysrhythmia.

▶ Caring for a family member at home is emotionally and physically stressful. This stress is greater when the family member is terminally ill. By guiding the client and family through the activities, and supporting them through the emotions associated with the terminal moments of life and the initial period after the death of a loved one, the nurse can help the family meet the challenge and reduce the stress associated with this period.

▶ A thorough assessment is imperative before beginning any intervention. Improperly performed postmortem techniques could result in serious legal, ethnic/cultural, or ethical/moral dilemmas.

▶ When there is a threatened or actual death, the care of significant others also becomes a nursing concern.

▶ Any exposure to body fluids presents a threat to the safety of the care-giver. Self-protective precautions, such as the use of gloves and gown in postmortem care, should be taken.

Nursing **P**rocedure **12.1**

Automatic Implantable Cardioverter Defibrillator (AICD) Management

☒ EQUIPMENT

- No equipment except gloves if contact with body fluids is likely.

Purpose

To maintain implant function so there is continuous monitoring of the heart rate and rhythm and deliver countershocks to the heart to terminate life-threatening recurrent ventricular dysrhythmias. Third-generation AICDs can also pace the heart.

Desired Outcomes (sample)

Maintenance of stable vital signs within the client's normal limit parameters.

Surgical incisions and abdominal pocket healing without signs of infection.

Client/caregiver verbalizes understanding of AICD maintenance and emergency management.

Assessment

Assessment should focus on the following:

Level of knowledge of the client and family related to the AICD and follow-up care.

Cardiovascular and pulmonary status

Signs of infection

Effects of antiarrhythmia medications

AICD activity diary

Environmental safety

Location of telephone

Client's or significant other's reliability to carry out home care instructions

Outcome Identification and Planning

Key Goals and Sample Goal Criteria

The client will:

Maintain adequate cardiac output and tissue perfusion
Regain skin integrity
Experience no infection of surgical sites
Articulate feelings of acceptance and adaptation to the AICD

The client and/or significant other will:

Demonstrate consistent ability to follow home care instructions
Verbalize when to call for assistance

Special Considerations

Anxiety and/or residual neurologic impairment as a result of an episode of sudden cardiac death can interfere with integration and processing of information. Repeated teaching sessions may be necessary before the client and significant other can demonstrate an acceptable level of understanding.

Touching the client when the AICD discharges will not cause harm.

Local emergency medical services (EMS) should be informed in advance that the client has an AICD.

If caregivers have not been taught how to administer cardiopulmonary resuscitation, arrangements should be made to schedule a session in which the caregivers can be instructed as soon as possible. It may be necessary to bring a mannequin into the home if no other arrangements can be made.

IMPLEMENTATION

Action	Rationale
1. Reinforce and complete teaching begun in the hospital.	*Fear and anxiety may interfere with processing of information*
2. Perform/instruct/observe the client and caregivers in the following steps:	
Clean incisions daily with soap and water. Inspect insertion and generator site daily for redness, swelling, excessive warmth or pain. The client may use a mirror to	*Decreases microorganisms* *Fever or signs of infection must be reported to the physician immediately*

Action	Rationale
examine the lower aspects of the device pocket.	
3. Instruct the client to avoid tight clothing.	*Prevents chafing the skin over the protruding generator box*
	Identifies malfunction of the AICD
4. Instruct the client to lie down when the AICD discharges.	*Psychological preparation decreases anxiety*
	Lying down will prevent falling
5. Instruct significant others to activate EMS and initiate CPR should cardiac arrest occur.	*In the event of cardiac arrest, the client will need basic life support until EMS arrive*
6. Instruct client to keep a diary of events resulting from each AICD discharge and examine diary of each visit.	
7. Assess for the effects of cardiac medications.	*Maximizes the chance of arrhythmia control*
8. Assess the home for environmental interference. Instruct the client to move away from any device that causes the AICD to emit a beeping tone.	*Electromagnetic sources may cause inappropriate firing or deactivation of the AICD*
	Beeping tones from the AICD are signaling AICD deactivation. Household appliances and microwave ovens will not interfere with the device.
9. Review any activity restrictions with client and caregiver.	*Any activity that involves rough contact that could damage the implant site or dislodge the device should be avoided*
10. Assess emotional adaptation to the AICD	*Negative thoughts may create unpleasant emotions; ongoing support may be needed*
11. Instruct the client to wear a Medic-Alert bracelet at all times and keep information about the AICD in the wallet.	*Provides others with necessary information to provide assistance in case of emergency*

Evaluation

Were desired outcomes achieved? Are additional services needed?

DOCUMENTATION

The following should be noted on the visit note:

- Teaching done and outcome of teaching
- Condition of the surgical sites and generator pocket
- Responses to AICD shocks and whether or not they are appropriate
- Plans for future visits
- Discharge planning

Sample Documentation

DATE	TIME	
9/26/98	0900	Left lateral thoracotomy and abdominal pulse generator pocket incisions without redness, drainage, swelling, or warmth. Temperature 99°F. Denies dizziness or chest pain. Has Medic-Alert necklace on. Reviewed instructions with client and spouse.

Nursing **P**rocedure *12.2*

Preparing for a Death in the Home

☒ EQUIPMENT

- Appropriate documentation to meet local regulations

Purpose

Prepares client and family for death in the home setting

Desired Outcomes (sample)

The client/caregiver will verbalize understanding of procedures to follow when an expected death occurs in the home.
The client/caregiver will be supported during this time.

Assessment

Assessment should focus on the following:

Client and family understanding of the dying process
Client and family wishes regarding death in the home
Possible need for transfer from home health services to hospice

Outcome Identification and Planning

Key Goals and Sample Goal Criteria

The client/caregiver will:

Recognize and accept the terminal nature of the illness
Verbalize wish to remain at home
Understand the procedures involved when a death occurs in the home
Be supported by agency staff during this time

Special Considerations

The transfer of a client to hospice services should always be considered when a home health nurse is caring for a client with a terminal illness who expresses a wish to die at home.

Hospice may provide specific and additional services to the client and family at this time.

Procedures, laws, and regulations regarding an expected death in the home vary from area to area. It is the responsibility of the nurse to know and comply with all current agency policy, nurse practice acts, and local law and regulation, particularly pertaining to pronouncement of death and notifications.

IMPLEMENTATION

Action	Rationale
1. Ascertain client and family understanding of terminal nature of disease.	*Allows ventilation of feelings*
2. Explore client's and family's wishes regarding death in the home.	*Allows all involved to express concerns*
3. Determine if client has an advance directive. Agency and physician should also have copy.	*Complies with law and regulations*
4. If client and family wish client to die at home, discuss with physician. Obtain Do Not Resuscitate (DNR) order	*Allows agency staff to not institute resuscitation measures if they are present at time of death*
5. Determine steps to be taken regarding notification of law enforcement, physician, funeral home at time of death. Provide written instructions for family.	*Ensures that proper procedures will be followed at time of death*
6. Utilize agency social worker or client support system for counseling during terminal phase of illness.	*Allows ventilation of feelings by client and family*
7. Assure client and family that if the client changes his or her mind and wishes more aggressive treatment, all decisions may be changed.	*Allows client to change his or her mind*
8. Review procedures with client and family fre-	*Provides support*

Action	Rationale
quently, and assure that agency support is available.	

Evaluation

Were desired outcomes achieved?

DOCUMENTATION

The following should be documented on the visit note:

- Copy of advance directive
- Do Not Resuscitate order signed by attending physician
- Location of advance directive and any other pertinent documentation in the home
- All instructions given to client and family
- Client and family response to instructions
- Assessment of client and family ability to follow instructions given

---

Sample Documentation

DATE	TIME	
5/21/99	1130	Reviewed significance of Do Not Resuscitate order with client and spouse. Both indicated understanding. Instructed in possible physical and mental changes as death approaches. Client and spouse indicate understanding. 24-hour agency phone number left in home with written instructions on whom to notify at time of death. Client and spouse appear prepared; daughter arriving today. Will visit in AM to assess client status and continue instruction with daughter present.

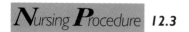

Nursing Procedure 12.3

🖑 *Postmortem Care*

⊠ EQUIPMENT

- Disposable gloves
- Clean linens
- Clean gown
- Wash basin
- Death certificate (situational)
- Isolation bags (optional)
- Cloth or disposable gown
- Two washcloths and towels
- 4 × 4-inch gauze or other dressing (optional)
- Moist cotton balls (optional)
- Identification bracelets or body tags
- Shroud (optional, unless agency policy)
- Dilute bleach mixture (optional)

Purpose

Provides proper preparation of body of deceased client for viewing by family members and for transport to funeral home or morgue with minimum exposure of family or staff to body fluids and excrement

Desired Outcomes (sample)

Body and environment are clean with a natural appearance.

Family views body with no signs of extreme distress at its physical appearance.

Body is prepared in accordance with local ordinances and policies.

There is no spread of disease.

Assessment

Assessment should focus on the following:

Agency policy regarding postmortem care and notification process

Need for autopsy (if death occurs as the result of suicide, homicide, or unknown causes; or if the family requests an autopsy)

Family or significant other's desires for preparation and viewing of the body

Outcome Identification and Planning

Key Goals and Sample Goal Criteria

The family will experience no excessive anxiety related to the
viewing of the deceased client's body
The body will appear clean and as natural as possible
The environment will appear clean and pleasant

Special Considerations

The bodies of deceased clients with known infections requiring
blood and body fluid precautions or isolation (eg, tuberculo-
sis, AIDS) should be tagged accordingly, and there should be
appropriate disposal of soiled items and cleaning of nondis-
posable items.

The client must be "pronounced dead" prior to removal of the
body from the home (unless being taken to hospital or health
facility). In some states and in some situations a nurse can
pronounce the client dead; consult state practice acts, laws,
and agency policy. Follow home-health agency policy for
recording the pronouncement on the client's chart.

When an autopsy is required or requested, the body must be
left basically undisturbed until transported to the medical ex-
aminer.

 Transcultural

Many religious rites and cultural practices may be employed by
a variety of cultures. It is important that the nurse demonstrate
respect for the deceased, as well as allow the family privacy.

Communicate with the family to determine what is important
before preparing the body. It may be important to summon a
priest, minister, rabbi, or other religious leader after the client
is deceased.

IMPLEMENTATION

Action	Rationale
1. Record time of death (cessation of heart function), notify physician, and time pronounced dead by physician or appropriate professional.	*Required for death certificate and all official records*

Action	**Rationale**
2. Notify family members that client has died and assist them from the room explaining your wish to prepare the body. Respect their desire to remain with the deceased and assist with cleaning the body.	*Provides privacy for family during initial grief.*
3. Close door to client's room.	*Prevents accidental viewing of body by family before body is prepared*
4. Don gloves and isolation gown (all persons involved).	*Protects nurse from body secretions*
5. Hold the deceased client's eyelids closed until they remain closed or place moist 4 × 4-inch gauze or cotton balls on lids.	*Fixes eyelids in a natural, closed position before rigor mortis onset*
6. Remove tubes, such as IV, nasogastric (NG) catheter, or urinary catheter, if allowed and no autopsy is to be done.	*Provides a more natural appearance for viewing by family members*
7. If unable to remove tubes: - Clamp IVs and tubes. - Coil NG and urinary tubes and tape them down. - Cut IV tubings as close to clamp as possible, cover with 4 × 4-inch gauze, tape securely.	*Retains secretions and provides as clean and natural an appearance for family viewing as possible*
8. Remove extra equipment from room.	*Allows free mobility around bed and improves appearance of environment*
9. Wash secretions from face and body.	*Improves appearance of body and decreases room odor*
10. Replace soiled linens and gown with clean articles.	*Provides clean appearance and decreases odor*
11. Place linen savers under body and extremities, if needed.	*Catches secretions and excrement escaping from open sphincters or oozing wounds*
12. Put soiled linens and pads in bag (isolation	*Decreases exposure to body fluids*

Action	Rationale
bag, if appropriate) and remove from room.	*Removes odor and improves appearance of environment*
13. Position body supine with arms at side, palms down.	*Provides a natural appearance*
14. Place dentures (if present) in mouth, put a pillow under head, close mouth, and place rolled towel under chin.	*Gives face a natural appearance and sets mouth closed before onset of rigor mortis*
15. Remove all jewelry (except wedding band, unless band is requested by family members) and give to family with other personal belongings; record the name(s) of receiver(s).	*Prevents loss of property during transfer of body and ensures proper disposal of belongings*
16. Place clean top covering over body leaving face exposed.	*Allows family to view client, and covers remaining tubes and dressings*
17. Place chair at bedside.	*Provides for family member unable to stand or if momentary weakness occurs*
18. Dim lighting.	*Makes atmosphere more soothing and minimizes abnormal appearance of body*
19. After body has been viewed by family and the funeral home attendants arrive, assist as they tag with appropriate identification (some agencies require that body be placed in a covering or shroud and that an outer covering identification tag be applied).	*Ensures proper identification of body before transfer to funeral home or morgue*
20. Send completed death certificate with body to funeral home or complete paperwork as required by agency and send body to morgue and medical director.	*Fulfills legal requirements for documentation of death*

Action	Rationale
21. Restore or dispose of equipment, supplies, and linens properly after the body is removed. Remove gown and gloves and wash hands.	*Reduces microorganism transfer* *Maintains clean and orderly environment*
22. Assist or instruct family with cleaning the room. Use special cleaning supplies if client had infection (eg, 1:10 chloride dilution for AIDS clients, special germicides for isolation situations).	*Prevents transfer of microorganisms*

Evaluation

Were desired outcomes achieved?

DOCUMENTATION

The following should be noted on the visit note and appropriate termination papers:

- Time of death and code information, if performed
- Notification of physician and family members
- Response of family members
- Disposal of valuables and belongings
- Time body was removed from room

Sample Documentation

DATE	TIME	
12/3/98	1200	No pulse, no spontaneous respirations. DNR order in home. Dr. Brown notified. Family present at the time of death. Body released to James Funeral Home. Watch and wedding ring removed by daughter in home.

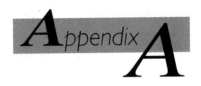

Stress Management Techniques

The following techniques can be taught to provide an individual with an opportunity to control his or her response to stressors and, in turn, to increase his or her ability to manage stress constructively. Suggested readings are listed at the end to provide more specific information.

Progressive Relaxation Technique

Progressive relaxation is a self-taught or instructed exercise that involves learning to constrict and relax muscle groups in a systematic way, beginning with the face and finishing with the feet. This exercise may be combined with breathing exercises that focus on inner body processes. It usually takes 15 to 30 minutes and may be accompanied by a taped instruction that directs the person concerning the sequence of muscles to be relaxed.

1. Wear loose clothing; remove glasses and shoes.
2. Sit or recline in a comfortable position with neck and knees supported; avoid lying completely flat.
3. Begin with slow, rhythmic breathing.
   a. Close your eyes or stare at a spot and take in a slow deep breath.
   b. Exhale the breath slowly.
4. Continue rhythmic breathing at a slow steady pace and feel the tension leaving your body with each breath.
5. Begin progressive relaxation of muscle groups.
   a. Breathe in and tense (tighten) your muscles and then relax the muscles as you breathe out.
   b. Suggested order for tension–relaxation cycle (with tension technique in parentheses):
      - Face, jaw, mouth (squint eyes, wrinkle brow)
      - Neck (pull chin to neck)
      - Right hand (make a fist)
      - Right arm (bend elbow in tightly)
      - Left hand (make a fist)
      - Left arm (bend elbow in tightly)

- Back, shoulders, chest (shrug shoulders up tightly)
- Abdomen (pull stomach in and bear down on chair)
- Right upper leg (push leg down)
- Right lower leg and foot (point toes toward body)
- Left upper leg (push leg down)
- Left lower leg and foot (point toes toward body)

6. Practice technique slowly.
7. End relaxation session when you are ready by counting to three, inhaling deeply, and saying, "I am relaxed."

Self-Coaching

Self-coaching is a procedure to decrease anxiety by understanding one's own signs of anxiety (such as increased heart rate or sweaty palms) and then coaching oneself to relax.

For example, "I am upset about this situation but I can control how anxious I get. I will take things one step at a time, and I won't focus on my fear. I'll think about what I must do to finish this task. The situation will not be forever. I can manage until it is over. I'll focus on taking deep breaths."

Thought Stopping

Thought stopping is a self-directed behavioral procedure learned to gain control of self-defeating thoughts. Through repeated systematic practice, a person does the following:

1. Says "stop" when a self-defeating thought crosses the mind (eg, "I'm not smart enough" or "I'm not a good nurse")
2. Allows a brief period—15 to 30 seconds—of conscious relaxation (because of an increased focus on negative thoughts, it may seem at first that self-defeating thoughts increase; however, eventually the self-defeating thoughts will decrease)

Assertive Behavior

Assertive behavior is the open, honest, empathetic sharing of your opinions, desires, and feelings. Assertiveness is not a magical acquisition but a learned behavioral skill. Assertive people do not allow others to take advantage of them and thus are not victims. Assertive behavior is not domineering but remains controlled and nonaggressive. An assertive person

Does not hurt others
Does not wait for things to get better
Does not invite victimization

Listens attentively to the desires and feelings of others
Takes the initiative to make relationships better
Remains in control or uses silences as an alternative
Examines all the risks involved before asserting
Examines personal responsibilities in each situation before as-
serting

Refer to suggested readings for specific techniques or participate in an assertiveness training course led by a competent in-
structor. Assertive behavior is best learned slowly in several
sessions rather than in one lengthy session or workshop.

Guided Imagery

This technique is the purposeful use of one's imagination in a
specific way to achieve relaxation and control. The person con-
centrates on the image and pictures himself involved in the
scene. The following is an example of the technique.

1. Discuss with person an image he or she has experienced that
   is pleasurable and relaxing, such as
   a. Lying on a warm beach
   b. Feeling a cool wave of water
   c. Floating on a raft
   d. Watching the sun set
2. Choose a scene that will involve at least two senses.
3. Begin with rhythmic breathing and progressive relaxation.
4. Have person travel mentally to the scene.
5. Have the person slowly experience the scene; how does it
   look? sound? smell? feel? taste?
6. Practice the imagery.
   a. Suggest tape recording the imagined experience to assist
      with the technique.
   b. Practice the technique alone to reduce feelings of embar-
      rassment.
7. End the imagery technique by counting to three and saying,
   "I am relaxed" (if the person does not use a specific ending,
   he or she may become drowsy and fall asleep, which defeats
   the purpose of the technique).

Bibliography

Alberti, R.E., & Emmons, L. (1974). *Your perfect right: A guide to
assertive behavior* (2nd ed.). San Luis Obispo, CA: Impact.
Bloom, L., Coburn, K., & Pearlman, J. (1976). *The new assertive
woman.* New York: Dell.

Chenevert, M. (1978). *Special techniques in assertiveness training for women in the health professions.* St. Louis: C. V. Mosby.

Chenevert, M. (1985). *Pro-nurse handbook.* St. Louis: C. V. Mosby.

Frisch, N.C., & Kelley, J. (1996). *Healing life's crisis: A guide for nurses.* Albany, NY: Delmar.

Gridano, D., & Everly, G. (1979). *Controlling stress and tension.* Englewood Cliffs, NJ: Prentice-Hall.

Herman, S. (1978). *Becoming assertive: A guide for nurses.* New York: Van Nostrand.

Hill, L., & Smith, N. (1985). *Self-care nursing.* Englewood Cliffs, NJ: Prentice-Hall (especially Part II, Self-care primarily associated with the mind).

McCaffery, M. (1979). *Nursing management of the patient with pain* (2nd ed.). Philadelphia: J. B. Lippincott (especially Chapter 9, Relaxation; Chapter 10, Imagery).

Rancour, P. (1991). Guided Imagery: Healing when curing is out of the question. *Perspectives in Psychiatric Care, 27*(4), 30–33.

From Carpenito LJ. (1997). Nursing Diagnosis, 7/e. Philadelphia: Lippincott-Raven, pp. 1118–1119.

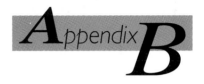

Appendix B

Pain Management

Basic Principles

- Pain is subjective and an individual experience; therefore, the client's report of pain characteristics must be considered accurate and valid.
- Pain tolerance is subjective and varies among individuals.
- Acute pain, by definition, generally lasts less than 6 months.
- Chronic pain, by definition, is pain lasting more than 6 months.
- Successful assessment and management of pain depends in part on a good nurse–client relationship.
- Prevention is better than treatment.

Pain Assessment

- Self-report of the client's perceptions regarding pain must be considered valid.
- Assess factors/characteristics of client's pain:
  Location (Where is the pain? Can you point to it?)
  Intensity (On a scale of 1–10, how bad is it? or use visual pain analog scale)
  Quality (Is it dull, sharp, nagging, burning?)
  Radiation (Does it radiate? Where does it radiate to?)
  Precipitating factors (What were you doing when it occurred?)
  Aggravating factors (What makes it worse?)
  Associating factors (Do you get nauseated or dizzy with the pain?)
  Alleviating factors (Do you know of anything that has made it better at times?)
- The following factors must be considered in assessing and managing the client's pain: medical diagnosis, age, weight, sociocultural affiliation (religion, race, gender)
- Self-management devices DO NOT exempt the nurse from performing frequent and careful client assessments.

General Pain Management Strategies

- Always assess pain first.
- Client/family teaching should be included as part of non-pharmacologic management to include factors such as what causes the pain, what the client can expect, what needs to be reported, instructions for reducing activity and treatment-related pain, relaxation techniques, etc.
- Consider general comfort measures such as client repositioning, back rub, pillows at lower back, bladder emptying, cool or warm washcloth to area, etc.
- Consider management of anxiety along with pain, using strategies of relaxation.
- Escalating and repetitive pain may be difficult to control. Early intervention is best, when needed.
- Unrelieved pain has negative physical and psychological consequences.
- Take into consideration what the client believes will help relieve the pain and the client's ability to participate in treatment.
- If pain cannot be realistically relieved completely, educate client as to what would be considered a tolerable level of pain of the condition.
- Nonsteroidal anti-inflammatory drugs and drugs which inhibit platelet aggregation should be used with caution in clients with bleeding tendencies and conditions such as thrombocytopenia or gastrointestinal ulceration.

Postoperative Pain Management

- Always check the general surgical area for manifestations of postoperative complications when the client complains of pain. Watch for problems such as compromised circulation, excessive edema, bleeding, wound dehiscence and evisceration, infection, etc.
- Goals of postoperative pain management regimens include attaining a positive client outcome and reducing immobility.
- Administering nonsedative pain medications before ambulation should be considered to facilitate early and consistent ambulation postoperatively.
- The Agency for Health Care Policy and Research (AHCPR) and American Pain Society (APS) guidelines for management of acute pain indicate that surgical clients should receive nonsteroidal anti-inflammatory drugs or acetaminophen around the clock, unless contraindications prohibit use.
- Opioid analgesics are considered to be the cornerstone for management of moderate to severe acute pain. Effective use of opioid analgesics may facilitate postoperative cooperation

in activities such as coughing and deep-breathing exercises, physical therapy, and ambulation.

- Intravenous administration is the parenteral route of choice after major surgery.
- Oral drug administration is primary choice of drug routes in the ambulatory surgical population.
- Oral administration of drugs should begin as soon as the client can tolerate oral intake.
- Acute or significant pain not explained by surgical trauma may warrant a surgical evaluation.

Complications of Drug Therapy

Watch for signs of narcotic overdose carefully—decreased respiratory rate and/or depth, decreased mentation, decreased blood pressure.

Administer naloxone as indicated by orders/agency policy immediately!

Major signs of drug dependence are client need for increased dosages of medication (after other methodologic and drug alternatives have been attempted), and client being consistently euphoric with narcotic administration (rather than just pain relief).

Pain Management in the Elderly

- Elderly clients often have complex pain because of multiple medical problems. Elderly clients are at a greater risk for drug-drug and drug-disease interactions.
- Elderly clients may experience a longer duration and higher peak effect of opioids. It is best to start with more conservative doses and increase as needed from that point.
- Some elderly clients may experience more severe post-surgical pain than other age groups. In these cases, consider options such as oral morphine or hydromorphone, if ordered.

Special Considerations

- As a routine, pain medications are not given to clients with acute neurologic conditions, because assessment of true neurologic status may be skewed with central or peripheral nervous system effects.
- The pain status of clients who have had recent vascular surgery should be monitored carefully. Excessive pain may result in increased blood pressure in response to stress, with subsequent rupture of newly grafted or anastamosed vessels.

- Note procedures on patient-controlled analgesia (PCA) management, transelectrical nerve stimulation (TENS) unit management, epidural catheter management, and application of heat/cold therapy in this procedure book.

Evaluation of Therapy

- Note verbal statement of pain decrease or increase.
- Note accompanying clinical indicators of pain increase or decrease.
- Note appearance of area of pain.
- Coping skills successfully used by client.
- Anxiety-reducing techniques successfully used.

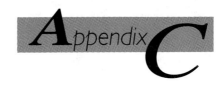

*A*ppendix *C*

Medication Interactions: Drug-Drug

(Most interactions included were those known to be severe(*), with some moderate interactions being noted. However, the degree of interaction for specific individuals may vary, thus this list is not all inclusive.) Attempts were made to eliminate duplicate listings.

Type of Drug (examples)	Interacting Drug Type (examples)	Common Interaction
Analgesics Acetaminophen	Alcohol	Increased risk of liver damage
Ketoprofen (Orudis) Aspirin	Methotrexate (for cancer chemotherapy)	Increased risk of methotrexate toxicity: fever, mouth sores, low white blood cell production
Aspirin Barbituates amobarbital (Amytal) phenobarbital (Luminal) pentobarbital (Nembutal) and others	Anticoagulants (oral) such as warfarin (Coumadin, Panwarfin)	Decrease in anticoagulation effect. *Note:* if dosage maintained and barbituates are discontinued, bleeding may occur.
Ibuprofen Indocin	Lithium	Elevated levels of lithium and risk of toxicity. Signs: nausea, slurred speech, muscle twitching.
Meperidine	Chlorpromazine	Increased sedation

Type of Drug (examples)	Interacting Drug Type (examples)	Common Interaction
(Demerol)	(Thorazine)	
Antihypertensives ACE inhibitors enalapril (Vasotec) lisinopril (Zestril) Atenolol (Tenorim) Thiazide drugs Bumex Lasix Hydralazine	Indomethacin (Indocin)	Inhibition of the antihypertensive drugs results in lack of control of hypertension
Anticoagulants Oral: dicumarol and warfarin (Coumadin Panwarfin)	Amiodarone (Cordarone) Aspirin Ibuprofen Diflunisal (Dolobid) Naproxin and other NSAIDs	Increased risk of bleeding; enhanced anticoagulant effect. Signs: hematemesis, blood in urine, stool, sputum.
Anticonvulsives Phenytoin (Dilantin)	Amiodarone (Cordarone) Disopyramide (Norpace)	Increased phenytoin levels and toxicity signs: confusion, rapid eye movement, lack of muscle coordination Dysrhythmia and anticholinergic signs: dry mouth, tachycardia.
Antidepressants Monoamine oxidase (MAO) inhibitors such as isocarboxazid (Marplan) phenelzine (Nardil) tranylcypromine (Parnate) and others	Meperidine (Demerol)	Severe hypotension or hypertension, impaired breathing, convulsions, coma and death
MAO inhibitors	Pseudoephedrine Phenylpropranola-mine Phenylephrine Metaraminol (Aramine)	(See respiratory drugs) Severe hypertension

Type of Drug (examples)	Interacting Drug Type (examples)	Common Interaction
Tricyclic drugs amitriptyline (Elavil) doxepin (Sinequan) and others	Guanethidine (Ismelin)	Hypertension due to the decreased antihypertensive effect of Ismelin
Heart medications Procainamide (Procan SR)	Pyridostigmine (Mestinon) for myasthenia gravis	Decreased effect of pyridostigmine with increased myasthenia gravis symptoms
Quinidine (Quinaglute)	Digoxin (Lanoxin) Digitoxin (Crystodigin)	Increased digoxin/digitoxin effect; risk for toxicity: poor appetite, visual abnormality, weakness, irregular heart beat.
Gastrointestinal meds Antacids	Anti-infection drugs: ketoconazole (Nizoral); Tetracyclines (Sumycin, Doxycycline, Vibramycin)	Reduced absorption with diminished effects of anti-infective drug
Acid inhibitors Cimetadine (Tagamet)	Theophylline (Theo-Dur, Primatene)	Increased levels of theophylline with risk for toxicity: nausea, tremor, diarrhea, tachycardia, seizures.
Cimetadine (Tagamet) Famotidine (Pepcid) Omeprazole (Prilosec) Rantidine (Zantac) Sulcrafate (Carafate)	Warfarin (Coumadin)	Increased risk of bleeding: blood in emesis, urine, stool.
Sulcrafate (Carafate)	Varied oral anti-infection drugs; Ciprofloxacin (Cipro); Norfloxacin (Noroxin)	Decreased effect of antiinfection drugs due to reduced absorption
Antidiabetic drugs Oral agents:	Sulfonamides	Increased effect of

Type of Drug (examples)	Interacting Drug Type (examples)	Common Interaction
chlorpropamide (Diabinese) glipizide (Glucotrol) glyburide (Micronase)	sulfamethoxazole (Bactrim)	antidiabetic drugs →hypoglycemia (signs: tachycardia, tremors, diaphoresis, nausea, convulsions →coma and death)
	phenylbutazone (Butazolidin)	Risk for hypoglycemia
	Alcohol	Increased hypoglycemic effect from antidiabetic agents with moderate-to-large intake of alcohol
	Nonselective beta blockers (Propranolol, Inderal); Pindolol (Viskin); Timolol (Blocadren); Carteolol (Cartrol); Nadolol (Corgard)	May decrease secretion of insulin, thus reducing effect of antidiabetic drugs and resulting in continued or increased hyperglycemia
Respiratory drugs Theophylline (Primatene, Theo-Dur)	propranolol (Inderal)	Increased theophylline risk for toxicity (signs: nervousness, tachycardia)
Asthma Drugs Epinephrine (Primatene, Epifrin) Isoproterenol (Isuprel)	Non-specific beta blockers: Propranolol (Inderal); Pindolol (Viskin); Timolol (Blocadren); Carteolol (Cartrol); Nadolol (Corgard)	Decreased effect of epinephrine and isoproterenol (signs: continued respiratory distress or anaphylaxis) Hypertension with systemic epinephrine treatment unrelated to allergy
Allergy or Cold/Cough Phenylephrine (Neo-Synephrine, Dristan, Night	Several tricyclic antidepressants: amitriptyline	Acute increase in blood pressure and cardiac

Type of Drug (examples)	Interacting Drug Type (examples)	Common Interaction
Relief and others)	(Elavil); doxepin (Sinequan)	contractility (signs: confusion, chest pain, palpitations, headache)
Phenylpropanolamine (Allerest, Comtrex, Contac, Triaminic, Dimetapp, Sinarest and others; *also diet aids Acutrim and Dexatrim)	Antidepressants, Monoamine oxidase (MAO) inhibitors such as isocarboxazid (Marplan); phenelzine (Nardil); tranylcypromine (Parnate) and others	Severe hypertensive reactions (signs: chest pain, flushing face, lightheadedness)
Ephedrine (Primatene, Broncholate and others) OR Pseudoephedrine (Actifed, Benedryl, Tylenol cold med)	MAO inhibitors (See above)	Severe hypertension (as above)
Antimicrobials Aminoglycosides: gentamicin (Garamycin), amikacin (Amikin), tobramycin (Nebcin)	Ethacrynic acid (Edecrin)	Increased risk for hearing loss
Chloramphenicol	Oral antidiabetic drugs (Tobutamide)	Increased effect of antidiabetic drug and hypoglycemia
Ciprofloxacin (Cipro)	Theophylline (Theo-Dur, Primatene)	Increased levels of theophylline toxicity: nausea, tremor, diarrhea, tachycardia
Erythromycin (E-Mycin)	Cyclosporine (Sandimmune)	Increased levels of cyclosporine and high risk of kidney damage
Ketoconazole (Nizoral) or troleandomycin (TAO)	Terfenadine (Seldane)	Increased levels of terfenadine toxicity: dysrhythmia, dizziness
Anti-tuberculosis drugs Rifampin (Rifadin)	Immune suppressant	Decreased effect of

Type of Drug (examples)	Interacting Drug Type (examples)	Common Interaction
	cyclosporine (Sandimmune)	cyclosporine
Rifampin (Rifadin) Tetracyclines	Estrogen-containing oral contraceptives (Ortho Novum)	Decreased effect of contraceptive; high risk of pregnancy
Tetracyclines (Achromycin, Sumycin)	Calcium supplements or medications containing calcium	Reduced absorption and effect of tetracycline

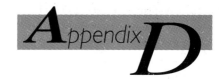

Appendix D

*Drug and Food Interaction Chart**

Drug	Interaction with Food	Action
Adenosine	Avoid food or drugs with caffeine	Avoid food or drugs with caffeine (Goody's®, Anacin®, Excedrin®)
Antibiotics		
Amoxicillin	No interaction with food	Take without regard to food
Ampicillin	Food decreases absorption	Take on empty stomach
Azithromycin	Better absorbed on empty stomach, do not give with antacids	Take on empty stomach
Cephalosporins	No interaction with food	Take without regard to food
Dicloxacillin	Food decreases absorption	Take on empty stomach
Erythromycin** (take PCE dispertab without food**)	Possible gastric distress	Best if taken on empty stomach but may be taken with food
Fluoroquinolones	Complexes formed when given with iron or dairy products	Avoid iron and dairy products within 2 hours of dose
Nitrofurantoin	Possible gastric distress; improved absorption with food	Should be taken with food
Penicillin	Food decreases absorption (50–80%)	Take on empty stomach
Sulfonamides		Take with plenty of fluid and on an empty stomach if possible

*From Drug Information Newsletter, Sept.-Oct. 1996, published by Drug Information Center, Pharmacy Department, Medical College of Georgia Hospital and Clinics.

Drug	Interaction with Food	Action
Tetracycline	Decreased absorption due to chelation by milk, dairy, iron, antacids	Take with plenty of fluid and avoid interacting products
Antihypertensives Propranolol, Metoprolol, HCTZ, and Hydralazine	Food enhances bio-availability	Take consistently with food
Atovaquone	Absorption of tablets increased 3–4 times when given with fatty foods	Can take with food
Bisacodyl	Milk breaks down protective coating which may lead to GI irritation	Avoid milk or antacids 1–2 hours before or after dose
Calcium Acetate	Food increases absorption	Best if taken on an empty stomach, avoid antacids
Captopril	Food decreases absorption	Take at a constant time in relation to meals
Carbamazepine	Food-induced bile secretions improve drug dissolution	Take with food
Didanosine	Food decreases absorption due to acid secretion	Take on an empty stomach
Estrogens	Administration with food decreases nausea	Take with food
Etidronate	Forms complexes with polyvalent cations in food, decreasing absorption	Avoid food within 2 hours of dose
Griseofulvin	High-fat foods increase absorption	Take with high fat meal or non-skim milk
Hypoglycemics Chlorpropamide Glipizide Glyburide Tolbutamide	Drug takes 30 minutes to be absorbed and become effective	Take 30 minutes before meals
Iron	Decreased absorption with antacids and certain foods (cheese, milk, ice cream)	Best if taken on empty stomach, but if taken with food, avoid interacting products

Drug	Interaction with Food	Action
Isoniazid	Food decreases and delays absorption	Take on an empty stomach
Ketoconazole	Antacids decrease absorption	May be taken without regard to meals, but not with antacids
Levadopa	Decreased absorption with high protein diet	Take on an empty stomach
Lithium	Sodium is exchanged with lithium which may lead to elevated lithium levels	Avoid abrupt changes in sodium intake or excretion
Lovastatin (excludes other HMGCoA drugs)	Food maximizes absorption and increases bio-availability	Take with meals
Methoxsalen	Food impairs absorption	May take with food if nausea occurs, but better absorption on an empty stomach
Metoprolol	Food enhances absorption	Should be taken in a consistent manner with relationship to meals to avoid fluctuations in drug levels
Mexiletine	Food enhances absorption	Take with food for stomach irritation associated with administration
Monoamine Oxidase Inhibitors Isocarboxazid Tranylcypromine Phenelzine	Potentially life-threatening hyper-tensive episode due to tyramine inter-action	Avoid cheeses, fermented meats, pickled herring, yeast, meat extracts, chianti wine
Moricizine	Food delays absorption	Best if taken on an empty stomach
Morphine	Food increases bio-availability	Take with food
Nifedipine	Food alters release properties of drug	Take on an empty stomach
NSAIDs Diflunisal, Fenopro-fen, Ibuprofen, Indo-methacin, Keto-profen, Meclofena-mate, Naproxen, Piroxicam, Salsalate, Sulindac, Tolmetin	Stomach irritation may occur	Take with food

Drug	Interaction with Food	Action
Olsalazine	Increases residence of drug in body	Take with food
Omeprazole	Food delays absorption	Take on an empty stomach
Ondansetron	Food increases absorption by 17%	Take with food
Phenytoin	May decrease absorption with food	May be taken with or without food, but take consistently with or without food
Potassium (oral)	Stomach irritation and discomfort	Take with plenty of fluid and/or food
Pravastatin		May be taken with or without meals; Avoid taking with high-fiber meals
Propafenone	Food increases absorption	Take with food
Quinidine	Possible stomach upset; increased absorption	May take with food if stomach upset occurs; avoid citrus fruit juices
Sotalol	Food decreases absorption	Take on empty stomach
Sucralfate	Food inhibits therapeutic effects of drug (coats stomach)	Take on an empty stomach 1 hour before meals with plenty of water; avoid antacids 1–2 hours before or after dose
Theophylline	Charcoaled meats cause decreased levels; high-fat foods increase absorption, raising levels	Avoid consumption of barbecued meats during therapy, avoid co-administration with high-fat food
Ticlopidine	High fat meals increase absorption; antacids decrease absorption	Take with food to decrease GI upset
Warfarin	Vitamin K-containing foods decrease the PT (green leafy vegetables, lettuce, broccoli, brussel sprouts)	Avoid large amounts of, or changes in, consumption of vitamin K-containing foods; avoid alcohol
Zalcitibine	Food decreases bioavailability by 14%	Avoid administration with food
Zidovudine	Food decreases concentration of drug	Take on an empty stomach

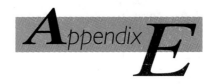

*A*ppendix *E*

Types of Isolation

There are two tiers of isolation precautions recommended by the Hospital Infection Control Practices Advisory Committee (HICPAC). The tiers include Standard Precautions and Transmission-based Precautions for clients with known or suspected infections with epidemiologically important pathogens. The major category of isolation involves the use of standard precautions, which combine the major features of universal precautions and body substance isolation. HAND WASHING IS REQUIRED WITH ALL CLIENT CONTACT AND WITH ALL FORMS OF ISOLATION.

Standard precautions (blood and body fluid) involve the use of protective coverings whenever contact with blood and certain other body fluids is a possibility. These precautions are intended to prevent contact of the skin and mucous membranes of health care workers with blood and body fluids of the client.

Standard precautions are applied to blood; and all body fluids, secretions, and excretions except sweat, regardless of the presence of visible blood; nonintact skin; and mucous membranes. If a client is known to have an infection involving highly transmissible pathogens, additional precautions are employed to interrupt transmission. Three types of precautions—airborne, droplet, and contact—are used. The appropriate disease-specific or transmission-specific isolation system is initiated (see table for protective barriers required).

Standard precautions involve the use of protective barrier coverings whenever contact with any body fluid is expected. These precautions are based on the principle that not all clients infected with blood-borne pathogens can be reliably identified prior to the possible exposure of health-care team members. Health-team members are instructed to use precautions with all clients and to add transmission precautions when indicated.

Precautions are posted in all clients' rooms. Gloves are used when handling any body secretion or secretion-soiled item. A gown is added when soiling of clothing is likely. A mask and goggles are worn whenever secretions are projectile or when an infection with a microorganism that is transmitted through air droplet transmission is suspected (an additional mask-precautions notice may be posted). All linens are handled with care to

CDC Isolation Guidelines *AJIC*, February 1996, pp. 32–52.

prevent contamination of the nurse's clothing. Reusable items used on clients known to be infected are tagged accordingly when sent for disinfecting.

Disease-specific transmission precautions involve the use of isolation precautions identifying required barrier coverings when caring for clients with diseases caused by specific microorganisms that are identified by the mode of disease transmission. Many facilities design isolation cards that identify the necessary precautions (eg, the use of gloves, gown, masks, goggles, or special disposal of contaminated materials) in a yes/no format. The table includes information found on most cards.

Precautions Used by Healthcare Team Members

Isolation/Precaution Systems	Gloves	Gown	Mask	Goggles	Special Handling of Reusable Equipment
Standard precautions	Y	With possible soiling	If splashing likely	Y with projectile secretions	Y if contaminated with body substances
Transmission-based precautions	D	D	D	D	D
Contact	Y	Y	Y	Y with secretions	Y
Droplet	Y	Y	Y	Y if splashing	Y if soiled
Airborne	N	Y/D	Y	Y with secretions	Y if soiled

D = depends on disease; N = no, item is not generally required; Y = yes, item is needed in most circumstances (some listed). Some agencies require double-bagging of soiled materials prior to removal from the room; isolation card should identify these requirements.

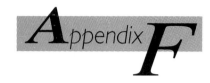

Appendix F

Equipment Substitution in the Home

Equipment	Substitution
Bed cradle, footboard	Folding tray table, cardboard box
Bedrail	Folding card table with legs under mattress
Male urinal	Liter plastic soda bottle, cut to enlarge opening, cut edge taped
Electric adjustable bed	1. Concrete block under corners of bed to elevate entire bed.
	2. Tightly rolled blankets under mattress to elevate head or foot of bed.
Heel and elbow protectors	Heavy-duty socks with padded heels, with the toe cut out
Hand mitts to prevent scratching	Heavy-duty socks
Ice collar, bag	Plastic bag of water frozen in desired shape
Linen protector	Large plastic bag with towel taped on surface touching client
Device to prevent foot drop	Well-fitted high top sneakers
IV pole	Cup hook
	Wire hanger
	Picture hanger
Trochanter roll	Large towels rolled and taped
Weights	Unopened food cans or bags of sugar/flour
Call bell	Soda can filled with small stones
Medicine organizer and dispenser	Egg carton, muffin tray

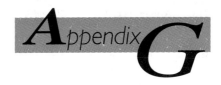

Common Clinical Abbreviations

*When multiple meanings are possible, consider context.

abd	abdomen	diab	diabetic
ac	before meals	diag, DX	diagnosis
ADLs	activities of daily living	DOA	dead on arrival
		dr	dram
ad. lib.	as desired	EENT	eye, ear, nose, throat
adm	admission	et	and
AKA	above the knee amputation	EKG	electrocardiogram
		exam	examination
alb	albumin	F	fahrenheit
amb	ambulate	FBS	fasting/fingerstick blood sugar
ant	anterior		
AP	anterior-posterior	FHT	fetal heart tones
ax	axillary	fl, fld	fluid
approx	approximately	ft	feet
b.i.d.	twice a day	fx	fracture/fractional
BKA	below-the-knee amputation	g/gm	gram
		gr	grain
BM	bowel movement	grav	gravida
BP	blood pressure	gt, gtt	drops
BRP	bathroom privileges	h, hr	hour
C	centigrade, celsius	hg	mercury
c̄	with	hct	hematocrit
Ca	calcium	hgb	hemoglobin
CA	cancer	HOB	head of bed
CC	chief complaint	hs	hour of sleep
cc	cubic centimeter	hx	history
C & S	culture and sensitivity	I & D	incision and drainage
c/o	complains of	I & O	intake and output
CVP	central venous pressure	ID	intradermal
		IM	intramuscular
cysto	cystoscopy	irriga	irrigation
DC	discontinue	IV	intravenous
K	potassium	RLQ	right lower quadrant
kg	kilogram	RO or r/o	rule out
L	liter	ROM	range of motion
L, lt	left	Rx	prescription
lat	lateral	s̄	without
lb	pound	SC/sub q	subcutaneous

659

lymph	lymphatic	sm	small
MAE	moves all extremities	SL	sublingual
m	minims	SOB	short of breath
mcg	microgram		*or*
mEq	milliequivalent		side of bed
mg, mgm	milligrams	sol	solution
MI	myocardial infarction	sp. gr.	specific gravity
ml	milliliter	S & S	signs/symptoms
neg	negative	stat	immediately
NKA	no known allergies	supp	suppository
noct	nocturnal	T, temp	temperature
NPO	nothing by mouth	T & A	tonsillectomy and
N & V	nausea and vomiting		adenoidectomy
OOB	out of bed	tab	tablet
oz	ounce	tbsp	tablespoon
OD	right eye	t.i.d.	three times a day
OS	left eye	tinc	tincture
OU	each eye	TKO	to keep open
p.c.	after meals	trach	tracheostomy
PO	by mouth, orally	tsp	teaspoon
pr	per rectum	TUR	transurethral
PRN	when needed		resection
q	every	tx	treatment
qAM	every morning	UA	urinalysis
qd	every day	UGI	upper gastro-
q.i.d.	four times a day		intestinal
q.o.d.	every other day	vag	vaginal
qs	quantity sufficient	vol	volume
R	rectal	VS	vital signs
RBC	red blood cell	WBC	white blood cell
rt, R	right	WNL	within normal limits
resp	respirations	wt	weight

Selected Abbreviations Used for Specific Descriptions

ASCVD	arteriosclerotic cardiovascular disease	DOE	dyspnea exertion
		DT's	gdelerium tremens
		D_5W	5% dextrose in water
ASHD	arteriosclerotic heart disease	FUO	fever of unknown origin
BE	barium enema	GB	gallbladder
CMS	circulation move-ment sensation	GI	gastrointestinal
		GYN	gynecology
CNS	central nervous system	H_2O_2	hydrogen peroxide
		HA	hyperalimentation or headache
	or		
	Clinical Nurse Specialist	HCVD	hypertensive cardio-vascular disease
DJD	degenerative joint disease	HEENT	head, ear, eye, nose, throat

HVD	hypertensive vascular disease	PI	present illness
ICU	intensive care unit	PM & R	physical medicine and rehabilitation
LLE	left lower extremity	Psych	psychology; psychiatric
LOC	level of consciousness; laxatives of choice	PT	physical therapy
LMP	last menstrual period	RL (or LR)	Ringer's lactate; lactated Ringer's
LUE	left upper extremity	RLE	right lower extremity
LUQ	left upper quadrant	RR	recovery room
Neuro	neurology; neurosurgery	RUE	right upper extremity
NS	normal saline	RUQ	right upper quadrant
NWB	non-weight bearing	Rx	prescription
OPD	outpatient department	STSG	split-thickness skin graft
ORIF	open reduction internal fixation	Surg	surgery, surgical
Ortho	orthopedics	THR; TJR	total hip replacement; total joint replacement
OT	occupational therapy		
PAR	post-anesthesia room	URI	upper respiratory infection
PE	physical examination	UTI	urinary tract infection
PERRLA	pupils equal, round, and react to light and accommodation	VD	veneral disease
		WNWD	well-nourished, well-developed
PID	pelvic inflammatory disease		

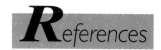
References

AHCPR Panel for the Prediction and Prevention of Pressure Ulcers in Adults (1992). *Prediction and Prevention of Pressure Ulcers in Adults: Clinical Practice Guideline No. 3.* (AHCPR Publication No. 92-0047). Rockville, MD: Agency for Health Care Policy and Research, Public Health Service, U.S. Department of Health and Human Services.

AHCPR Panel for the Treatment of Pressure Ulcers in Adults (1992). *Treatment of Pressure Ulcers in Adults: Clinical Practice Guideline No. 15.* (AHCPR Publication No. 95-0652). Rockville, MD: Agency for Health Care Policy and Research, Public Health Service, U.S. Department of Health and Human Services.

Beyea, S. & Nicoll, L. H. (1996). Back to Basics: Administering IM Injections the Right Way. *American Journal of Nursing* 96(1): 34–35.

Carr, D. B., Jacox, A. K., Chapman, C.R., et al. (Feb. 1992). *Acute Pain Management: Operative or Medical Procedures and Trauma: Clinical Practice Guideline No. 1.* AHCPR Pub No. 92-0032. Rockville, MD: Agency for Health Care Policy and Research, Public Health Service, U.S. Department of Health and Human Services, Feb. 1992.

Carroll, P. (1995). Chest tubes made easy. *RN* 58(12), 46–48, 50, 52–56.

Clarke, L. (1995). A critical event in tracheostomy care. *British Journal of Nursing* 4(12), 676, 678–681.

Cofield, V. (1995). *Percutaneous Nephrostomy Tubes: Nursing Care. Urologic Nursing* 15(4): 128–130.

Copnell, B., Fergusson, D. (1995). Endotracheal suctioning: time worn ritual or timely intervention? *American Journal of Critical Care* 4(2), 100–105.

Craven, R. F., & Hirnle, C. J. (1996). *Fundamentals of Nursing: Human Health & Function.* Philadelphia: Lippincott-Raven Publishers.

Diagnostic Ultrasound Corporation (1996). Product Brochures for BV1 5000 and BV1 2500.

Drug Information Center at the Medical College of Georgia Hospital and Clinics. (1996). *Drug–Food Interactions: What You Should Know.* Drug Information Newsletter 22(4): 1–6.

Earnest, V. (1993). *Clinical Skills in Nursing Practice, 2nd ed.* Philadelphia: Lippincott-Raven Publishers.

Greene, L. M., & Gerlach, C. J. (1994). Central lines have moved out. *RN* 57(5):26–30.

Hospital Infection Control Practices Advisory Committee, Centers for Disease Control and Prevention, Public Health Service, U.S. Department of Health and Human Services (1996). *Guideline for isolation precautions in hospitals — Part II: Recommendations for Isolation Precautions in Hospitals. American Journal of Infection Control* 24(1): 32–52.

Humphrey, C. J. (1994). *Home Care Nursing Handbook, 2nd ed.* Gaithersburg, Maryland: Aspen.

Jacox, A., Carr, D. B., Payne, R., et al. (March, 1994). *Management of Cancer Pain. Clinical Practice Guideline No. 9.* AHCPR Publication No. 94-0592. Rockville, MD: Agency for Health Care Policy and Research, U.S. Department of Health and Human Services, Public Health Service.

Levins, T. T. (1996). Central intravenous lines: Your role. *Nursing96* 26(4), 48–49.

Lewis, & Collier (1992). Assessment and management of clinical problems. *Medical-Surgical Nursing 3rd ed.* St. Louis: Mosby.

Masoorli, S. (1995). When IV practice spells malpractice. *RN* 58(8), 53–55.

Metheny, N., Reed, L., Berglund, B., & Wehrle, M. A. (1994). Visual characteristics of aspirates from feeding tubes as a method for predicting tube location. *Nursing Research* 43(5), 282–287.

Pasero, C. L., and McCaffery, M. (1996). Pain in the Elderly. *American Journal of Nursing* 96(10): 39–45.

Petrosky-Pacini, A. (1996). The Automatic Implantable Cardioverter Defibrillator in Home Care. *Home Healthcare Nurse* 14(4): 238–243.

Rice, R. (1995). *Home Health Nursing Procedures.* St. Louis: Mosby.

Schein, J. R., & Hansten, P. (1993). *The Consumer's Guide to Drug Interactions.* New York: Collier Books–Macmillan Publishing Company.

Urinary Incontinence Guideline Panel (March, 1992): *Urinary Incontinence in Adults Clinical Practice Guideline.* AHCPR Pub. No. 92-0038. Rockville, MD: Agency for Health Care Policy and Research, Public Health Service, U.S. Department of Health and Human Services.

Webber-Jones, J. (1991). Performing clean intermittent self-catheterization. *Nursing91* 21(8): 56–59.

Wolf, Z. (1996). Updating your practice: Verifying NG tube placement. *Nursing96* 26(1), 10.

*I*ndex

Page numbers followed by *f* indicate illustrations; *t* following a page number indicates tabular material.